William T. O'Donohue · Crissa Draper
Editors

Stepped Care and e-Health

Practical Applications to Behavioral
Disorders

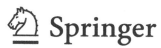 Springer

Editors
William T. O'Donohue
Department of Psychology
University of Nevada, Reno
NV 89557-0062, USA
wto@unr.edu

Crissa Draper
Department of Psychology
University of Nevada, Reno
NV 89557-0062, USA
crissa.draper@gmail.com

ISBN 978-1-4899-9157-7   ISBN 978-1-4419-6510-3 (eBook)
DOI 10.1007/978-1-4419-6510-3
Springer New York Dordrecht Heidelberg London

Printed on acid-free paper

Springer is part of Springer Science+Business Media (www.springer.com)

Stepped Care and e-Health

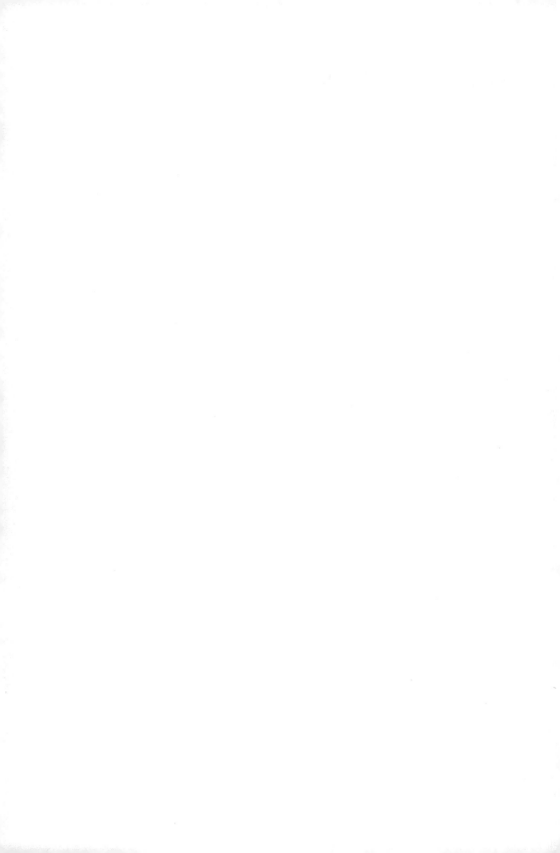

Contents

Contributors

Gerhard Andersson Department of Behavioural Sciences and Learning, Linköping University, Linköping, SE 581 83, Sweden, gerhard.andersson@liu.se

Joaquin Borrego Department of Psychology, Texas Tech University, Lubbock, TX 79409, USA, joaquin.borrego@ttu.edu

Lucas A. Broten Department of Psychology, Western Michigan University, 1903 W. Michigan Ave, Kalamazoo, MI 49008, USA, lucas.a.broten@wmich.edu

Per Carlbring Department of Psychology, Umea University, SE-901 87 Umea, Sweden, per@carlbring.se

Crissa Draper Department of Psychology, University of Nevada-Reno, Mail Stop 0298, Reno, NV 89557, USA, crissadraper@gmail.com

Bruce M. Gale BehaviorTech Solutions, Inc, 6430 Ventura Blvd, Suite 107, Encino, CA 91436, USA, bgale@behaviortech.net

Scott T. Gaynor Department of Psychology, Western Michigan University, 1903 W. Michigan Ave, Kalamazoo, MI 49008, USA, scott.gaynor@wmich.edu

Matthew Ghiglieri Department of Psychology, University of Nevada-Reno, Mail Stop 0298, Reno, NV 89557, USA, mattghiglieri@aol.com

Holly Hazlett-Stevens Department of Psychology, University of Nevada-Reno, Mail Stop 0298, Reno, NV 89557, USA, hhazlett@unr.edu

Alyssa H. Kalata Department of Psychology, Western Michigan University, 1903 W. Michigan Ave, Kalamazoo, MI 49008, USA

Chelsea Klinkebiel Department of Psychology, Texas Tech University, Lubbock, TX 79409, USA

Michael E. Levin Department of Psychology, University of Nevada-Reno, Mail Stop 0298, Reno, NV 89557, USA, levinm2@gmail.com

Jason Lillis Department of Psychology, University of Nevada-Reno, Mail Stop 0296, Reno, NV 89557, USA, jasonlillis22@gmail.com

Brett Litz National Center for Post-Traumatic Stress Disorder (116-B2) Boston Department of Veterans Affairs Medical Center, 150 South Huntington Ave (Room 13-B-74), Boston, MA 02130, USA, brett.litz@med.va.gov

Victoria Mercer Department of Psychology, University of Nevada-Reno, Mail Stop 0298, Reno, NV 89557, USA, vicmercer@gmail.com

Brie A. Moore University of Nevada, Reno Pinecrest Children's Behavioral Health, 6490 S. McCarran Blvd. Ste. D1-28, Reno, NV 89509, drmoore@pinecresthealth.com

Amy E. Naugle Department of Psychology, Western Michigan University, 1903 W. Michigan Ave, Kalamazoo, MI 49008, USA, amy.naugle@wmich.edu

Ronald R. O'Donnell Director, Behavioral Health Program, School of Letters and Sciences, Arizona State University, P.O. Box 37100, Mail Code 3252, Phoenix, AZ 85069, USA, ronald.odonnell@asu.edu

William T. O'Donohue Department of Psychology, University of Nevada-Reno, Mail Stop 0298, Reno, NV 89557, USA, wto@unr.edu

Anthony Papa Department of Psychology, University of Nevada-Reno, Mail Stop 0298, Reno, NV 89557, USA, apapa@unr.edu

M. Todd Sewell Department of Psychology, University of Nevada-Reno, Mail Stop 0298, Reno, NV 89557, USA, toddsewell@aol.com

Michele P. Steever VA Sierra Nevada Health Care System, 1000 Locust St., Reno, NV 89502, USA, michele.steever@va.gov

Chapter 1
The Case for Evidence-Based Stepped Care as Part of a Reformed Delivery System

William T. O'Donohue and Crissa Draper

Healthcare is in crisis in the United States (Cummings and O'Donohue, 2008). Most view healthcare as too costly, of uneven quality, difficult to access, and inefficient. Behavioral healthcare is no different. Practitioners often charge 10–20 times the minimum wage (and sometimes argue that even this price is insufficient) and provide assessment and therapies of unknown quality or those that are obviously deficient (e.g., Rorschach, rebirthing, drum circles) (Lilienfeld et al., 2008). Waits for child psychiatrists can be from months to half a year, and services are unevenly distributed geographically. The poor and the rural people have a difficult time gaining access to any healthcare, let alone quality healthcare. Finally, there has been too little emphasis on improving the value proposition behavioral healthcare providers give to their consumers (both clients and third-party payers). Industries grow and become profitable as they become more productive and efficient. Behavioral healthcare still relies on a delivery model that is at least a 100 years old—private practitioners in their private offices seeing one client every hour. The computer industry has Moore's law—that computing power doubles every 2 years and price halves. We have witnessed nothing like this gain in productivity in behavioral healthcare delivery.

Most innovation in behavioral healthcare centers around treatment development—deriving a new therapy and running efficacy and effectiveness trials. This is reasonable but it does not address a major problem in behavioral healthcare—problems in healthcare delivery noted above. As a field, we need to recognize that we also need to redesign our healthcare delivery to make it more efficient, more accessible, safer, more consumer centric, and more transparent. We submit that a major problem in the field—perhaps the major problem in the field—is problems in the design of behavioral healthcare delivery, not just a lack of a therapy. However, the vast majority of attention is in new therapy development, not in new delivery design. This needs to change to address the problems in access, affordability, safety, efficiency, and stakeholder satisfaction with healthcare.

W.T. O'Donohue (✉)
Department of Psychology, University of Nevada-Reno, Mail Stop 0298, Reno, NV 89557, USA
e-mail: wto@unr.edu

W.T. O'Donohue, C. Draper (eds.), *Stepped Care and e-Health*,
DOI 10.1007/978-1-4419-6510-3_1, © Springer Science+Business Media, LLC 2011

Evidence-based stepped care has this potential. A stepped-care delivery system is one in which treatment options are organized in a hierarchy of intensity (which usually correlates with cost). Patients then can be triaged based on some relevant criteria (e.g., severity, cost, or choice) to a certain step. It is also generally recognized that it is acceptable to "fail upward," i.e., that a certain step can be tried and if the problem is refractory at this step, then a more intense step can be attempted next.

"Evidence based" is a more widely known construct. It simply relies on the notion that there are reasonably designed scientific studies, especially randomly controlled trials of the efficacy, effectiveness, consumer satisfaction, and safety of the intervention. Process studies are also useful as are studies that show the generalizability to key populations (e.g., the elderly, Spanish-speaking clients).

An example might be useful of evidence-based stepped care. For major depressive episode, the steps might be as follows:

1. Watchful waiting (for mild cases, perhaps tending toward improvement, no suicidal ideation or history, patient is willing to wait a few weeks to see for improvements). But patient can call in immediately for other steps if condition worsens.
2. Psychoeducation—materials such as pamphlets that give information about depression and what might be done (e.g., behavioral activation, exercise, and gaining increased social support).
3. Bibliotherapy. Books such as David Burns' (1999) excellent *Feeling Good* that have outcome research (Scogin et al., 1987; Ackerson et al., 1998; Jamison and Scogin, 1995) that are accessible quickly and cheaply that essentially are cognitive-behavioral interventions put in a self-help format.
4. E-health. Web sites such as moodgym.com that have more involved therapies (that may be inexpensive or free) that also instantiate cognitive-behavioral treatments.
5. Group therapy. Group therapies are more efficient than individual therapy and often have similar outcome and patient satisfaction.
6. Individual outpatient therapy. This is of course the modal form of intervention in specialty mental health and has its place in stepped care. Stepped-care approaches though assume that it is overused given that the delivery system is not properly structured to demonstrate alternatives.
7. Medication. One of the most utilized interventions because most depression is treated in the primary care medical setting (Katon et al., 1997). Part of the reform has to be to design evidence-based stepped-care systems for primary care so that primary care physicians can give alternatives to their patients.
8. Inpatient therapy. Expensive and costly in terms of altering patients' life but sometimes necessary due to severity of the problem, especially given suicidal behavior.

Again, it is beyond the scope of this chapter to discuss the evidence base of each of these steps but this will be done in Chapter 2 of this book. More research is needed regarding triage: Is there some sort of patient matching that would be predictive of best outcomes? Currently, we believe that professionals should show patients all these options and engage in conjoint decision making to decide upon an initial step. Then patient progress should be closely monitored (by patient or professional) to decide whether another step should be considered. At times, multiple steps can be tried together (bibliotherapy plus medication).

The Myth That Intervention Intensity Correlates with Intervention Efficacy

It is also very important to note that intervention intensity does not correlate with intervention efficacy. In other words, more intense treatments are not necessarily more effective treatments. In the example above, there is little evidence that individual therapy for depression is more effective than group therapy and no evidence that inpatient therapy is more effective than outpatient therapy. In fact, there is some evidence that bibliotherapy is as effective as individual and group therapies (Gould et al., 1993; Floyd et al., 2004).

Clinicians need to be mindful of the costs of increased intensity of interventions. They need to be mindful that they are doing their patients some sort of favor by giving them a more intense intervention. Financial costs (to the patient and to the system) do increase as intensity increases. In addition, factors such as stigma, social disruption, and possible iatrogenic effects also increase with treatment intensity. An important value of stepped-care approach is that it seeks to minimize these costs while maximizing benefits.

Stepped Care and Ethics: The Tyranny of Outpatient Therapy

Stepped care is potentially much more consistent with the ethical imperative of choosing the least intrusive intervention for one's patient. The adage is often learned in graduate school and either forgotten or sloppily applied. Most practitioners' default value is once a week outpatient psychotherapy. The thinking must be "outpatient treatment is less intrusive than inpatient, thus I am ethically compliant." However, a stepped-care model which explicates many more steps allows a refined approach to choosing the least intrusive intervention.

Stepped Care and Public Health: Increasing Access

Stepped care is a more viable approach to many mental health problems as it is more scalable. The major rhetorical move in the introductions of journal articles and dissertations is to document that huge (and often growing) incidence of the problem of interest—millions are currently suffering and many more millions will be suffering soon. But then, given our clinical orientation, some therapy is examined. The question becomes how do these two relate to one another, i.e., How does one-on-one therapy translate to being a viable treatment for millions of clients? How does one train sufficient therapists (and make sure they adhere to the protocol)? How does one structure a delivery system so that these millions have access to this therapy? How does one make all this affordable?

The answer of course is that it is not a viable option. The field needs to realize the limitations of a sole reliance on a clinical approach. The steps of an evidence-based stepped-care approach allow more access and more efficient treatment for the large number of individuals suffering from a particular problem.

Stepped Care and Patient Choice

Providing a patient with informed consent about treatment alternatives and the advantages and disadvantages of each is ethically required before treatment is started. An explicit system of evidence-based stepped care provides this better than the current model. Patients can see all their options; read or discuss each until they understand each, particularly the evidence base, cost, and effect size for each; and then participate in the decision regarding which they prefer. This empowers the consumer much more than the current system.

There are critical areas for improvement to create a second generating stepped-care system. We believe that outcomes and costs should be more transparent at each step. Each delivery system can use benchmarks (what effectiveness trials have produced in terms of costs, outcomes, satisfaction), and then their own outcomes can be continuously tracked compared to these. This would be a sort of transparent report card for each step, which would further enable consumers to make informed decisions. Patient comments can also be included (e.g., "Chapters 4 and 6 were the most helpful" or "Dr X was warm and supportive").

Stepped Care and Integrated Care

The primary care medical setting is the de facto mental health delivery system in the United States. Most patients seek help for their mental health concerns in this setting. However, this setting is not set up to adequately address these concerns. Many primary care physicians do not want to treat these sort of problems or are not sufficiently trained to do so. Thus, often they are ignored, missed, or treated with the hammer that these healthcare professionals have: medications. However, increasingly the limitations and safety of this treatment option have been understood (Antonuccio et al., 1995). Evidence-based stepped care should be the basis for integrated care services, in which primary care physicians educated in stepped-care models work with collocated behavioral health providers who comprise an important part of a treatment team. More information on this approach can be found in O'Donohue et al. (2004) and James and O'Donohue (2008).

Structure of This Book

This book is set up to have different disorders or clinical presentations provide a model for what the empirical data would suggest in putting together a stepped-care model for that problem. There are additionally two chapters (Chapters 14 and 15) that review issues essential for consideration concerning the implementation of a stepped-care model. The chapters in this book provide information on specific problems and tend to include the following information:

1. Assessment and Triage—This information can be used to determine which step is the best step for an individual in beginning treatment, and some chapters also consider how there can be a stepped-care model within the assessment process. For example, some chapters consider more and less intense screening and assessment modules and those that can be used with and without a trained therapist or varying degrees of using therapist time.
2. Watchful Waiting—This information can be used to determine which disorders may show a natural return to baseline and disappear without specific intervention. Additionally, some chapters discuss the idea that immediate treatment after the incident may actually be iatrogenic and give empirical guidelines in terms of when an individual may want to seek the next level of care.
3. Psychoeducation—This type of low-intensity intervention includes several modalities of providing simple information about disorders, treatment for disorders, or other expectations. This can be delivered via web sites, books, pamphlets, groups and classes, or any other mode of information delivery.
4. Bibliotherapy—Bibliotherapy, or self-help, is broadly the use of text to implement behavior change or to see movement on a given disorder. The most widely used form of bibliotherapy is self-help books, but some chapters also examine the use of noninteractive web sites and occasionally even videos. Bibliotherapy generally provides consumers with an active intervention including homework (usually in the form of workbooks) and many aspects that would be present in individual treatment of the given disorder.
5. E-Health—E-health is a broad term, which in this text refers to the use of technology to provide tailored or interactive modules in addition to the treatment that may be used in bibliotherapy. This includes both computer-based interventions (CBIs), in which there is little or no therapist contact, and computer-assisted interventions (CAIs), in which a therapist plays a role in the treatment, although the treatment is delivered largely via computer and may also include adjuncts including the use of electronics such as palm devices or text messaging to enhance other modalities of treatment.
6. Group Therapy—This form of therapy may vary greatly in where it falls in the stepped-care model, depending on the structure and purpose of the group. Groups can range from support groups led by nontherapists to psychoeducational groups delivered between one or several meetings, to treatments similar to individual treatments, but minimizing therapist time by providing the same information and intervention for multiple people at once.

7. Individual Therapy—This step is what we usually would refer to as simply "therapy" and is the portion in the model that has received by far the most research. This step is commonly among the first step for most people who seek treatment (along with medication), and many practitioners accept this and do not triage to lower levels when indicated. As this book will show, this norm is not necessarily the most practical and does not necessarily provide better outcomes.
8. Medical and Medication—This step is, for some disorders, often found to be the first line of treatment even when this is counter-indicated by current research. In the treatment of many disorders, this may actually be considered among the last steps of a fail-forward attempt, generally due to side effects and often showing higher cost in the long-term.
9. Inpatient Treatment—This step is widely seen as the highest step in the treatment of any disorder and is often only indicated in the event of failures of previous steps, particularly when previous steps have not helped the consumer to address suicidal ideation.

Chapters also address consumer preference data where available, as well as both dissemination and research agenda. Multiple chapters in this book alter the steps included to accommodate the existing data and relevant factors for the specific problem. Many different disorders or presenting problems also have information on adjunctive modalities, which may maximize outcomes while minimizing therapist time.

Additionally, Chapters 14 and 15 provide additional insight into issues important to the implementation of stepped care. Chapter 14 provides information regarding cost and cost offset of using different modalities of treatment and has information regarding how managed care companies are already using the stepped-care system. Chapter 15 provides information on how minorities in the United States who do decide to seek treatment are often not satisfied with mental health services and are increasing in numbers and percentages. Author Borrego provides information on what is being done and what can be done to address this ever-growing problem.

In the following sections, we will review the highlights of the information listed above, giving an overview of the important issues in implementing a stepped-care model, as viewed between disorders.

As authors Levin and Lillis point out in Chapter 7 in this volume, "There is a tendency to overuse more invasive and costly interventions, such as individual outpatient therapy and inpatient/residential programs, even when less intense treatments, including brief therapies, bibliotherapy, and e-health may be successful." Author O'Donnell points out in Chapter 14 that companies are largely turning to the use of advanced algorithms to figure out which individuals need more intensive treatment to minimize costs to the system, due to the fact that a very small minority of individuals make up the large majority of health care costs in the United States, and that there is some evidence that integrated care administered to the individuals who need it and in the way they need it may actually serve to lower overall costs in the long term. This may also be true for the mental disorders and other presenting problems that have less empirical data on a system-level or long-term cost level and should be considered.

Assessment and Triage

Several chapters in this volume provide evidence that assessment can often be provided with equal or nearly equal reliability through less-invasive and less costly or time-consuming modalities, including telephone, videoconferencing, and online assessments (Chapters 2, 4–7). Some chapters further report on research stating that assessments administered with relative privacy, such as those done online, may actually be more accurate due to a tendency of increased reporting due to anonymity when dealing with stigmatizing issues (Chapters 5 and 12). This provides evidence that there can be a variety of steps even within the chosen assessment or assessment modality. Even in disorders where different modalities of assessment would not be ideal, such as autism, there are instruments available that can screen people into a more intense assessment of the problem (Chapter 11).

Client collaboration in deciding what treatment should be used and in what way to suit them has been shown in several instances (Chapters 2 and 14). In both cases, the authors describe systems which provide the essential element of an informed consumer, who then makes the decision himself or herself what treatment would be best, with positive results. Other chapters discuss what predictive variables indicate the best 'step' fit for an individual, including data suggesting that more severe anxiety problems predict need for a higher level of care (Chapters 3 and 4), and that complex algorithms determining which individual presentations can help medical companies predict who would be best suited for behavioral healthcare or integrated healthcare can provide better client outcomes and medical cost offset.

When providing assessment within the context of a stepped-care model, one may also want to consider subclinical presentation (Chapters 2, 3, and 5), and therefore assessments may be less useful when thinking that they provide a "there" or "not there" forced choice result and may prove more useful in this model when viewed as a continuum. One may also want to consider the fact stated in several chapters that a more severe presentation is not necessarily more effective in a higher level of care (Chapters 7 and 14), and that the level of care needed should be determined by regular monitoring (Chapters 2, 9, 10, and 12). Mercer states in Chapter 9 that "A stepped care treatment plan for each patient should include a decision tree that includes specific thresholds that should be used … to guide patient outcome monitoring and move the patient between levels of care."

Watchful Waiting

Watchful waiting is often helpful in disorders in which a natural return to baseline is somewhat likely (Chapter 2) or in which problems that do not interfere with daily life are not likely to get worse, as is the case with mild problem drinking (Chapter 7). In some instances, watchful waiting is seen as an important first step, as is the case with PTSD and complicated grief. In these instances, a triggering event leads to levels of dysfunction that are normative in the short term, and early treatment of these symptoms or presentations may prove iatrogenic (Chapters 5 and 12). Additionally, several chapters provide data that consumers prefer watchful waiting (Chapters 2, 4, and 8) even when it is sometimes not the recommended course of action, as is the case with obesity and autism. A few presenting problems provide guidelines or successful outcomes using more specific forms of monitoring (Chapter 2), but even for those without specific guidelines, the idea would be that self-monitoring would be a necessary part of most watchful waiting periods, and this alone has been found to have some treatment effects for some disorders (Chapter 7).

Some presenting problems, such as autism, may not ever be appropriate for watchful waiting following a reliable assessment, and waiting may even have long-term negative consequences in this case; or, as is the case with obesity, this waiting may reduce the effectiveness of eventual therapy.

Psychoeducation

Psychoeducation is included as a part of nearly all comprehensive treatment packages, but can be provided as the primary or sole basis as indicated for some presenting problems, and as mentioned earlier in this chapter, it can be delivered in various modalities. Different forms of psychoeducation have proved successful in decreasing symptoms in a few disorders including depression, generally with moderate effect sizes (Chapter 2). Psychoeducation programs may also show smaller drop-out rates (Chapter 2), which may prove to provide more of an impact even with small or moderate effect sizes than other interventions with higher effect sizes but higher drop-out rates (Chapter 14). In treating PTSD, there is some evidence to suggest that even psychoeducation may prove iatrogenic when used in the early stages after treatment (Chapter 5).

As with most modalities, psychoeducation is better suited to manage some presenting problems over others and seems particularly well-suited to Chronic Disease Management. Psychoeducation may also prove particularly important in a different form in educating parents of children with recent autism diagnoses to ensure obtaining treatment quickly and based on empirical standards (Chapter 11).

Bibliotherapy

Self-help books are commonly published but relatively rarely studied. However, studies in several domains show that some of these books may be particularly successful in combating presenting problems and in some cases may even be relatively comparable to face-to-face therapy (Chapters 2–4 and 6). As author Gale points out, there are some individual factors that might determine whether an individual might benefit as much from bibliotherapy as from higher modalities, as is the case with parent training for ODD when parents show inconsistent attendance to live meetings (Chapter 10). Several chapters point out what appears to be a significant problem in the implementation of self-help books—while the data generally look positive, it is consistently noted that attrition is higher for these test groups (Chapters 2, 4, and 6). In some cases, however, this can be mitigated by brief contact through phone or e-mail (Chapters 2–4 and 6).

Bibliotherapy is often prescribed as an adjunct to individual therapy (Chapter 2) and has data to attest to its usefulness as an adjunct to medical care with many behavioral medicine issues (Chapter 9). Author Pasquale also discusses a set of parent-training video tapes as a form of bibliotherapy in Chapter 11 due to the fact that the videos are informational and not interactive, but provide more detailed information than just psychoeducation.

E-Health

Computer-based interventions (CBIs) or computer-based cognitive-behavioral therapy protocols (CCTB programs) are an up-and-coming stage of research for many disorders; however, there are good data to support that they can be useful in different ways. Some chapters report overall low effect sizes compared to controls (Chapter 2), although some other CBIs prove competitive with face-to-face therapy, usually for low-to-moderate levels of the presenting problem (Chapters 2–5). Some programs have shown additional movement on the disorder process when using a CBI (Chapter 2). As is the case with bibliotherapy, CBI programs often show a high attrition rate, and multiple programs have seemingly tried to combat this issue with brief therapist contact, such as telephone calls or e-mail contact (Chapters 4, 6, and 7), which generally returned less attrition. In several cases, however, it was found that the inclusion of additional personal contact did not find better outcomes than the CBI alone (Chapters 6 and 14).

As E-health is a broad term referring generally to the addition of technology to reduce time-intensive treatments, some chapters also report on novel uses, such as bibliotherapy in combination with automated phone technology, or other uses of telephone or live computer interventions, or even psychoeducational video games (Chapters 2, 7, and 9). In one such case, it appears that a stepped-care intervention between providing individuals with phone call sessions when needed based on their movement in the CBI provided similar outcomes to a condition which gave the full intervention of phone calls plus CBI, but reduced staff time in half (Bischof et al., 2008; Chapter 7), although in another case data showed that more intensive treatments were correlated with more positive outcomes (Wylie-Rosett et al., 2001; Chapter 14). This of course could make perfect sense in light of the fact that this case randomly assigned individuals to a step instead of attempting a stepped-care triage like the previous study. Several chapters also provide information on CBIs that show significant gains, but do not have a control condition (Chapters 9, 11, and 14).

As mentioned earlier, even though CBIs often have medium or occasionally small effect sizes, these would be very meaningful—even against conditions with better effect sizes—in the event that they were reaching a population otherwise unreachable by stronger interventions, or if they led to less dropout in some populations. Further research needs to be done to determine whether these interventions are actually reaching a different treatment-seeking population, but it is hypothesized by many chapters that this might be so due to the decreased stigma in seeking online treatments and to the ability to reach rural locations or those with other barriers that may prevent them from more intensive face-to-face contact (Chapters 2, 5, 7, and 12). Further research may also explore if some people, such as those who experience significant stigma, may actually show lower drop-out rates even if the overall attrition is high.

Group Therapy

Group therapy can vary in intensity and therefore vary in its placement on the stepped-care model. However, it is placed here with the assumption that it is usually less intensive to the practitioner and more cost-effective for all (and may even provide medical cost offset for the system in general as author Mercer reports in Chapter 9), but may be similar in intensity to individual therapy for the consumer. Group therapy may be as effective in some cases as individual therapy, while saving this therapist time and cost (Chapter 2) but may also have higher drop-out rates (Chapters 2, 4, and 6). Additionally, some cases show positive gains, but do not provide a control group (Chapter 3). Groups may also show unique opportunities, such as learning from the presenting problems of others, normalizing reactions, and providing an exposure element to speaking in front of people (Chapters 6 and 12). As authors Papa and Litz point out in Chapter 12, support groups may also at times be offered in the form of online forums (Chapter 12), although there is little research in this area to determine whether such groups are useful.

Individual Therapy

Individual therapy has often been tested against psychopharmacology for given disorders and has generally found equal or better results and often reports longer term gains (Chapters 2 and 6). While it may be common to think that more severe cases of problems like depression and anxiety may require medication, it has also been shown that cognitive-behavioral therapy techniques can combat even these severe problems for many individuals (Chapters 2 and 3).

Individual therapy can also vary in its intensity or use of system resources. For example, there may be a dosing effect by which a certain number of sessions show optimal gains; additionally, some forms of therapy may be more simplistic and require less specialized training, which may lead to increased access to empirically supported treatments (Chapters 2 and 3).

While individual therapy is often what we think of as the treatment of choice, it has been found to be ineffective for some groups, specifically polysubstance users

(Chapter 7). This information is important as it likely means that medication interventions are the lowest step for some complex problems. In other groups, however, it is likely the highest step needed only for the most severe or complex cases, as is the case with Chronic Disease Management, and individual therapy may only be needed (or provide the outcome worth the resources put in) on a broad scale for things like small doses of CBT for adherence (Chapter 9). In autism, however, intensive individual treatment seems to be the only largely empirically supported treatment, and previous steps may be seen as adjunctive enhancements to receiving this care (Chapter 11).

Medication or Medical Interventions

The use of medications or psychopharmacology is an interesting step in the model, in that they are generally widely available, which gets at the access issues that many other steps address. However, we tend to place it at a higher level because these interventions do not appear sustainable after the treatment has ended, leading to higher long-term costs, and because of the side effects that many of these interventions entail. While these treatments may be considered a lower step in terms of time and effort, they may be considered a higher step in other respects due to high financial costs and adverse side effects (see Antonuccio et al., 1995), in a cost/benefit analysis (as discussed in Antonuccio et al., 1995), they may be considered a higher step to some due to the high cost and adverse side effects. However, for individuals who are treatment resistant or who have been unsuccessful in lower steps, these costs may tip the scale in weighing against the benefits. Several standards of care and national guidelines have concluded a similar idea that medications may be seen as the last option considered or would be recommended to be used only on top of individual treatments (Chapters 2 and 5). Individuals are also likely to see psychopharmacology as a non-preferred option (Chapters 2 and 9). Because psychopharmacology is often used as a first line of defense in real-world settings, it is interesting to note that in Chapter 2, authors Broten et al. note a stepped-care model in which individuals start with depression and then fail to individual therapy. As is noted in Chapter 7, there are varying steps within the medication step as well; for example, nicotine replacement therapy may be seen as a low step for smoking cessation, whereas medications such as disulfiram (Antabuse) for problem drinking or methadone replacement for heroin addiction may be much higher. In Chronic Disease Management, therapies at this level may not necessarily include psychopharmacology, but instead may be things like meal replacements or bariatric surgery.

Inpatient Treatment

Inpatient treatment is often seen with much less variability as the highest step in the stepped-care model. In the case of depression, an average stay for depression needing inpatient treatment ranged from $5,000 to $7,000 (Chapter 2). The most common reason for inpatient stays is to address concurrent suicidal ideation with any disorder (Chapters 2 and 12), but can also be recommended when individuals are so overcome by their presenting problem that they cannot manage their daily lives (Chapters 5 and 12). In the case of more complicated and severe substance abuse, inpatient treatment may be among the best places to begin therapy (Chapter 7). As is pointed out by Levin and Lillis in Chapter 7, the cost and inconvenience of inpatient treatment may prove to be logistically difficult verging on impossible for some clients, and this may be considered when there is not an immediate safety issue in deciding whether triage leads to inpatient care. In any case, when this step is implemented, it appears to be essential to step down after the inpatient period has ended into a lower step to either continue working on the presenting problem or to maintain any progress made (Chapters 2 and 7).

Treatment can vary greatly at inpatient settings (Chapter 2), and different techniques that fall along the model (mainly brief therapy, group therapy, individual therapy, and medication) may be used in conjunction with the invasive but relatively safe setting (Chapters 2 and 5).

Other Therapies

Virtual reality therapy may be seen as a step in the treatment of any disorder that is likely to benefit from imaginal exposure protocols and occasionally to teach skills through virtual practice (Chapters 5, 6, and 11). This therapy may be seen as the step between individual therapy and medication, as it generally requires the same amount of resources as individual therapy, but adds on the price of equipment and the time and cost of developing the program. This type of therapy has been shown to fit in well in this model, due to the fact that individuals who may previously have failed in imaginal exposure as treatment for PTSD can show successful treatment in this more intensive therapy. In some cases, such as virtual practice for real environments in high-functioning autism, it may prove more cost-effective in time, as the same program would be likely to benefit multiple children.

Many adjunctive treatments have been mentioned earlier, but it is notable that nearly any two steps may prove a good fit in maximizing gains while minimizing resources for some problem and in some way for some people. For example, many chapters touch on brief therapies (Chapters 5 and 7) or the addition of brief therapy with the use of a self-help book or web site (Chapters 7, 9, and 14) with successful data. Studies have also proved successful in pairing group with individual treatment (Chapters 5, 7, and 9). Case management is often paired with other treatments, such as inpatient care and medication (Chapter 7).

For some presenting problems, there may be other ways to reach the goals of stepped care even when the data suggest that only higher steps are worthwhile. For example, in the treatment of autism, only intensive individual therapy is currently recommended by the research; however, author Pasquale notes that there are data to show that parents can be trained to act as the individual therapists to their child, thereby limiting need to system resources and limiting costs. This is especially important in the treatment of a disorder in which the costs are so high—reportedly $101,445 for the first 3 years of treatment, which is a deal when you look at the $940,118 this may save over a lifetime (Chapter 11).

Integrated care, or a multimodal treatment usually involving mental health as an adjunct to what usually would be seen as a medical issue, is another topic worth noting and can be seen as addressing the problems holistically (Chapters 7, 9, and 14). Integrated care has been shown to create significant medical cost offset when costs are viewed in the long term, with medical services being 50–100% higher for individuals seeking medical treatment with co-occurring depression (Chapter 14). Thinking about problems holistically and including stepped-care approaches is certainly important to implementing any new services in the medical field, but may also be an important way to think about and understand the system from a mental health standpoint.

Consumer Preferences, Dissemination, and Research Agenda

Consumer preferences are an often overlooked part of the system, but are essential for the overall working of the system as it is intended. The mental health system has a good start on developing treatments supported for some disorders, and even on implementing these treatments in large-scale ways, but this would not be at all helpful if no one shows up for treatment. The mental health system may be seen as a cycle by which researchers come up with new treatments, practitioners give treatments to consumers, and consumers seek treatments that work. However, each piece has a needed link between the cycle. For example, researchers can do all the work in the world, but if they do not learn to be efficient and aim for scalability in dissemination of these new treatments to practitioners, the utility is lost. Practitioners may be torn between different angles including their egos/wallets (which may make it difficult for them to implement a stepped-care model), complex research-based treatments, and trying to deliver what they think people want, which may lead to less scientific therapy and less successful outcomes. Consumers can want to seek treatment, but with a lack of information regarding what options are available, what the science says about different treatments, and what practitioners might offer these treatments, they too fall out of the game.

In short, the mental health field needs to start attending to consumer preference, disseminability, and research that will be helpful in real-life settings to make things work. This book intends to address this issue by looking at these issues as well as the scientific basis for the model among different presenting problems and disorders.

As we would assume, clients often do not seek treatment if they cannot receive their preferred treatment (Chapters 2 and 3). Drop-out rates are high, and treatment-seeking rates are low (Chapters 2, 4, 5, 7, and 10). There is research to show that people would tend to prefer the treatments with the most research backing (PTSD), but also research to show that the general public is not well informed about mental health (Chapter 10). Some research suggests that permitting consumer choice and providing interventions tailored to the individual do in some cases promote higher consumer preference ratings and better outcomes (Chapters 7 and 9).

Consumer preference is often messy and regularly asks people who have already completed a given treatment if the treatment was acceptable and then reports this as high satisfaction. Unfortunately, if attrition did not already answer the question for them, cognitive dissonance would be likely to do so. As we would expect given this interpretation, nearly all interventions from each chapter mentioned reported high satisfaction ratings. Several chapters discuss comparative treatment consumer preference, but often only between medication and individual therapy, often finding that individual therapy is preferable (Chapters 2 and 3). Nonclinical samples have reported similar findings, preferring individual therapy or therapy with the most empirical backing (Chapters 2, 3, and 5). Research on consumer preference should focus on the future of clinical samples actually comparing active treatments at different steps. It is also interesting to note that some consumers find Internet treatments lacking in credibility (Chapters 4 and 6).

Chapter 14 also touches on the idea that some treatments need to meet the client where they are to promote treatment seeking, providing information for motivational techniques delivered via the Internet to increase seeking a next level of treatment and basically moving consumer preference for treatment (Chapters 7 and 14).

Dissemination

Several chapters point out the gap between the demand for services and the resources available to deliver empirically based services (Chapters 2, 5, and 11). There is a clear need for the research side of the system to be considering and testing scalable dissemination practices as a part of any intervention meant to be disseminated, lest the treatment remain an academic practice.

Even in the event that some treatments are well documented as being empirically supported, these treatments are not often used in clinical settings (Chapters 5 and 7). As is the case with PTSD, exposure therapy is known as the gold standard of care for the treatment of the disorder, but 83% of licensed clinical psychologists have *never* used exposure to treat posttrauma symptoms (Becker et al., 2004; Chapter 5).

O'Donnell and Broten et al. discuss the implementation of algorithms to determine which patient best fits which program of treatment in Chapters 2 and 14. These algorithms have been used by managed care companies to attempt to weed out what individuals might need more intensive care and what that care might look like based on their presenting factors and the extent literature.

The dissemination of implementing better screenings within the medical system may also be an important area of future research. For example, in Chapter 11, author Pasquale cites that very few pediatricians actually screen for autism, even though 1 out of 150 children will be diagnosed with a disorder in the autism spectrum.

This is especially troublesome due to the fact that early diagnosis and treatment are essential to the disorder (Chapter 11). This field has attempted to address the problem with video training available to professionals to administer a brief screening for the disorder, but there does not appear to be any data regarding the outcome of this dissemination (Chapter 11). It is, however, an example that other sections within the mental health field may want to attend to help address the issue of getting empirically supported treatment and assessment where it needs to be: to the practitioners.

Some research on working with adjunctive treatments such as web sites or bibliotherapy has provided evidence that it may help a given treatment disseminate in theory, and this would be a face valid assumption that this might be helpful (Chapters 2, 5, and 7).

Research Agenda

We believe this book will give a good overview of the information we currently have on a broad spectrum of disorders and issues within the mental health field; however, nearly every chapter highlights the fact that there is a great need for further information. Few studies have been done on the stepped-care system. While there have been a dozen or so therapies reported that have compared modalities and intensities, they generally stick to one or two. Gordon Paul asked the big question over 40 years ago—"What treatment, by whom, is most effect for this individual with that specific problem under which set of circumstances, and how does this come about?" (Paul, 1967, p. 44). Forty years later, we are not too much closer to answering the question as a whole, but now have even more to add—And how do we do this with the financial, time, and logistical resources available to both the consumers and the practitioners? And what treatments under what circumstances and for what individuals will they be willing to seek, adhere to, and complete? We as a system need to start answering system-level questions with system-level problems. We need to start looking at less-intensive treatments more carefully and comparing moderators and individual barriers to provide treatment matching information. We need to lower costs, improve treatment seeking, improve treatment adherence, and improve the implementation of evidence-based therapy. How to do all of these things are empirical questions, so there you have a research agenda.

References

Ackerson J, Scogin F, McKendree-Smith N, Lyman RD. Cognitive bibliotherapy for mild and moderate adolescent depressive symptomatology. J Consult Clin Psychol. 1998;66(4):685–90.
Antonuccio D, Danton W, DeNelsky G. Psychotherapy versus medication for depression: challenging the conventional wisdom with data. Prof Psychol: Res Pr. 1995;26(6):574–85.

Becker CB, Zayfert C, Anderson E. A survey of psychologists' attitudes towards and utilization of exposure therapy for PTSD. Behav Res Therapy. 2004;42(3):277–92. doi:10.1016/S0005-7967(03)00138-4

Bischof G, Grothues JM, Reinhardt S, Meyer C, John U, Rumpf HJ. Evaluation of a telephone-based stepped care intervention for alcohol-related disorders: a randomized controlled trial. Drug Alcohol Dependence. 2008;93:244–51.

Burns D. Feeling good: the new mood therapy revised and updated. New York: HarperCollins; 1999.

Cummings NA, O'Donohue WT. Eleven blunders that cripple psychotherapy in America: a remedial unblundering. New York: Routledge; 2008.

Floyd M, Scogin F, McKendree-Smith NL, Floyd DL, Rokke PD. Cognitive therapy for depression: a comparison of individual psychotherapy and bibliotherapy for depressed older adults. Behav Modif. 2004;28(2):297–318.

Gould RA, Clum GA, Shapiro D. The use of bibliotherapy in the treatment of panic: a preliminary investigation. Behav Ther. 1993;24(2):241–52.

James LC, O'Donohue WT. The primary care toolkit: practical resources for the integrated behavioral care provider; 2008.

Jamison C, Scogin F. The outcome of cognitive bibliotherapy with depressed adults. J Consult Clin Psychol. 1995;63(4):644–50.

Katon W, Korff MV, Lin E, Unützer J, Simon G, Ludman E, et al. Population-based care of depression: effective disease management strategies to decrease prevalence. Gen Hosp Psychiatry. 1997;19(3):169–78.

Lilienfeld SO, Lynn SJ, Lohr JM (Eds.). Science and pseudoscience in clinical psychology. New York: Guilford; 2008.

O'Donohue WT, Byrd MR, Cummings N, Henderson DA. Behavioral integrative care: treatments that work in the primary care setting. 1st ed. New York, NY: Routledge; 2004.

Paul GL. Strategy of outcome research in psychotherapy. J Consult Psychol. 1967;31(2):109–18.

Scogin F, Hamblin D, Beutler L. Bibliotherapy for depressed older adults: a self-help alternative. Gerontologist. 1987;27(3):383–7.

Wylie-Rosett J, Swencionis C, Ginsberg M, Cimino C, Wassertheil-Smoller S, Caban A, et al. Computerized weight loss intervention optimizes staff time: the clinical and cost results of a controlled in a managed care setting. J Am Diet Assoc. 2001;101:1155–62.

Chapter 2
Depression and a Stepped Care Model

Lucas A. Broten, Amy E. Naugle, Alyssa H. Kalata, and Scott T. Gaynor

Given the public health significance of depression and the limited resources available for providing evidence-based treatment, there is a need to develop effective models of care to reduce the personal and societal costs of the disorder. Within stepped care service provisions, all patients presenting with symptoms of depression generally are first offered the lowest intensity and least intrusive intervention deemed necessary following assessment and triage. Only when patients do not show improvement do they move to higher, more intensive levels of care. However, stepped care models also provide information to aid clinicians in decision making regarding selection of treatment strategies that are most appropriate for an individual patient. For some individuals, lower levels of care would never be appropriate or may not be preferred by the consumer. Thus, stepped interventions offer a variety of treatment options to match the intensity of the patient's presenting problem as well as potential patient preference. In this chapter, we discuss various strategies for treating depression consistent with a stepped model of care beginning with least intensive treatment and then moving up through the hierarchy of steps of care. While this is not a comprehensive review of all available treatments for depression, the chapter is designed to make clinicians aware of specific strategies for addressing depressive symptoms and to provide guidance about resources available at the various levels of care.

Step 1: Assessment and Monitoring

Assessment and Triage

Assessment in a stepped care model should assist in ideographically informing treatment decision making. The assessment process should guide decisions regarding

L.A. Broten (✉)
Department of Psychology, Western Michigan University, 1903 W. Michigan Ave, Kalamazoo, MI 49008, USA
e-mail: lucas.a.broten@wmich.edu

W.T. O'Donohue, C. Draper (eds.), *Stepped Care and e-Health*, DOI 10.1007/978-1-4419-6510-3_2, © Springer Science+Business Media, LLC 2011 level of care appropriate for an individual patient and should typically involve administration of self-report instruments as well as a clinical interview. One commonly used self-report screening measure of depressive symptoms in adults is the Beck Depression Inventory-II (Beck et al., 1996). The BDI-II has high 1-week test–retest reliability ($r = 0.93$) as well as internal consistency finding an alpha coefficient of 0.91 (Beck et al., 1996). The Montgomery–Asberg Depression Rating Scale (MADRS; Davidson et al., 1986) is another commonly used screening measure of depression. It has been found to have excellent inter-rater test–retest reliability ($r = 0.93$). One interesting consideration of the MADRS is that similar indices of reliability have been examined when administered via telephone, videoconference, as well as face to face (Williams and Kobak, 2008). Other commonly used measures are the Hamilton Rating Scale for Depression (Hamilton, 1980) and the lengthier Structured Clinical Interview for DSM-IV. For young children, the Children's Depression Inventory (Kovacs, 1992) is widely used and may be a helpful measure; however, there have been some concerns that it may lack appropriate specificity to be used as a stand-alone diagnostic tool (Carey et al., 1987). For adolescents, some inventories developed for adults may be appropriate. In particular, the BDI-II and the BDI-SF have been shown to be a valid screening tool for inpatient adolescents 11 years and older even in the presence of comorbid conditions (Bennet et al., 1997). The Reynolds Adolescent Depression Scale (Reynolds, 1987) may be used in cases where the BDI-II is deemed a poor fit. This measure has been found to have acceptable test–retest reliability and high concurrent validity with other measures of depression in both clinical and community samples (Masip et al., 2008). The semi-structured clinical interview, the Children's Depression Rating Scale-Revised (CDRS-R; Poznanski and Mokros, 1996), may be used with both children and adolescents to provide a more ideographic approach to assessment of depression. This measure has been found to have acceptable internal consistency and 2-week test–retest reliability of 0.80 (Poznanski and Mokros, 1996). Finally, the Geriatric Depression Scale is commonly used for screening of depression in an older population (Yesavage et al., 1983). The advantage of these screening instruments is that they offer indicators for different degrees of depressive symptomatology (i.e., mild, moderate, severe symptom presentations) as well as allow for monitoring of suicidality. These indicators may assist healthcare providers in determining whether and when a higher level of care is warranted.

In addition to initial screening and assessment, ongoing monitoring of symptoms allows a clinician to determine whether a higher level of care is warranted at any stage in the treatment process. This practice also allows for regular assessment of suicidality or self-harm behaviors that may warrant inpatient or more intensive care. Such monitoring of suicidality in patients who present with depressive symptoms should occur throughout the course of care. In addition to the symptoms monitoring forms mentioned previously, there are a number of specific suicide assessments that can be used if a clinician is concerned about a patient's risk for self-harm (e.g., The Modified Scale for Suicidal Ideation; Joiner et al., 1997). Such assessment should include questions about frequency, intensity, and duration of suicidal ideation; specificity of plan; access to a plan; any preparatory behaviors; reasons for living; self-control strategies; and intent to die (Joiner et al., 1999). Acute assessment should also include family and personal history of suicide, attempts, mental illness as well as an evaluation of protective factors, strengths, and vulnerabilities with supplementary data being provided from those close to the individual when possible (APA, 2003).

An innovative approach to assessment and treatment that incorporates several useful aspects of stepped care model has been described in the Wilford Hall model of outpatient treatment (Kelleher et al., 1996). In an effort to streamline treatment, an orientation period was implemented in a group format where initial assessment, psychoeducation, and treatment alternatives were presented. After initial assessment, the client and the group facilitators collaboratively decided on the most appropriate treatment option based on available assessments, treatment goals, and client preferences. The Wilford Hall model also includes continual monitoring using a computer-based data management system (COMIS; Clinical Outcome/Management Information System). This system provides ongoing assessment of the presenting problem and treatment satisfaction. This is a valuable information for managed care providers on the efficacy of treatments delivered using objective outcome measures, an increasing necessity for reimbursement (Ciarlo et al., 1986; JCAHO, 1993). This particular model is designed to be used in a military setting with a variety of different presenting problems and corresponding assessments to help inform treatment. The one consistent assessment is an ideographic functional assessment, which may be an important tool in identifying the appropriate step for the patient. This model of assessment could be a useful tool in a stepped care model as it incorporates several important aspects of the decision-making process (severity, preference, ongoing assessment) that will be discussed throughout the remainder of the chapter.

Watchful Waiting

There is some evidence to suggest that spontaneous remission may occur in individuals seeking treatment with minor symptoms of depression (Peterson and Halstead, 1998). It has been found that many people naturally recover from major depressive episodes as well, especially within the first 3 months of occurrence (Posternak et al., 2006). For this reason, a watchful waiting period is often considered a first-line, low-intensity level of care for individuals with low levels of depressive symptoms. Watchful waiting involves repeated assessment or monitoring of symptoms without any other active treatment (i.e., medication, psychotherapy; Meredith et al., 2007) and is usually a collaborative decision between the clinician and the patient (Hegel et al., 2006). Data collected by the Canadian Community Health Survey has shown that 16% of those that had their first major depressive episode recovered within 2 weeks and 30% recovered within 4 weeks, which would support the use of a watchful waiting period (Patten, 2006). Additional evidence supporting use of watchful waiting emerged from investigations of cognitive behavior therapy (CBT) for depression. In these studies, time-course investigations have revealed that a significant amount of change in CBT occurs within the first 4 weeks of treatment

(Ilardi and Craighead, 1994) before any explicit CBT strategies are introduced, suggesting that supportive therapy may also be a low-level, first-step intervention. This rapid response to treatment is maintained over time and occurs regardless of treatment condition (Busch et al., 2006; Gaynor et al., 2003; Renaud et al., 1998). Watchful waiting has been effective across populations, including with older adults (Williams et al., 2000) and adolescents (Bridge et al., 2007; Cheung et al., 2005; Renaud et al., 1998). However, it should be noted that watchful waiting has not produced significant results in all studies (Hegel et al., 2006). In addition to efficacy data, there are data to suggest that watchful waiting may be preferred by some patients. In one clinic-based survey, 16% of individuals indicated a preference for watchful waiting over active treatment and were subsequently less likely to seek alternate, more active, treatments (Dwight-Johnson et al., 2006). Given that treatment dropout rates can reach up to 50% for psychotherapy and medication treatment (Marks, 2002), patient treatment preferences may be critical (Institute of Medicine, 2001), particularly if patients are not likely to pursue options other than the one they prefer.

Watchful waiting has several advantages and may be a cost-effective, time-efficient first step of care. Watchful waiting periods may be accomplished without requiring patients to present at a healthcare facility. Scogin and colleagues (2003) suggested telephone- and Internet-based monitoring systems (such as the COPE program detailed later in this chapter) may be useful strategies for tracking depressive symptoms in a stepped care model. Additionally, these may be implemented by clinicians without a high degree of specialized training, including counselors, social workers, and case managers. Such care providers may be more readily available, especially in geographic areas or settings where access to more intensive, evidence-based treatments is limited. Given the potential for improvement during watchful waiting periods, it seems like systematic monitoring of symptoms during waitlist periods when a more intensive treatment is not yet available for a patient is warranted.

Watchful waiting can be implemented in different forms. Typically, watchful waiting involves a non-directive approach to care and begins with a clinical interview and/or self-report measures providing an initial assessment of depressive and other mental health symptoms in a supportive, empathic encounter. In addition to a clinical interview, self-report assessment of depressive symptoms may be most useful for ongoing monitoring. There are instances where watchful waiting is contraindicated and an alternate treatment strategy may be recommended. These contraindications include moderate to severe levels of depressive symptomatology and cases where a patient is considered to be at risk for harming self or others.

A period of at least 4 weeks is recommended as a standard watchful waiting period. When sudden gains or early treatment response occurs, it generally happens within this time frame (Gaynor et al., 2003; Ilardi and Craighead, 1994). During this 4-week period, patient symptoms are monitored on a weekly basis. If at the end of the watchful waiting period symptoms have failed to achieve clinically significant improvement, patients typically progress into a more intensive intervention. Individuals who respond effectively to watchful waiting may benefit from a continued period of monitoring as a strategy for preventing and/or addressing worsening of symptoms should this occur.

Step 2: Interventions Requiring Minimal Practitioner Involvement

Psychoeducation

Psychoeducation is a part of nearly all comprehensive evidence-based treatments for depression. However, it may also be delivered as a stand-alone strategy that requires minimal specialized training, if a therapist is needed at all, and is thus considered a lower level of intervention in the stepped care model. Despite presumed clarity about the definition of the term "psychoeducation," descriptions of this intervention in the research literature vary considerably. Most definitions of psychoeducation for depression describe it as a form of treatment that emphasizes instruction and education on a variety of topics relating to depression, including symptoms, the expected clinical course and prognosis, treatment options and strategies, and signs of relapse (Dowrick et al., 2000; Lin et al., 2008; Ong and Caron, 2008). Psychoeducation can be provided through verbal communication between a patient and mental health service provider, in either an individual or group format, through written materials, such as pamphlets or books or through computer programs and web sites (Christensen et al., 2004; Cuijpers, 1998; Dowrick et al., 2000). Computerized psychoeducation may be relatively comparable to the written material found in pamphlets or books or it can be quite complex and include animation and video clips. Treatment approaches that utilize psychoeducation may involve a single session of varying length, from a couple of hours to an entire day, or may take place through numerous sessions attended over the span of a number of weeks. This approach has a number of intended purposes, including providing informational material that assists patients in understanding their symptoms, increasing appropriate treatment seeking, encouraging compliance with and participation in psychological and pharmacological treatments, increasing the speed of recovery, and enhancing the repertoire of skills that patients have to help them cope. Psychoeducation has been applied successfully to individuals experiencing subclinical and clinical levels of depression (Christensen et al., 2004; Cuckrowicz and Joiner, 2007; Cuijpers, 1998; Dowrick et al., 2000). Furthermore, it has been used with a number of age groups, including adolescents, adults, and the elderly, as well as caregivers of the elderly and family members of children, adolescents, and adults suffering from depression (Cuijpers, 1998; Ong and Caron, 2008). Psychoeducation has also been applied successfully with more specific populations, low-income women in a group format as well as individual education supplemented by a pamphlet, and women experiencing postnatal depression in a non-directive group format (Honey et al., 2002; Lara et al., 2003).

Although numerous studies examining the efficacy of psychoeducation have been completed, only one meta-analysis of the existing data on psychoeducation has been conducted. This meta-analysis examines a specific cognitive-behavioral psychoeducational course titled "Coping with Depression" (Cuijpers, 1998). The results of the meta-analysis found that when compared to control groups, the mean effect size of the "Coping with Depression" course was 0.65, which is considered to be a moderate effect size. When calculated based on change from pretest to posttest, the mean effect size of the "Coping with Depression" course was 1.21, which is considered to be a large effect size, suggesting that psychoeducation is an effective option for treating depression. Furthermore, Cuijpers (1998) noted that there was some evidence to suggest that individuals who receive psychoeducation continue to demonstrate improvement over post-treatment follow-up periods, although additional research on the post-treatment effects of psychoeducation is needed.

Although psychoeducation is a treatment approach that is very adaptable to computer-based formats, only one study has been conducted to date examining the efficacy of non-interactive computer-based psychoeducational program. Christensen and colleagues (2004) compared the efficacy of a psychoeducational web site, titled BluePages (www.bluepages.anu.edu.au), and an interactive cognitive-behavioral therapy web site, titled MoodGYM (www.moodgym.anu.edu.au), to an attention placebo condition as a treatment for individuals in the general community exhibiting symptoms of depression. Both programs were found to have moderate effect sizes when intent-to-treat analyses were done as well when only those who completed the full course of treatment were examined. It was also found that there were significantly fewer dropouts in the psychoeducation program (15%) compared to the CBT program (25%). This suggests that both psychoeducation and cognitive-behavioral therapy administered through the Internet are efficacious treatments for the symptoms of depression, particularly for individuals exhibiting clinical levels of symptoms. A subsequent study conducted by Cukrowicz and Joiner (2007) also supports a CBT-based program of psychoeducation. They examined the comparative efficacy of a brief computerized cognitive-behavioral psychoeducational program, titled the Cognitive-Behavioral Analysis System of Psychotherapy (CBASP), to a computerized psychoeducational program, in a college student population. The results of the study indicated that at 2-month follow-up, individuals in the CBASP group had moderate effect sizes in their symptoms of anxiety and depression and greater improvement than those in the computerized psychoeducational program group. Cukrowicz and Joiner (2007) concluded that computer-based psychoeducational programs may be useful treatment options for individuals experiencing depression, particularly given their user-friendly, time-efficient, and cost-effective nature.

Psychoeducational approaches may appeal more to certain populations. It has been suggested that computer-based psychoeducational approaches may be particularly beneficial when used with populations that have had more exposure and training in the use of computers. Psychoeducational approaches to treatment may also be acceptable in instances where patients live too far away from mental health service providers to receive regular therapy services, do not have the financial means to receive regular therapy services, or are currently on a waitlist to receive therapy services. There are also some patients for whom psychoeducational approaches are not indicated, in including individuals with comorbid disorders (e.g., psychosis, substance abuse) and individuals with severe concentration or attention difficulties (Cuijpers, 1998). Controversy exists about whether psychoeducational approaches are appropriate for populations with severe symptoms of depression. Some research exists suggesting that psychoeducational approaches may be effective for individuals with severe symptoms of depression, including those individuals with histories of depression-related hospitalization and symptoms that are unresponsive to antidepressant medications (Swan et al., 2004). There is some evidence that may support a more intensive intervention for those suffering from more severe depressive symptomology including three to six times higher prevalence for relapse for those that have residual symptoms (Tranter et al., 2002), and findings from large-scale studies that have indicated that more severe depressive symptoms may benefit from medication plus active treatment as an initial step (Elkin et al., 1989, 1995). However, further research is necessary to determine the populations for which psychoeducation is most likely to be an effective treatment approach.

Bibliotherapy

Bibliotherapy has been used as a preventive intervention for individuals at high risk for depression and for individuals exhibiting elevated symptoms of depression and as an adjunct to traditional forms of therapy (Stice et al., 2006). Mains and Scogin (2003) reported that as many as 60–97% of psychologists prescribe bibliotherapy as a component of their treatment to enhance the learning of strategies discussed in therapy and to increase the degree of behavioral change outside of session (Gregory et al., 2004).

While bibliotherapy can be completed without the assistance of a mental health service provider, many individuals have advocated for minimal mental health service provider contact as part of a bibliotherapy regimen. Cuijpers (1997) and Mains and Scogin (2003) recommend that mental health service providers conduct a thorough assessment of candidates for bibliotherapy, provide a brief introduction to bibliotherapy in a separate session, and schedule 5–15 min phone contacts with the patient on a weekly basis. The rationale for this contact is to mitigate risks which may contribute to the failure of the treatment. One risk is that of misdiagnoses. In the absence of a formal diagnosis of a trained professional, an individual may run the risk of using a treatment that is inappropriate (e.g., a depression protocol for the treatment of bipolar) (Cuijpers, 1997). Additionally, it has been found that treatment dropout may be more likely in bibliotherapy (Rosen et al., 1976) than in face-to-face interventions. Weekly contact may help with adherence and can also help provide alternatives if dropout is deemed appropriate. A weekly check-in may also allow for monitoring of symptoms and suicidality to quickly move a client into a more intensive step of care if necessary. The efficacy and necessity of these measures await further empirical investigation as other research suggests that entirely self-administered treatments are equally as effective as those treatments in which mental health service providers give additional assistance during the treatment process (Gregory et al., 2004).

The most recent meta-analysis of bibliotherapy, conducted by Gregory and colleagues in 2004, examined 29 treatment outcome studies of cognitively oriented forms of bibliotherapy, 17 of which were judged to be particularly methodologically rigorous. When considering all 29 studies, bibliotherapy had an effect size of 0.99, but when including only those studies deemed to be of higher quality in terms of their research design, bibliotherapy had an effect size of 0.77. The authors compared these effect sizes to those obtained in a meta-analysis of controlled studies of individual therapy for depression and a meta-analysis of controlled studies of cognitive therapy for depression and determined that the effect size of bibliotherapy is relatively comparable to these therapeutic approaches. Gregory et al. (2004) also found no significant differences in effect sizes between group-administered bibliotherapy and self-administered bibliotherapy, which is further support that either modality is acceptable.

Two examples of books that are commercially available and have empirical support are *Feeling Good* (Burns, 1980) and *Control Your Depression* (Lewinsohn et al., 1986). *Feeling Good* is cognitively oriented and focuses primarily on identifying and altering distorted or problematic thinking, although some behaviorally oriented techniques such as activity scheduling are included in the book. *Control Your Depression* is behaviorally oriented and focuses primarily on pleasant activities, developing social skills, and relaxation strategies, although cognitive techniques are also included in the book. In addition to these two commonly used books, many other books are commercially available that have a solid theoretical basis such as *Overcoming Depression One Step at a Time: The New Behavioral Activation Approach to Getting your Life Back* (Addis and Martell, 2004) and *The Mindfulness and Acceptance Workbook for Depression: Using Acceptance and Commitment Therapy* (Strosahl and Robinson, 2008). These treatments have been shown to be efficacious when administered by a therapist, but that have not yet been empirically tested in a bibliotherapy format. Additionally, as with psychoeducational approaches to the treatment of depression, bibliotherapy can also be easily adapted to computerized formats that have the distinct advantages of being easily updated and free to the public (Cuijpers, 1997).

As with psychoeducation and watchful waiting, bibliotherapy may be an appropriate intervention for patients who do not have the means to access traditional therapy services or for patients who are currently on a waiting list to receive traditional therapy services. Bibliotherapy may also be a particularly appealing intervention for individuals who may otherwise avoid seeking treatment because of the stigma associated with traditional psychotherapy (Mains and Scogin, 2003). The current research literature has only examined bibliotherapy as an intervention for individuals suffering from mild to moderate depression (Cuijpers, 1997; Gregory et al., 2004). The risks of suicide and challenges in motivation and attention that often accompany severe depression make bibliotherapy an inappropriate recommendation for this population (Gregory et al., 2004; Mains and Scogin, 2003). Additional patient characteristics that should be taken into account when considering bibliotherapy as a treatment option include the cultural relevance of a specific bibliotherapy program such as treatment goals that are explicitly contradicted by the patient's culture or values. Additionally, the patient's expectations and preferences for treatment, the patient's attitude toward bibliotherapy as a treatment option, the patient's reading level and/or disabilities that might impair comprehension of the material, and the patient's history and preferences for school-like tasks (Gregory et al., 2004; Mains and Scogin, 2003) should be considered.

Computer-Based Intervention/E-Health

Computer-based intervention, also known as computer-aided cognitive-behavioral therapy (CCBT), is defined as "any computing system that aids cognitive-behavioral therapy by using patient input to make at least some computations and treatment decisions" (Marks et al., 2007). CCBT includes cognitive-behavioral therapy programs delivered through the Internet, CD-ROMs, DVDs, PDAs, telephone systems, and virtual reality devices, but does not include treatments in which a mental health service provider makes all treatment decisions, while treatment is being provided through the use of technology (e.g., over the telephone, in an Internet chat room) (Marks et al., 2007). Most CCBT programs use multimedia technology and include textual components, audio voice-overs, video clips, and interactive components, including multiple-choice questions and short-answer responses boxes that patients use to input information (Cavanagh and Shapiro, 2004). Many of the CCBT programs also include weekly homework assignments, measures tracking patient symptoms, and opportunities for patients to provide consumer satisfaction feedback (Cavanagh and Shapiro, 2004). Because of the portability of CCBT technology, treatment can take place in a variety of settings, including the homes of patients, outpatient clinics, inpatient units, schools, and public locations, such as libraries (Marks et al., 2007). Some CCBT programs may require large amounts of mental health service provider contact (e.g., virtual reality exposure CCBT) while other CCBT programs may require no contact with a mental health service provider (e.g., those accessed from the home of the patient over the Internet, with no initial consultation from a mental health service provider).

One meta-analysis has been conducted examining the efficacy of CCBT programs for depression. Cavanagh and Shapiro (2004) analyzed the data from five available CCBT treatment outcome studies that utilized the Beck Depression Inventory as a treatment outcome measure. The results of their meta-analysis showed a large (1.38) pretest to posttest effect size for CCBT, but only a small (0.34) effect size for CCBT when compared to waitlist controls. Furthermore, they found a medium (0.63) effect size favoring therapist-administered CBT over CCBT, although this effect size was calculated based on only two studies with 18 participants in the two CCBT conditions.

Since the Cavanagh and Shapiro (2004) meta-analysis, a number of important CCBT treatment outcome studies have been completed and several commercially available CCBT programs have emerged with adequate empirical support as measured by improvement on the BDI-II in relation to standard care. Two large-scale studies conducted by Proudfoot and colleagues (2004) and Cavanagh and colleagues

(2006) found that completion of the *Beating the Blues* (www.beatingtheblues.co.uk) CCBT program led to significant decreases in measures of anxiety and depression and significant increases in measures of well-being and work and social adjustment. These improvements were maintained at up to 6 months following treatment, leading the National Institute for Clinical Excellence (NICE) to recommend it as a treatment for mild to moderate depression (Marks et al., 2007).

The most recent iteration of the *Overcoming Depression* (www.overcoming-depression.com) was tested by Whitfield and colleagues (2006) with a group of individuals who were on a waitlist to receive therapy services for their depression. Whitfield et al. (2006) found that participants who completed the entire six-session program demonstrated significant decreases in their symptoms of depression and expressed high degrees of satisfaction with the program.

Good Days Ahead: The Multimedia Program for Cognitive Therapy (www.mindstreet.com) is an eight-session multimedia computer program that has been tested in one randomized controlled trial where participants were assigned to computer-assisted cognitive therapy, standard cognitive therapy, or a waitlist control condition (Wright et al., 2005). Unlike in previous studies, participants assigned to the computer-assisted therapy condition spent half of each of their 50-min sessions receiving standard individual cognitive therapy and the other half of each of their sessions completing the *Good Days Ahead* program. Computer-assisted cognitive therapy and standard cognitive therapy both led to significant improvements in symptoms of depression that were maintained at 6-month follow-up. Furthermore, participants in the computer-assisted cognitive therapy condition had experienced significant decreases in negative core beliefs and automatic thoughts, whereas individuals in the standard cognitive therapy condition only experienced significant decreases in negative automatic thoughts. This finding suggests that there may be some advantages to having computer programs supplement traditional therapy approaches.

As previously mentioned, Christensen and colleagues (2004) compared the efficacy of a psychoeducational web site, titled BluePages, and a free interactive cognitive-behavioral therapy web site, titled MoodGYM, to an attention placebo condition as a treatment for individuals in the general community exhibiting symptoms of depression with positive results. In addition, further examination into the efficacy of MoodGYM has found it to be effective at decreasing depressive symptomology at 6- and 12-month follow-up (Christensen et al., 2006; Mackinnon et al., 2008). The makers of Mood Gym have also released a version for adolescents, e-Couch (www.ecouch.anu.edu.au), which is still awaiting empirical testing.

In addition to these promising programs, other types of computer-based and e-health interventions currently exist that seek to incorporate new, innovative additions to computer-based treatments. For example, *COPE* (www.healthtechsys.com) utilizes a combination of treatment booklets and telephone calls to treat depression (McKendree-Smith et al., 2003). The telephone calls are routed to a computer system that uses interactive voice response technology to provide individualized feedback to patients as they complete the treatment program or record messages for clinicians if necessary (McKendree-Smith et al., 2003). Additional computer-based treatment programs are also currently in the development and testing stage. Researchers at Western Michigan University have recently developed a 10-session computer-based behavioral activation treatment for depression, titled *Building a Meaningful Life Through Behavioral Activation* (Spates and Naugle, 2009). The first six sessions of this treatment focus on helping patients to track their day-to-day behaviors and bring their behaviors more in line with their values and goals. The remaining four sessions of the treatment are guided ideographically based on the problems described by individual patients. This program is not yet available for public dissemination and preliminary efforts investigating the effectiveness of the program are underway.

Certain individuals have suggested that specific populations may prefer computer-based interventions, including those who would rather work with a computer than a therapist or those with schedules or life circumstances that may interfere with regular therapy attendance (e.g., irregular work schedules or homelessness). Additionally, individuals who have difficulties with the stigma associated with seeking therapy services may be more inclined to participate in a computer-based protocol (e.g., Mood Gym and Blue Pages) as personal stigma has been demonstrated to be significantly reduced (Griffiths et al., 2004). However authors also found an increase in perceived stigma associated with the use of the programs. Considering that the most cited reason for avoiding psychological treatment is stigma (Corrigan, 2004), further investigation into computerized treatment and stigma is warranted. Computer-based interventions may be appropriate for individuals who have employment obligations that make seeking therapy services difficult (Marks et al., 2007), for those who are currently on a waitlist for services (Cavanagh and Shapiro, 2004) or for individuals who cannot seek therapy because of their location in rural areas. There are other populations for which computer-based interventions may not be recommended. Wright et al. (2005) note that computer-based interventions have only been tested with individuals displaying mild to moderate symptoms of depression and as such, computer-based interventions may not be appropriate for individuals experiencing severe levels of depression. Other authors have suggested that computer-based interventions may not be appropriate for individuals who cannot read or write in the language of the intervention or for individuals who have diagnoses of active substance abuse or psychosis (Cavanagh and Shapiro, 2004). As with psychoeducation and bibliotherapy, further research is needed to determine more specific populations for which computer-based approaches may and may not be indicated.

Step 3: Interventions Requiring More Intensive Care and Specialized Training

Group Treatment for Depression. Group interventions are a form of psychotherapy in which one or more therapists treat a group of clients simultaneously. Although it is well established that psychological interventions are effective treatments for depression with adults as well as children and adolescents (Weisz et al., 2006), it has not been definitively determined whether group treatments are as effective as individual treatments (Cuijpers et al., 2008). Managed care companies perceive the cost of treatments of depression to be excessive (Henk et al., 1996) which has promoted a shift in research from determining the best treatment to the best treatment at the best value (Yates, 1995). Given that group treatments allow many people to receive a therapeutic intervention simultaneously, it may be a viable option for reducing the burden on the strained healthcare system; however, it is still a more intensive level of care than the models discussed previously. Group interventions may also maximize cost-effectiveness as the costs of group therapy are about half that of individual treatment (Vos et al., 2005) depending on the length of time, number of therapists involved, and size of the group (Scott and Stradling, 1990). The apparent cost-effectiveness of group interventions has led to certain health management organizations to encourage its use as the treatment of choice by raising financial incentives for the use of group therapy (Jeffery, 1999). A recent meta-analysis comparing treatment outcomes of individual versus group treatments for depression found small but significant differences in acute treatment outcome in favor of individual therapy (Cuijpers et al., 2008). However, the effect size was 0.20, which is considered to be small and may not be of clinical significance. Additionally, the post-treatment outcomes favoring individual treatment did not persist at 1- or 6-month follow-up, indicating that individual treatment may be slightly more beneficial in the short term but of equal effectiveness after the conclusion of treatment. Other research has also suggested that group treatments can be equally efficacious as an individual treatment of depression (McDermut et al., 2001).

Similar results have been found in adolescent treatment of depression. Clarke et al. (1999) conducted a randomized clinical trial with depressed adolescents comparing group CBT, group CBT plus a separate parent group, and a waitlist control. CBT groups had higher depression recovery rates (66.7%) and a greater reduction in self-reported depression than the waitlist group, which achieved 48.1% recovery rate. Lockwood et al. (2004) conducted a meta-analysis which found group and individual CBT were equally efficacious for the treatment of moderately depressed adolescents.

It has been found that group cognitive behavior therapy also appears to be an effective treatment when delivered in a community setting (Peterson and Halstead, 1998; Satterfield, 1998). These positive findings, while not as large as those obtained in research settings coupled with its cost-effectiveness, led Peterson and Halstead to recommend that group CBT may be a first-line treatment in a stepped care approach. In addition, it has been postulated that group therapy may address factors that individual treatment cannot (McDermut et al., 2001). For example, interpersonal relationship functioning and social support have been shown to predict the subsequent course of depression, both of which are potentially available in, and could be targeted by group therapy (Brown and Moran, 1994; Hammen, 1991; Keitner and Miller, 1990).

Consideration must be given to suicidality of severely depressed patients when administering group interventions. Individuals may be less likely to report suicidality in a group setting than in individual psychotherapy or with their personal physician. It may be beneficial to add a brief individual suicide assessment as a first step to a group therapy format as a precautionary measure. In addition, for more severe patients, semi-regular concurrent individual therapy sessions (possibly at a reduced frequency compared to standard individual therapy) could be incorporated as an augment to the group therapy where careful suicide assessments could be conducted in a one-on-one format.

Treatment acceptability may play an important role in determining if an individual is better suited to individual or group interventions. Group interventions have consistently had higher dropout rates when compared to individual psychotherapy (Cuijpers et al., 2008). Furthermore, there is some evidence that dropout may be directly related to the fact that the treatment was implemented in a group (Meresman et al. 1995; Steuer et al., 1984). There are several possible reasons for these findings. Group treatments are less flexible than individual psychotherapy and are often only available at a specified time; thus, a conflict in scheduling may arise leading to the discontinuation of therapy. Also, individuals may be uncomfortable or unwilling to disclose important personally relevant information in group therapy. Thus, those with variable schedules or strong preference against group interventions may be particularly suited for a treatment that provides relative anonymity and flexibility such as the Internet-based applications mentioned previously. An assessment of treatment preference and willingness may be useful in determining treatment selection.

Individual Psychotherapy

Individual psychotherapy is typically considered a more intensive and costly level of stepped care. However, in spite of the greater initial cost of psychotherapy, the cumulative cost of medications may prove to be more expensive. It has been reported that a large proportion of patients with Major Depressive Disorder suffer a chronic (25%) or recurrent (75%) course (Rush et al., 2008), and there is no evidence that antidepressants alter the course of depression (Dimidjian et al., 2006). Since antidepressants do not appear to have enduring effects after use is discontinued, patients may be at significant risk for relapse and recurrence (Hollon et al., 2005). The current recommendation for the treatment of chronic or recurrent episodes of depression is prescription of antidepressants indefinitely (American Psychiatric Association, 2000). Given that some psychotherapeutic interventions have been proven to have enduring effects and to be equally efficacious for the treatment of depression in adults as medication (Dimidjian et al., 2006), using psychotherapy as a first-line treatment of depression with antidepressants in adjunct or in response to a lack of improvement or relapse may provide significant long-term savings.

In a stepped care model, individual intervention may be appropriate for individuals who do not benefit from lower levels of care, have moderate to severe symptom presentation, have a strong preference for individual therapy, or are considered treatment resistant. Individual psychotherapy is delivered by mental health specialists and requires specialized training in the form of psychotherapy that is delivered. It is delivered in a one-on-one format most typically in an outpatient care setting. There is great variability in the length, theory, and technique of treatment in individual psychotherapies. Cognitive Behavior Therapy (CBT) and Interpersonal Psychotherapy (IPT) are the treatments that have received the most attention and support in the literature for the treatment of depression, however, investigations have shown Behavioral Activation (BA) to be equally effective.

CBT has been shown to be effective in the treatment of depression in more randomized controlled trials than any other psychosocial treatment (Persons et al., 2001). In general, it has been found that CBT is more effective than waitlist and placebo, and marginally more effective than other bona fide psychotherapeutic interventions (Dobson, 1989; Gloaguen et al., 1998). The Treatment of Depression Collaborative Research Project (TDCRP) found CBT to be an effective treatment for mild to moderate depression but recommended medication management for those suffering from more severe depression (Elkin et al., 1989). However, more recent studies have shown CBT to be equally effective as medication for moderate to severe depression (DeRubeis et al., 2005). One strength of CBT is that its effects appear to be maintained after treatment is discontinued, with maintenance effects that compare favorably to ongoing antidepressant treatment (Hollon et al., 2005).

CBT is a result of a merger of cognitive psychology based on the practice and research of Aaron T. Beck (1976) and behavior therapy. Beck proposed that depressive symptoms result when stressful external life events activate maladaptive schema or cognitive structures that bias the interpretation of experiences (Beck et al., 1979). These maladaptive schemas influence overt behaviors, cognitions or automatic thoughts, and emotions. The interactions among these elements are believed to be reciprocal and causal in nature, with a change in one affecting the others. In the context of a structured therapy session, CBT uses several interventions that are aimed at changing maladaptive schemas that influence overt behaviors, cognitions or automatic thoughts, and emotions in combination with behaviorally based treatment objectives aimed at increasing contact with naturally reinforcing contingencies through goal setting and homework assignments. The reader is referred to Essential Components of Cognitive-Behavioral Therapy for Depression (Persons et al., 2000) for a more detailed explanation of this therapeutic approach.

Interpersonal psychotherapy (IPT) is another time-limited approach to the treatment of depression with substantial empirical support (Weissman et al., 2007). In a meta-analysis by Cuijpers et al. (2008) comparing the efficacy of treatments for depression, IPT was found to be slightly more efficacious than other psychological treatments, including CBT. However, it should be noted that other meta-analyses have found IPT to be equally or less effective than CBT (Dobson, 1989; Gloaguen et al., 1998). A meta-analysis conducted by Kotova (2005) examining efficacy of IPT specifically for women suffering from depression found that when compared to no treatment, IPT achieved large effect sizes (0.60–0.73). Direct comparisons between IPT and CBT yielded roughly equivalent results with a slight favor for IPT for severely depressed individuals (Elkin et al., 1989). When compared to placebo or psychoeducation, IPT achieved moderate effect sizes (0.37–0.48) and was slightly less effective than medication (–0.15). These results were reported to maintain their efficacy over time.

Although IPT has no specific theoretical origin it was originally designed in an attempt to specify (manualize) the practice of supportive therapy and was based on the work of Sullivan, Meyer, and Bowlby. The main focus of IPT is to attempt to understand and address depressive symptoms in the context of close interpersonal attachments and explore how these interactions are currently causing problems in the patient's personal and social context. Additionally, IPT seeks to build interpersonal skills and improve communication through the use of role play and experimentation in close relationships. The specific goals of IPT are based on which of the four common problem areas (grief, roles disputes, role transitions, or interpersonal deficits) seem to be the primary concern for the patient (Weissman et al., 2007).

For a detailed description of the most recent iteration, the reader is directed to *Comprehensive Guide to Interpersonal Psychotherapy* (Weissman et al., 2000).

CBT and IPT require specialized training and are delivered primarily by mental health specialists who tend to be more expensive, less widely available, and often are not located in places where the greatest need for services reside. Thus, it may be recommended that treatments that are shorter in duration and simpler to train and implement while maintaining efficacy may be a more effective use of resources and time as a first-line individual treatment for depression. Delivery of these interventions using computer or telehealth mechanisms as addressed above may be one cost-effective alternative.

Behavioral activation (BA) is another viable option. There is now solid empirical support for using a purely behavioral model among depressed adults (Jacobson et al., 1996), including older adults (Scogin et al., 1989). Jacobson et al. (1996) describes BA as "the application of behavioral principles such as goal setting, self-monitoring, activity scheduling, problem solving, and graded task assignment" to alter the avoidance and rumination behaviors that are characteristic of depression. Furthermore, BA seeks to increase behaviors that put the participant in contact with natural reinforcing contingencies that will ultimately become self-maintained and to decrease activities that promote depressive symptoms. This is accomplished by performing an ideographic functional analysis to identify problematic avoidance behavior and alternative coping strategies to produce higher rates of meaningful response contingent positive reinforcement (Kanter et al., 2007). For a full account of BA, the reader is referred to *Depression In Context*: *Strategies for Guided Action* (Martell et al., 2001). Dimidjian et al. (2006) found that BA was as effective as antidepressant medications and superior to CBT in the acute treatment of moderately to severely depressed adults and maintained effects over time. Further support comes from the component analysis conducted by Jacobson et al. (1996) demonstrating that 20 sessions of the purely behavioral component of CBT was equal in efficacy to the full CBT package described by Beck et al. (1979). As suggested by Jacobson, BA is a more parsimonious treatment than CBT and could be more easily trained and implemented by clinicians with less specialized expertise. People who are poor, on welfare, less educated, unemployed, or from certain minority groups may be at greater risk for depression. These individuals are also at the greatest risk for having restricted access to assessment and treatment, especially individual treatment, due to those same circumstances. As suggested by Dimidjian et al. (2006), BA is meant to be more exportable and easier to train than cognitive therapy, IPT, and other complex interventions. This would allow more professionals at a larger variety of locations to deliver an empirically supported manualized treatment, especially to the aforementioned at-risk populations. Thus, if it could be shown that BA can be effectively trained and implemented by lower level therapist, it may expand options for implementing evidence-based treatments in settings where more intensive levels of care are not otherwise available (i.e., community-based centers, school settings, primary care, specialty clinics) and for wider dissemination of treatment to at-risk populations (US Department of Health and Human Services, 2002) while lessening the burden on an overwhelmed healthcare system. Additionally, given BA's straightforward theory and implementation, it may lend itself well to bibliotherapy and the computer-based interventions listed previously. These strategies currently await further empirical investigation.

Assessing treatment preference may be important in deciding which intervention is best as an initial step. In a meta-analysis of studies that investigated treatment preferences, it was consistently found that subjects preferred psychotherapy and counseling over medication (van Schaik et al., 2004). It has also been found that more patients enter treatment when their preference of treatment is discussed and supported and in cases they could not receive their preferred treatment, they were more likely to go with no treatment altogether (Dwight-Johnson et al., 2001). If it is found that lower level therapist can effectively deliver BA, it may allow greater access to an empirically based intervention for those that may prefer individual therapy but currently do not have access.

Medication

While this chapter is primarily focused on psychosocial interventions within a stepped care model, pharmacotherapy for depression is often a first-line treatment and warrants some discussion. In most instances access to antidepressant medication is readily available in primary care settings, unlike evidence-based psychosocial interventions which generally require a specialized therapist. However, compliance with medication can often be an issue and therefore should be given consideration within a behavioral health care stepped care model. In addition, medication management often requires inclusion of elements of care discussed elsewhere in this chapter. Indeed, the American Psychiatric Association suggests that psychiatric management consist of a "broad array" of services including a diagnostic evaluation, evaluation of safety (suicide/homicide), establishment and maintenance of the therapeutic alliance, monitoring of symptoms, psychoeducation, and efforts to enhance treatment adherence (APA, 2000). This certainly places additional burden on prescribing physicians, some of which may be more efficiently accomplished using technology-based mechanisms.

The treatment of children and adolescents has even more complicating factors. The National Institute of Mental Health (NIMH)-funded Treatment for Adolescents with Depression Study (TADS, 2003) found that CBT plus fluoxetine (Prozac) is "the most favorable trade-off between benefit and risk for adolescents with major depressive disorder." The TADS study indicates that CBT plus fluoxetine is the most effective treatment for adolescent depression as this combination provided the greatest improvement in symptoms of major depressive disorder (MDD) while moderating risk of harm-related adverse events. In spite of this recommendation, antidepressants alone are routinely given as a first-line treatment for depressed youth (Safer, 1997) which may be due to the fact that CBT combined treatment is often not feasible for financial or other reasons. Adding to these concerns, in 2004 the US Food and Drug Administration (FDA) issued a black box warning for antidepressants used with pediatric populations due to concerns regarding suicidality leaving many clinicians and patients wary of psychopharmacological interventions. There are also significant other risks for side effects including agitation, sleep disruption, gastrointestinal and sexual problems (Antonuccio et al., 1999). Additionally, there is a lack of investigation into potential effects of antidepressants on development. This is especially concerning considering case reports that SSRIs may be linked to growth suppression (Weintrob et al., 2002). SSRIs also have troubling withdrawal symptoms upon abrupt discontinuation, which may be more prevalent in children and adolescents given their passive involvement in treatment. When long-term efficacy is examined, CBT alone appears to have equal efficacy as fluoxetine at 18-week follow-up and combination treatment at 36 weeks without the significant risk involved with psychotropic medications (TADS, 2007).

It has been argued that due to the significant risk for side effects as well as the difficulty in implementation and high cost of CBT plus fluoxetine, other scientifically supported interventions may be determined to be preferable as a first-line intervention for certain populations. Antonuccio (2008) suggests that using the TADS studies as a guide, it may be possible to tailor treatment decisions to patient and parent preferences after education about the various risks and outcomes. This may play a vital role in treatment selection in a stepped intervention. For those whom safety is a priority or those suffering from less severe depressive symptoms, some of the interventions mentioned previously in this chapter may the best initial step. For those for whom short-term efficacy is prioritized, CBT plus fluoxtine or fluoxtine alone may be warranted. For a more thorough discussion and a summary handout meant to assist in patient education, the reader is referred to Antonuccio (2008).

Pharmacotherapy has also been addressed and investigated using a stepped care model in adult populations. The Sequenced Treatment Alternatives to Relieve Depression (STAR*D; Rush et al., 2008) study was designed to investigate the impact of sequenced treatment strategies. The study implemented a SSRI antidepressant (citalopram) as the first step in the model of treatment. Those who failed to respond to this initial step were then given the option of changing medications, changing to cognitive psychotherapy, augmenting medication with cognitive therapy, or augmenting with another medication type. In total, 70% of those that completed the stepped protocol achieved remission (Fawcett, 2008). However, many of the participants needed several steps to achieve remission and those who required more steps showed higher intolerance for treatment and higher relapse rates (Rush et al., 2008).

Expert panels have also identified approaches that take the best evidence for medication treatment for depression into account and have developed sets of algorithms for administering and monitoring medication for depression (i.e., Texas Implementation of Medication Algorithm, Michigan Implementation of Medication Algorithm). The medication algorithm guidelines are directed to primary care practitioners rather than specialists. The algorithms aid those with prescriptive authority in making evidence-based decisions about adjustment of medication regimens based on patient improvement or worsening. Investigators at Western Michigan University have developed an interactive multimedia technology to disseminate information about medication algorithms to prescribing physicians as well as to increase the efficiency and use of the algorithms in guiding decisions about patients. This technology allows medical staff to regularly monitor depressive symptoms using well-established symptom questionnaires and to make evidence-based decisions about medication regimens.

Step 4: Most Restrictive and Intensive Forms of Care

Inpatient Care

Inpatient care for depression is considered among the highest, most restrictive, and most intensive levels of care. It is costly and requires extensive resources. Cotterill and Thomas (2004) found the typical cost per case in inpatient treatment was between US $5000 and 7000 for an average of $410–638 per day. In addition to these concerns are concerns of stigma, risk of damage to the therapeutic alliance, as well as the fact that those that are hospitalized may lose their jobs as a result of time missed. Although there are forms of inpatient care that are meant to be intensive and long term, the purpose of the section is to discuss brief hospitalization as a safety measure for severely depressed individuals as the final measure in a stepped protocol. In cases of severe depression where acute suicidality or homicidally is present, inpatient care via voluntary or mandated commitment to a hospital setting may be considered. This practice currently accounts for 50–60% of all psychiatric hospitalizations (Sullivan et al., 2005).

The APA's Practice Guidelines for Selecting a Treatment Setting for Patients at Risk for Suicide (2004) suggest that for those whom suicidality is a reaction to a precipitating event, have a plan that is low in lethality or intent, have a stable and supportive living environment, and are agreeable to follow-up recommendations, an outpatient safety plan may be the best course of action. The safety plan should be a collaborative effort designed to provide immediate safety, ensure adequate monitoring, provide social support, and draw upon individual resources to problem solve upcoming times that may be especially problematic. Utilization of a safety plan may ameliorate the weakness of "no-harm contracts" (Paladino and Minton, 2008; Shea, 2002), as these have not been found to reduce the risk of suicide (APA, 2003).

For those with stronger indicators of suicide risk, it may be best to directly discuss options of care with the client, recommending voluntary placement in an inpatient facility. In cases where it is determined that the client is a great risk to themselves but refuses voluntary placement, involuntary commitment to an institutionalized setting where their behavior can be careful monitored and intensive short-term treatment can be implemented should be used.

Treatment that is received in inpatient settings may vary greatly (Brabender, 1993), yet very few outcome studies have been conducted to evaluate short-term treatments in these settings (Jarrett, 1995). Given the expense and personal cost in time and freedom to an individual that has been hospitalized, briefer and more effective treatments are always being sought. This is especially important considering that depressive symptom severity at discharge is associated with risk of future hospitalization (Lieberman et al., 1998). Currently, antidepressant medications are the "mainstay" in treatment with suicidal patients with acute, recurrent, or chronic depression. However, there is little evidence to suggest that antidepressants reduce suicide risk (APA, 2003). In fact, as discussed previously, there is some evidence that antidepressants may increase suicidality in adolescent populations. This finding also has support in the adult literature. An increased risk for completed suicide of about twice that of the base rate for an at-risk population was found in the first 12 weeks following the beginning of antidepressant treatment (Valenstein et al., 2009). These concerns necessitate further research into brief inpatient interventions. A promising new treatment for those in inpatient care is Brief Behavioral Activation Treatment for Depression (BATD; Hopko, et al., 2003; Lejuez et al., 2001a, b, 2002). Based on the behavioral activation treatment described previously, BATD provides a brief, manualized approach for intervention in a hospital setting. In a small trial, BATD plus antidepressant medication when compared to supportive treatment as usual plus antidepressant medication achieved favorable outcome with a large effect size of 0.73 after only a 2-week treatment period (Hopko et al., 2003). This preliminary evidence seems to support this approach as a brief intervention for severely suicidal inpatients.

It has been suggested that one of the most critical times to intervene with a patient that has had a history of suicidal behavior is at the point of discharge (Goldacre et al., 1993; Jacobs, 1999). There is significant evidence that taking a proactive or broad-based community approach to prevention is indicative of improved outcomes for suicidal patients (e.g., King et al., 2003; Knox et al., 2003; Motto and Bostrom, 2001). In a literature review of suicide prevention, Goldney (2005) suggested that community-based approaches should be emulated on a large scale as they are promising interventions for suicide prevention. Certainly discharge planning should involve recommendations and resources to provide evidence-based care in a less restrictive setting once the patient is released from inpatient care.

Research Agenda for Stepped Care

A fully realized stepped care model would maximize client outcomes while mini-mizing provider costs. Demand for services far outnumbers the availability of those who have been trained to deliver effective mental health services (Haaga, 2000). Effective stepped interventions may ease this burden while maximizing the quality of care. Given the high incidence of depression, as well as the high rate of those who suffer yet go unrecognized and treated, an organized national stepped care plan is essential. To reach this goal will require a dedicated and systematic research agenda. Data from existing sequenced care trials (e.g., STAR*D and TORDIA—Treatment Of Resistant Depression In Adolescents; Brent et al., 2008) began to shed light on the potential benefits of augmenting (adding another medication or CBT) or switch-ing (to another medication or CBT) treatment after an initial sub-optimal response to selective serotonin reuptake inhibitor pharmacotherapy. These trials are a valuable beginning, but they only look at a few possible steps. Many other sequences remain open to empirical investigation. For instance, is pharmacotherapy the best first step? There is some evidence that antidepressant medication may reduce symptoms more quickly and, thus, may be more cost-effective as an acute treatment compared to CBT (Domino et al., 2008; Elkin et al., 1989). However, an initial response to pharmacotherapy may not be as sustained as in CBT (Hollon et al., 2005; Rohde et al., 2008). Lengthier remission/recovery periods and lower recurrence/relapse rates may enhance the cost-effectiveness of CBT when calculated over longer time spans (Dobson et al., 2008). Furthermore, given that depressive episodes are typi-cally recurrent, treatments that produce sustained recovery and reduced relapse rates may ultimately be more cost-effective than even watchful waiting (which appears unlikely to have any preventative effect on future episodes). Thus, in addition to exploring a range of steps and sequences, research allowing for analysis of short-term and long-range clinical outcomes and additional service utilization is needed to examine these possibilities empirically.

Furthermore, other interventions beyond medication and CBT warrant investi-gation. As reviewed earlier, both IPT and BA have solid empirical support in the treatment of depression. How should these interventions be incorporated into a com-prehensive stepped model that cuts across modalities? In addition, how should they be sequenced within the domain of psychotherapeutic interventions? Should they be delivered in person by a therapist or via the computer? Should there simply be a menu of empirically supported psychosocial treatment options from which patients choose, either in person or on the computer? Should IPT or BA replace, precede, or post-date CBT and on what grounds? These remain important open questions. To illustrate, consider BA. Conceptually BA could be readily used in sequence with CBT, as the first part of most CBT protocols typically incorporates components of BA, such as activity scheduling (see Beck et al., 1979). If a substantial percentage of patients would respond to a Step 1 involving straightforward activity schedul-ing and, thus, not need to progress to more individualized functional analysis-based behavioral activation or cognitive therapy techniques this would be the beginning of a theoretically logical *and* empirically sensible stepped model. Furthermore, might there be some interventions that are so broadly applicable and easy to implement by a therapist or computer program (e.g., activity scheduling) that they may be more cost-effective than even watchful waiting?

Current models of evidenced-based psychological practice emphasize treatment planning based on a combination of empirical evidence, provider expertise in treatment delivery, and client variables such as treatment preferences (Spring, 2007). Thus, it is important to explore how a therapist's expertise in treatment and client preferences can be best incorporated into stepped care models. To illustrate, consider that despite its strong empirical track record, only a minority of patients in the STAR*D trial chose to switch to, or receive augmentation with, CBT (Thase et al., 2007). These data suggest we need research focused not only on treatment outcome but on treatment decision making and how treatment options are presented to clients. Furthermore, in several of the large trials of CBT versus medication there have been findings of site differences—that is, at some centers CBT outcomes were better than at other centers within the same study—possibly related to expertise in delivery of CBT (DeRubeis et al., 2005; Jacobson and Hollon, 1996). If most depressed patients do not opt for comprehensive CBT and its effects are variable even across academic centers conducting funded treatment trials using integrity protocols, these are important considerations that must be studied as stepped care models are developed.

It is important not only to investigate multiple stepped care models to examine differential immediate and long-range outcomes, but also to consider variables that moderate outcome. That is, are there intake (clinical or demographic) characteristics of clients that predict which step or sequence of steps is most likely to be helpful? For instance, do the most severely depressed clients do best if provided combined pharmacotherapy and psychotherapy as the first step? Should clients with a history of prior episodes of depression receive a different series of steps, skip potential initial steps like watchful waiting, or progress through the steps more rapidly, compared to those receiving treatment for first depressive episode? These questions suggest that even if there is convergence on a generally applicable set of steps, one size is unlikely to fit all. Thus, identification of variables that predict treatment response among subgroups of patients would be important to determine.

Finally, it is important to note that the stepped care research agenda is tied to developments in the broader depression intervention research arena. It is still unclear exactly why many of our most empirically supported treatments work. Determining the mechanisms of action in effective intervention may allow for more targeted and effective intervention, which would be critical to maximizing the potential efficacy of a given step in a stepped care model. Furthermore, in psychotherapy it is important not only to determine the variables that mediate outcome at the level of a treatment package (e.g., a 20 session CBT protocol) but also to determine which techniques within packages are "active ingredients" so as to also amass empirically supported techniques (O'Donohue and Fisher, 2009). Progress in this area may benefit from research examining whether specified techniques produce change in a theoretically identified variable, which then mediates subsequent changes in symptomatic functioning. Stepped care models could then be crafted to emphasize techniques, tied to specific process variables, that appear most active in the change process.

References

Addis M, Martell C. Overcoming depression one step at a time: the new behavioral activation. Oakland, CA: New Harbinger Publications; 2004.

American Psychiatric Association. Practice guidelines for the treatment of patients with major depressive disorder (revision). Am J Psychiatry. 2000;157:1–45.

American Psychiatric Association. Practice guideline for the assessment and treatment of patients with suicidal behaviors. Am J Psychiatry. 2003;160:1–50.

Antonuccio D. Treating depressed children with antidepressants: more harm than benefit? J Clin Psychol Med S. 2008;15:92–7.

Antonuccio DO. Tailoring treatment to parental values: a comment on TADS. Arch Gen Psychiatry. 2008;65:723.

Antonuccio DO, Danton WG, DeNelsky GY, Greenberg RP, Gordon JS. Raising questions about antidepressants. Psychother Psychosom. 1999;68:3–14.

Beck AT. Cognitive therapy and the emotional disorders. New York: International Universities Press; 1976.

Beck AT, Rush AJ, Shaw BF, Emery G. Cognitive therapy of depression. New York: Guilford Press; 1979.

Beck AT, Steer RA, Brown GK. Manual for the BDI-II. San Antonio, TX: Psychological corporation; 1996.

Beck AT, Steer RA, Ball R, Ranieri W. Comparison of beck depression inventories -IA and -II in psychiatric outpatients. J Pers Assess. 1996;67:588–97.

Bennett DS, Ambrosini PJ, Bianchi M, Barnett D, Metz C, Rabinovich H. Relationship of Beck depression inventory factors to depression among adolescents. J Affect Disord. 1997;45: 127–34.

Brabender V. Inpatient group psychotherapy. In: Kaplan HI, Sadock BJ, editors. Comprehensive group psychotherapy. 3rd ed. Baltimore: Williams & Wilkins; 1993. p. 607–19.

Brent D, Emslie G, Clarke G, et al. Switching to another SSRI or to venlafaxine with or without cognitive behavioral therapy for adolescents with SSRI-resistant depression: the TORDIA randomized controlled trial. J Am Med Assoc. 2008;299:901–13.

Bridge JA, Iyengar S, Salary CB, et al. Clinical response and risk for reported suicidal ideation and suicide attempts in pediatric antidepressant treatment: a meta-analysis of randomized controlled trials. J Am Med Assoc. 2007;297:1683–96.

Brown GW, Moran P. Clinical and psychosocial origins of chronic depressive episodes: a community survey. Br J Psychiatry. 1994;165:447–56.

Burns DD. Feeling good. New York: Avon; 1980.

Busch AM, Kanter JW, Landes SJ, Kohlenberg RJ. Sudden gains and outcome: a broader temporal analysis of cognitive therapy for depression. Behav Ther. 2006;37:61–8.

Carey MP, Faulstich ME, Gresham FM, Ruggiero L, Enyart P. "Children's depression inventory: construct and discriminant validity across clinical and nonreferred (control) populations": correction to Carey et al. J Consult Clin Psychol. 1987;55(6):845.

Cavanagh K, Shapiro DA. Computer treatment for common mental health problems. J Clin Psychol. 2004;80(3):239–51.

Cavanagh K, Shapiro DA, Van Den Berg S, et al. The effectiveness of computerized cognitive behavioural therapy in routine care. Br J Clin Psychol. 2006;45:499–514.

Christensen H, Griffiths KM, Jorm AF. Delivering interventions for depression by using the internet: randomised controlled trial. Br Med J. 2004;328:265.

Christensen H, Griffiths KM, Mackinnon AJ, Brittliffe K. Online randomized controlled trial of brief and full cognitive behavior therapy for depression. Psychol Med. 2006;36:1737–1746.

Cheung AH, Emslie GJ, Mayes TL. Review of the efficacy and safety of antidepressants in youth depression. J Child Psychol Psychiatry. 2005;46:735–54.

Ciarlo JA, Brown TR, Edwards DW, Kiresuk TJ, Newman EL. Assessing mental health treatment outcome measurement techniques. Department of Health and Human Services Publication Number (ADM), 86-1301. Washington, DC: U.S. Government Printing Office, 41; 1986. p. 159–64.

Clarke GN, Rohde P, Lewinsohn PM, Hops H, Seeley JR. Cognitivebehavioral treatment of adolescent depression: efficacy of acute group treatment and booster sessions. J Am Acad Child Adolesc Psychiatry. 1999;38:272–79.

Corrigan P. How stigma interferes with mental health care. Am Psychol. 2004;59:614–25.

Cotterill PG, Thomas FG. Prospective payment for medicare inpatient psychiatric care: assessing the alternatives. Health Care Financ R. 2004;26:85–101.

Cuijpers P. Bibliotherapy in unipolar depression: a meta-analysis. J Behav Ther Exp Psychiatry. 1997;28:139–47.

Cuijpers P. A psychoeducational approach to the treatment of depression: a meta-analysis of Lewinsohn's "Coping With Depression" course. Behav Ther. 1998;29:521–33.

Cuijpers P, van Straten A, Warmerdam L. Are individual and group treatments equally effective in the treatment of depression in adults? A meta analysis. Eur J Psychiat. 2008;22:38–51.

Cukrowicz KC, Joiner TE. Computer-based intervention for anxious and depressive symptoms in a non-clinical population. Cognitive Ther Res. 2007;31:677–93.

Davidson J, Turnbull CD, Strickland R, Miller R, et al. The Montgomery-Asberg depression rating scale: reliability and validity. Acta Psychiat Scand. 1986;73:544–48.

DeRubeis RJ, Hollon SD, Amsterdam JD, et al. Cognitive therapy vs. medications in the treatment of moderate to severe depression. Arch Gen Psychiatry. 2005;62:409–16.

Dimidjian S, Hollon SD, Dobson KS, Schmaling KB, Kohlenberg RJ, Addis M. Randomized trial of behavioral activation, cognitive therapy, and antidepressant medication in the acute treatment of adults with major depression. J Consult Clin Psychol. 2006;74:658–70.

Dobson KS. A meta-analysis of the efficacy of cognitive therapy for depression. J Consult Clin Psychol. 1989;57:414–19.

Dobson KS, Hollon SD, Dimidjian S, et al. Randomized trial of behavioral activation, cognitive therapy, and antidepressant medication in the prevention of relapse and recurrence in major depression. J Consult Clin Psychol. 2008;76:468–77.

Domino ME, Burns BJ, Silva SG, et al. Cost-effectiveness of treatments for adolescent depression: results from TADS. Am J Psychiatry. 2008;165:588–96.

Dowrick C, Dunn G, Ayuso-Mateos JL, et al. Problem solving treatment and group psychoeducation for depression: multicentre randomised controlled trial. Br Med J. 2000;321:1–6.

Dwight-Johnson M, Meredith L, Hickey S, Wells K. Influence of patient preference and primary care clinician proclivity for watchful waiting on receipt of depression treatment. Gen Hosp Psychiat. 2006;28:379–86.

Dwight-Johnson M, Unutzer J, Sherbourne C, Tang L, Wells KB. Can qualityimprovement programs for depression in primary care address patient preferences for treatment? Med Care. 2001;39:934–44.

Elkin I, Gibbons RD, Shea MT, Sotsky SM, Watkins JT, Pilkonis PA, Hedeker D. Initial severity and differential treatment outcome in the national institute of mental health treatment of depression collaborative research program. J Consult Clinical Psychol. 1995;63(5):841–7.

Elkin I, Shea MT, Watkins JT, et al. National institute of mental health treatment of depression collaborative research program: general effectiveness of treatments. Arch Gen Psychiatry. 1989;46:971–82.

Fawcett J. Is the current state of the treatment of depression satisfactory? Psychiat Ann. 2008;37:172.

Gaynor ST, Weersing VR, Kolko DJ, Birmaher B, Heo J, Brent DA. The prevalence and impact of large sudden improvements during adolescent therapy for depression: a comparison across cognitive-behavioral, family, and supportive therapy. J Consult Clin Psychol. 2003;71:386–93.

Gloaguen V, Cottraux J, Cucherat M, Blackburn IM. A meta-analysis of the effects of cognitive therapy in depressed patients. J Affect Disord. 1998;49:59–72.

Goldacre M, Seagroatt V, Hawton K. Suicide after discharge from psychiatric inpatient care. Lancet. 1993;342:283–6.

Goldney RD. Suicide prevention: a pragmatic review of recent studies. Crisis: The J Crisis Intervention and Suicide Prevention. 2005;26:128–40.

Gregory RJ, Canning SS, Lee TW, Wise JC. Cognitive bibliotherapy for depression: a meta-analysis. Prof Psychol-Res Pr. 2004;35:275–80.

Griffiths KM, Christensen H, Jorm AF, Evans K, Groves C. Effect of web-based literacy and cognitive-behavioral therapy interventions on stigmatizing attitudes to depression: a randomized controlled trial. Br J Psychiatry. 2004;185:342–9.

Haaga DAF. Introduction to the special section on stepped care models in psychotherapy. J Consult Clin Psychol. 2000;68(4):547–8.

Hamilton M. Rating depressive patients. J Clin Psychiatry. 1980;45:21–4.

Hammen C. Depression runs in families: the social context of risk and resilience in children of depressed mothers. New York: Springer; 1991.

Hegel MT, Oxman TE, Hull JG, Swain K, Swick H. Watchful waiting in primary care: Remission rates and predictors of improvement. Gen Hosp Psychiatry. 2006;28:205–12.

Henk H, Kazelnick D, Kobak K, Griest J, Jefferson J. Medical cost attributed to depression among patients with high medical expenses in a health maintenance organization. Arch Gen Psychiatry. 1996;53:899–904.

Hermens MLM, van Hout HPJ, Terluin B, et al. The prognosis of minor depression in the general population: a systematic review. Gen Hosp Psychiatry. 2004;26:453–62.

Hollon SD, DeRubeis RJ, Shelton RC, et al. Prevention of relapse following cognitive therapy versus medications in moderate to severe depression. Arch Gen Psychiatry. 2005;62:417–23.

Honey KL, Bennett P, Morgan M. A brief psycho-educational group intervention for postnatal depression. Br J Clin Psychology. 2002;41:405–9.

Hopko DR, Lejuez CW, LePage JP, Hopko SD, McNeil DW. A brief behavioral activation treatment for depression: A randomized pilot trial within an inpatient psychiatric hospital. Behav Modif. 2003;27(4):458–69.

Ilardi SS, Craighead WE. The role of nonspecific factors in cognitive behavior therapy for depression. Clin Psychol Sci Practice. 1994;1:138–56.

Institute of Medicine. Committee on quality health care in America: crossing the quality chasm. Washington, DC: National Academic; 2001.

Jacobs D. The Harvard medical school guide to suicide assessments and interventions. San Francisco, CA: Josey Bass Inc; 1999.

Jacobson NS, Dobson KS, Truax PA, et al. A component analysis of cognitive-behavioral treatment for depression. J Consult Clin Psychol. 1996;64:295–304.

Jacobson NS, Hollon SD. Cognitive-behavior therapy versus pharmacotherapy: now that the jury's returned its verdict, it's time to present the test of the evidence. J Consult Clin Psychol. 1996;64:74–80.

Jarrett RB. Comparing and combining short-term psychotherapy and pharmacotherapy for depression. In: Beckham EE, Leber WR, editors. Handbook of depression. 2nd ed. New York: Guilford; 1995. p. 435–64.

Jeffery NA. HMOs face questions over push for group therapy. Wall Street J. 1999;Jan 11:A25, A28.

Joiner Jr TE, Rudd MD, Rajab MH. The modified scale for suicidal ideation among suicidal adults: factors of suicidality and their relation to clinical and diagnostic indicators. J Abnorm Psychol. 1997;106:260–5.

Joiner T, Walker R, Rudd MD, Jobes D. Scientizing and routinizing the outpatient assessment of suicidality. Prof Psychol-Res Pr. 1999;30:447–53.

Joint commission on accreditation of healthcare organizations. Overview of the indicator measurement system. Oakbrook Terrace, IL: JCAHO; 1993.

Kanter JW, Mulick PS, Busch AM, Berlin KS, Martell CR. The behavioral activation for depression scale (BADS): psychometric properties and factor structure. J Psychopathol Behav. 2007;29:191–202.

Keitner GI, Miller IW. Family functioning in major depression: an overview. Am J Psychiatry. 1990;147:1128–37.

Kelleher WJ, Talcott GW, Haddock CK, Freeman RK. Military psychology in the age of managed care: The Wilford Hall model. Appl Prev Psychol. 1996;5:101–10.

King R, Nurcombe B, Bickman L, Hides L, Reid W. Telephone counseling for adolescent suicide prevention: changes suicidality and mental state from beginning to end of a counseling session. Suicide Life-Threat. 2003;33:400–11.

Knox KL, Litts DA, Talcott GW, Feig JC, Caine D. Risk of suicide and related adverse outcomes after exposure to a suicide prevention programme in the US air force: Cohort study. Br Med J. 2003;327:1376–80.

Kotova E. A meta-analysis of interpersonal psychotherapy. Dissertation abstracts international: section B: Sciences and Engineering. 2005;66(5-B):2828.

Kovacs M. The children's depression inventory. Los Angeles, CA: Western Psychological Services; 1992.

Lara MA, Navarro C, Rubí NA, Mondragón L. Two levels of intervention in low-income women with depressive symptoms: compliance and programme assessment. Int J Soc Psychiatry. 2003;49:43–57.

Lejuez CW, Hopko DR, Hopko SD. A brief behavioral activation treatment for depression: treatment manual. Behav Modif. 2001a;25:255–86.

Lejuez CW, Hopko DR, LePage JP, Hopko SD, McNeil DW. A brief behavioral activation treatment for depression. Cogn Behav Pract. 2001b;8:164–75.

Lejuez CW, Hopko DR, Hopko SD. The brief behavioral activation treatment for depression (BATD): a comprehensive patient guide. Boston, MA: Pearson Custom Publishing; 2002.

Lewinsohn PM, Munoz R, Youngren M, Zeiss A. Control your depression. Englewood Cliffs, NJ: Prentice-Hall; 1986.

Lieberman PB, Wiitala SA, Elliott B, McCormick S, Goyette SB. Decreasing length of stay: are there effects on outcomes of psychiatric hospitalization? Am J Psychiatry. 1998;155: 905–9.

Lin M, Moyle W, Chang H, Chou M, Hsu M. Effect of an interactive computerized psycho-education system on patients suffering from depression. J Clin Nurs. 2008;17:667–76.

Lockwood C, Page T, Conroy-Hiller T. Comparing the effectiveness of cognitive behavior therapy using individual or group therapy in the treatment of depression. Adelaide, Australia: Joanna; 2004.

Mackinnon A, Griffiths KM, Christensen H. Comparative randomised trial of online cognitive-behaivoural therapy and an information web site for depression: 12-month outcomes. Br J Psychiatry. 2008;192:130–4.

Mains JA, Scogin FR. The effectiveness of self-administered treatments: a practice-friendly review of the research. J Clin Psychol/In Session: Psychother Pract. 2003;59:237–46.

Masip AF, Campos JAA, Olmos JG. Psychometric properties of the Reynolds child depression scale in community and clinical samples. Span J Psychol. 2008;11:641–9.

Marks IM. The maturing of therapy: some brief psychotherapies help anxiety/depressive disorders but mechanisms of action are unclear. Br J Psychiatry. 2002;180:200–4.

Marks IM, Cavanagh K, Gega L. Computer-aided psychotherapy: revolution or bubble? Br J Psychiatry. 2007;191:471–3.

Martell CR, Addis ME, Jacobsen NS. Depression in context: strategies for guided action. New York: W. W. Norton & Company, Inc; 2001.

McDermut W, Miller IW, Brown RA. The efficacy of group psychotherapy for depression: a meta-analysis and review of the empirical research. Clin Psychol Sci Pract. 2001;8:98–116.

McKendree-Smith NL, Floyd M, Scogin FR. Self-administered treatments for depression: a review. J Clin Psychol. 2003;59(3):275–88.

Meredith LS, Cheng WJY, Hickey SC, Dwight-Johnson M. Factors Associated with primary care and clinician's choice of watchful waiting approach to managing depression. Psychiat Serv. 2007;58:72–8.

Meresman JF, Horowitz LM, Bein E. Treatment assignment, dropout, and outcome of depressed patients who somaticize. Psychother Res. 1995;5:245–57.

Motto JA, Bostrom AG. A randomized controlled trail of a post crisis suicide intervention. Psychiatr Serv. 2001;52:828–33.

O'Donohue W, Fisher JE. General Principles and Empirically Supported Techniques of Cognitive Behavior Therapy. Wiley; 2009.

Ong SH, Caron A. Family-based psychoeducation for children and adolescents with mood disorders. J Child and Family Studies. 2008;17:809–22.

Paladino D, Minton CAB. Comprehensive college student suicide assessment: application of the BASIC ID. J Am Coll Health. 2008;56:643–50.

Patten SB. A major depression prognosis calculator based on episodeduration. Clin Pract Epidemil Ment Health. 2006;2:13.

Persons JB, Davidson J, Tompkins MA. Essential components of cognitive behavioral therapy for depression. American Psychological Association. Washington, DC; 2000.

Persons JB, Davidson J, Tompkins MA. Essential components of cognitive behavior therapy for depression. American Psychological Association. Washington, D.C; 2001.

Peterson AL, Halstead TS. Group cognitive behavior therapy for depression in a community setting: a clinical replication series. Behav Ther. 1998;29(1):3–18.

Posternak MA, Solomon DA, Leon AC, Mueller TI, Shea MT, Endicott J, Keller MB. The naturalistic course of unipolar major depression in the absence of somatic therapy. J Nerv Ment Dis. 2006;194:324–9.

Poznanski EO, Mokros HB. Children's depression rating scale, revised. Los Angeles, CA: Western Psychological Services; 1996.

Proudfoot J, Ryden C, Everitt B, et al. Clinical efficacy of computerised cognitive behavioural therapy for anxiety and depression in primary care: randomized controlled trial. Br J Psychiatry, 2004;185:46–54.

Renaud J, Brent DA, Baugher M, Birmaher B, Kolko DJ, Bridge J. Rapid response to psychosocial treatment for adolescent depression: a two-year follow-up. J Am Acad Child and Adolesc Psychiatry. 1998;37:1184–90.

Reynolds WM. Reynolds adolescent depression scale. Odessa, FL: Psychological assessment resources; 1987.

Rohde P, Silva SG, Tonev ST, et al. Achievement and maintenance of sustained response during TADS continuation and maintenance therapy. Arch Gen Psychiatry. 2008;65:447–55.

Rosen GM, Glasgow RE, Barrera M. A controlled study to assess the clinical efficacy of totally self-administered systematic desensitization. J Consult Clin Psychol. 1976;44:208–17.

Rush JA, Kilner J, Fava M, et al. Clinically relevant findings from STAR*D. Psychiat Ann. 2008;38:188–93.

Safer DJ. Changing patterns of psychotropic medications prescribed by child psychiatrists in the 1990s. J Adolesc Psychopharmacology. 1997;26:267–74.

Satterfield JM. Cognitive behavioral group therapy for depressed, low-income minority clients: retention and treatment enhancement. Cogn Behav Pract. 1998;5:65–80.

Scogin F, Jamison C, Gochneaur K. Comparative efficacy of cognitive and behavioral bibliotherapy for mildly and moderately depressed older adults. J Consult Clin Psychol. 1989;57:403–7.

Scogin FR, Hanson A, Welsh D. Self-administered treatment in stepped care models of depression treatment. J Clin Psychol. 2003;59:341–9.

Scott MJ, Stradling SG. Group cognitive therapy for depression produces clinically significant reliable change in community-based settings. Behav Psychotherapy, 1990;18(1):1–19.

Shea SC. The practical art of suicide assessment: a guide for mental health professionals and substance abuse counselors. New York: Wiley; 2002.

Spring B. Evidence-based practice in clinical psychology: what it is, why it matters; what you need to know. J Clin Psychol. 2007;63:611–31.

Steuer JL, Mintz J, Hammen CL, et al. Cognitive-behavioral and psychodynamic group psychotherapy in treatment of geriatric depression. J Consult Clin Psychol. 1984;52:180–9.

Stice E, Burton E, Bearman SK, Rohde P. Randomized trial of a brief depression prevention program: an elusive search for a psychosocial placebo control condition. Behav Res Ther. 2006;45:863–76.

Strosahl K, Robinson P. The mindfulness and acceptance workbook for depression: using acceptance and commitment therapy to move through depression and create a life worth living. Oakland, CA: New Harbinger Publications; 2008.

Sullivan AM, Barren CT, Bezmen J, Rivera J, Zapata-Vega M. The safe treatment of the suicidal patient in an adult inpatient setting: a proactive preventive approach. Psychiat Quart. 2005;76:67–83.

Swan J, Sorrell E, MacVicar B, Durham R, Matthews K. "Coping with depression": an open study of the efficacy of a group psychoeducational intervention in chronic, treatment-refractory depression. J Affect Disord. 2004;82:125–9.

Thase ME, Friedman ES, Biggs MM, et al. Cognitive therapy versus medication in augmentation and switch strategies as second-step treatments: A STAR∗D report. Am J Psychiatry. 2007;164:739–52.

Tranter R, O'Donovan C, Chandarana P, Kennedy S. Prevalence and outcome of partial remission in depression. J Psychiatry Neurosci. 2002;27(4):241–7.

Treatment for Adolescent Depression Study (TADS) Team. Fluoxetine, cognitive-behavioral therapy, and their combination for adolescents with depression. Treatment for Adolescents of Depression Study (TADS) randomized controlled trial. J Am Med Assoc. 2004;292:807–20.

Treatment for Adolescents with Depression Study (TADS). Treatment for adolescents with depression study: long term effectiveness and safety outcomes. Arch Gen Psychiatry. 2007;64:1132–44.

U.S. Department of Health and Human Services. National ambulatory medical care survey: 2002 Summary.

Valenstein M, Kim HM, Ganoczy D, McCarthy JF, Zivin K, Austin KL, et al. Higher-risk periods for suicide among VA patients receiving depression treatment: prioritizing suicide prevention efforts. J Affect Disord. 2009;112:50–8.

Van Schaik DJF, Klijn AFJ, van Hout HPJ, et al. Patient preferences in the treatment of depressive disorder in primary care. Gen Hosp Psychiatry. 2004;26:184–9.

Vos T, Corry J, Haby MM, Carter R, Andrews G. Cost-effectiveness of CBT and drug interventions for major depression. Aust NZ J Psychiat. 2005;39:683–92.

Weissman MM, Markowitz JC, Klerman GL. Comprehensive guide to interpersonal psychotherapy. New York: Basic Books; 2000.

Weissman MM, Markowitz JC, Klerman GL. Clinicians' quick guide to interpersonal psychotherapy. New York: Oxford Press; 2007.

Weintrob N, Cohen D, Klipper-Aurbach Y, Zadik Z, Dickerman Z. Decreased growth during therapy with selective serotonin reuptake inhibitors. Arch Pediat Adol Med. 2002;156:696–791.

Weisz JR, McCarty CA, Valeri SM. Effects of psychotherapy for depression in children and adolescents: a meta-analysis. Psychol Bull. 2006;132:132–49.

Williams JW, Barrett J, Oxman T, et al. Treatment of dysthymia and minor depression in primary care: a randomized controlled trial in older adults. J Am Med Assoc. 2000;284:1519–26.

Williams JW, Kobak KA. Development and Reliability of the Structured Interview Guide for the Montgomery-Asberg Depression Rating Scale. Br J Psychiatry. 2008;192:52–8.

Whitfield G, Hinshelwood R, Pashely A, Campsie L, Williams C. The impact of a novel computerized CBT CD Rom (Overcoming Depression) offered to patients referred to clinical psychology. Behav Cogn Psychoth. 2006;34:1–11.

Wright JH, Wright AS, Albano A, et al. Computer-assisted cognitive therapy for depression: maintaining efficacy while reducing therapist time. Am J Psychiatry. 2005;162:1158–64.

Yates BT. Cost-effectiveness analysis, cost-benefit analysis, and beyond: evolving models for the scientist-manager-practitioner. Clin Psychol-Sci Pr. 1995;2:385–98.

Yesavage JA, Brink TL, Rose TL, et al. Development and validation of a geriatric depression screening scale: a preliminary report. J Psychiatr Res. 1983;17:37–49.

Chapter 3
Anxiety

Holly Hazlett-Stevens

Numerous assessment instruments and treatments for anxiety are feasible to administer in primary care settings. Available treatment delivery formats include psychoeducation, bibliotherapy, and computer-based interventions, all of which provide cost-effective alternatives to intensive outpatient individual psychotherapy. A growing body of empirical research supports the effectiveness of these interventions. After a brief review of the available research, specific interventions are described and recommendations for triage are made. Finally, directions for future research and dissemination are discussed.

Assessment/Triage

Anxiety disorders traditionally were diagnosed following lengthy, in-depth clinical interviews. Many specialty anxiety disorder treatment centers and large-scale treatment research programs still utilize protocols such as the Anxiety Disorders Interview Schedule for DSM-IV (ADIS-IV; Brown et al., 1994) or the Structured Clinical Interview for DSM-IV Axis I Disorders (SCID-I/P; First et al., 2001). However, brief diagnostic assessment measures have been developed specifically for use in primary care medical settings where extensive clinician-administered interviews are not feasible. Alternative clinical interviews designed for primary care clinicians are quite short, averaging only 8–15 min to administer. In addition, brief diagnostic screening questionnaires can be completed by patients in the waiting room, saving valuable clinician contact time. Both types of measures are reviewed next.

The Mini International Neuropsychiatric Interview for DSM-IV (MINI; Sheehan and Lecrubier, 2002) is a widely used brief clinician-administered diagnostic interview. The close-ended question format allows for assessment of several prevalent Axis I disorders, yet takes approximately 15 min to administer. Sheehan and

H. Hazlett-Stevens (✉)
Department of Psychology, University of Nevada-Reno, Mail Stop 0298, Reno, NV 89557, USA
e-mail: hhazlett@unr.edu

W.T. O'Donohue, C. Draper (eds.), *Stepped Care and e-Health*,
DOI 10.1007/978-1-4419-6510-3_3, © Springer Science+Business Media, LLC 2011

colleagues (1998) found evidence of good diagnostic reliability and validity as well as good sensitivity, specificity, and predictive utility for the MINI.

Another measure known as the PRIME-MD (Primary Care Evaluation of Mental Disorders; Spitzer et al., 1994) combines a diagnostic screening questionnaire, the Patient Health Questionnaire (PHQ), with a brief interview in which the clinician reviews only those modules endorsed on the questionnaire. The clinical interview portion was completed in an average of 8.4 min in the original study conducted by Spitzer and colleagues. The PHQ fits on a single page, containing only 26 "yes" or "no" items that patients easily can complete in the waiting room. When used alone, the PHQ might serve as a reliable and valid screening tool that 80% of primary care physicians found useful to include in their practice (Spitzer et al., 1999). An alternate computer-administered telephone version of the PRIME-MD also has received some empirical support, and this instrument might be particularly useful in detecting alcohol abuse (Kobak et al., 1997).

The Psychiatric Diagnostic Screening Questionnaire (PDSQ; Zimmerman and Mattia, 2001a) contains 126 items screening for 13 separate Axis I disorders. Patients complete this questionnaire within 10–15 min in the waiting room before meeting with a clinician. Although this measure requires more time for patients to complete than the PHQ, the PDSQ does not require any further administration by the clinician. A body of research provided evidence of discriminate and convergent validity, good internal consistency, and high test–retest reliability for the individual PDSQ scales (Zimmerman and Mattia, 1999, 2001a, b).

Each of the diagnostic assessment instruments described above screens for an array of psychological disorders in addition to the anxiety disorders. In contrast, three additional questionnaire measures screen for generalized anxiety disorder (GAD), panic disorder, or social phobia specifically. The Generalized Anxiety Disorder Questionnaire-IV (GAD-Q-IV; Newman et al., 2002) is a diagnostic screening measure originally developed for research purposes. The Social Phobia Diagnostic Questionnaire (SPDQ; Newman et al., 2003) and the Panic Disorder Self-Report (PDSR; Newman et al., 2006) also were developed to screen individuals for subsequent research participation. Each measure contains straightforward "yes" or "no" format items and Likert rating scale items that map onto DSM-IV diagnostic criteria. Therefore, each short questionnaire can be completed by patients within minutes without the need for clinician administration. Despite this ease of administration, evidence of good reliability and validity was found for each measure. Furthermore, the sensitivity and specificity rates reported for each of these measures reflected excellent agreement between diagnosis obtained via the questionnaire and diagnosis obtained from a comprehensive clinical interview. Although these three diagnostic measures provide a promising alternative to more extensive diagnostic procedures, none have been studied or validated in primary care patient samples.

Clinicians consider these diagnostic measures worthwhile largely because available empirically supported interventions were developed for individuals diagnosed with a specific anxiety disorder. As such, the vast majority of research investigations supporting these interventions included only those individuals who met a certain set of diagnostic criteria. Consequently, an array of separate treatment protocols for each specific anxiety disorder emerged, requiring extensive clinician training to incorporate these protocols into practice (Allen et al., 2007). Newer cognitive-behavioral therapies for clinical anxiety problems address this obstacle by adopting a transdiagnostic conceptual model and intervention approach. Examples include the "unified protocol" for emotional disorders developed by Barlow and colleagues (Barlow et al., 2004) and the transdiagnostic cognitive-behavioral therapy (CBT) for anxiety disorders developed by Norton and colleagues (see Norton, 2008). In accord with this transdiagnostic approach, several reliable and valid self-report questionnaires measure common anxiety-related clinical features along a dimension. An excellent resource for clinicians contains descriptions and reprinted versions of several such measures for each anxiety disorder: *The Practitioner's Guide to Empirically Based Measures of Anxiety*, edited by M.M. Antony, S.M. Orsillo, and L. Roemer (published in 2001 by Kluwer Academic/Plenum Publishers).

Stepped Care Options

When working from a stepped care delivery approach, clinicians begin with the least intrusive form of treatment. If the need for treatment persists, a slightly more intensive alternative is provided. This process continues until a variety of cost-effective treatment options have been exhausted. Only then would traditional individual psychotherapy or inpatient treatment be recommended, reserving these services for the most treatment-resistant cases. A variety of treatment delivery options exist for the anxiety disorders, ranging from self-administered bibliotherapy and computer-based psychoeducation programs to medication and/or intensive outpatient and inpatient psychotherapy protocols. Preliminary patient acceptance data support the use of less traditional delivery formats. Furthermore, consideration of primary care patient preferences may complement the triage process. A growing body of research supports the effectiveness of some self-administered and minimal-contact therapies for anxiety, allowing primary care clinicians to incorporate a stepped care approach in their practice. Less invasive treatments are offered as alternatives to the more expensive and time-consuming options, all of which are briefly described below.

Consumer Preferences

Stepped care models include a variety of treatment delivery options other than traditional outpatient individual psychotherapy, presenting current patients with more choices than they may have had in previous years. Based on the assumption that matching services to patient preferences may increase treatment compliance and eventual treatment outcomes, researchers have begun to explore the nature of patient preferences. Indeed, patients may not begin treatment at all if they are not offered their preferred type of treatment (Eisenthal et al., 1979). Even when such patients do begin treatment, they may be less inclined to finish: primary care patients in need of treatment for depression were less likely to complete treatment when they did not receive their preferred treatment type (Schulberg et al., 1996).

Most available research on this topic examined depression treatment preferences in primary care settings, and most studies found that primary care patients preferred psychotherapy or counseling to antidepressant medication (see van Schaik et al., 2004 for a review of this literature). These consumer preference findings may not generalize to veterans, however. One investigation conducted in a VA primary care setting found that patients most often preferred antidepressant medication (32% of patients) compared to individual counseling (19%), both of these treatments combined (18%), and group counseling (7%; Dobscha et al., 2007). Interestingly, an additional 25% preferred watchful waiting. However, the offering of preferred treatment type was not associated with receiving treatment or with improved depression severity over time. Such null findings have appeared in other studies as well. In their review of this small literature, Raue and Schulberg (2007) concluded that this line of research is inconclusive; thus far researchers have failed to document the assumed benefits of accommodating patient preferences with measures of subsequent treatment adherence and clinical outcomes.

It remains unknown how well these depression treatment preference findings generalize to patients presenting with anxiety-related complaints, as far less empirical information exists regarding anxiety treatment preferences in primary care. We (Hazlett-Stevens et al., 2002) examined patient preferences among more than 1000 primary care patients indicating a recent panic attack episode. Patients who screened positive for panic were asked two follow-up treatment questions: "Would you be willing to take medication to help with these spells or attacks?" and "Would you be willing to meet with a specialist six times over 8 weeks to learn how to control these spells or attacks?" Patients responded with either "Not at all willing" or "Would consider it" for each question. In response to the medication question, 64% of the patient sample indicated willingness and 36% reported they would not be willing to consider medication. In response to the behavior specialist question, 67% indicated willingness and 33% were not willing. Thus, while each treatment type appeared acceptable to the majority of primary care patients, each type was also unacceptable to a significant minority. Future research examining preferences for primary care patients endorsing other anxiety problems is certainly needed. In addition, patient preference research investigating treatment alternatives other than medication and brief psychotherapy would have important implications for triage and stepped care practices.

An indirect way to examine patient treatment preferences is to assess the degree to which patients report acceptance of or satisfaction with a treatment after it has been offered or provided. Primary care treatment researchers increasingly are including such acceptance/satisfaction measures in their studies. For example, a large group psychoeducation intervention for anxiety disorders yielded not only clinical improvements but also high patient satisfaction ratings (Houghton and Saxon, 2007). Favorable patient acceptance and satisfaction ratings also were reported for less intensive forms of effective stepped care anxiety interventions, including assisted bibliotherapy (Reeves and Stace, 2005) and computer-based therapy programs (Proudfoot, 2004). While clinicians need to realize that patient satisfaction variables do not measure therapy outcomes or treatment effectiveness, offering treatments that tend to be well accepted may increase the likelihood that patients will access and complete appropriate treatments.

Outcome Data

A large body of randomized controlled trials support the efficacy of CBT for anxiety disorders. These investigations typically utilized strong methodological designs to maximize internal validity and delivered 12–16 sessions of individual psychotherapy (or group psychotherapy in the case of social phobia) to clinical research participants. Several diagnosis-specific psychotherapy protocols have received strong empirical support in this fashion, including panic control treatment (PCT) for panic disorder (with and without agoraphobia), exposure with response/ritual prevention (EX/RP) for obsessive compulsive disorder, and cognitive-behavioral group therapy (CBGT) for social phobia/social anxiety disorder. CBT protocols for specific phobias, GAD, and posttraumatic stress disorder (PTSD) also have received considerable empirical support. The reader is referred to the *Clinical Handbook of Psychological Disorders, 4th ed.*, edited by D.H. Barlow (published in 2007 by Guilford) for detailed therapy protocols. However, this intensive individual outpatient psychotherapy delivery format may not be feasible in primary care settings. Furthermore, this form of treatment may not be desired by all primary care patients struggling with anxiety.

Clinical researchers since have streamlined original CBT protocols by reducing the number of sessions and/or adapting individual treatments to a group therapy format. In our review of the abbreviated CBT outcome literature (Hazlett-Stevens and Craske, 2002), we defined brief CBT as fewer than 10 sessions. Individual brief CBT appeared effective for panic disorder (with and without agoraphobia) and specific phobias and also may yield some improvement in cases of GAD, social phobia, and PTSD. Some of these studies delivered brief CBT in a group format, supporting the effectiveness of this approach in the treatment of panic disorder, generalized anxiety disorder, and social phobia. Several other studies supported the efficacy of individual single-session CBT for a variety of phobias, including fears of flying, spiders, blood/injury stimuli, injection, and claustrophobia, even when single-session treatment was directly compared to longer length treatments. With the exception of single-session specific phobia treatment, these brief CBT protocols were supplemented with self-help adjunct materials.

One brief CBT protocol was developed specifically for panic disorder patients in the primary care setting. This Collaborative Care for Anxiety and Panic (CCAP) intervention provided on-site assessment and treatment consisting of six individual CBT sessions with a behavioral health specialist and six follow-up phone contacts. Expert medication consultation also was provided to patients' primary care physicians. Indeed, patients randomized to CCAP treatment reported greater improvements than a treatment as usual control group, and these treatment gains continued for 12 months (Roy-Byrne et al., 2005).

Another brief CBT treatment was investigated with patients reporting a variety of anxiety problems including panic/agoraphobia, specific phobias, social anxiety, generalized anxiety, posttraumatic stress, obsessive compulsive disorder, and hypochondriasis (Houghton and Saxon, 2007). This treatment was delivered in a large group (i.e., up to 24 patients per group) psychoeducation class format over four 90-min weekly classes. Results from follow-up outcome data suggested that almost half (20 of 44 patients) of those who returned for follow-up assessment enjoyed reliable improvement from the classes. Patient satisfaction data were promising as well. This intervention approach was designed for use in a stepped care delivery model and might be helpful to a large proportion of patients who choose to attend classes.

CBT interventions for anxiety disorders have been streamlined even further by providing patients with self-help materials designed for use with minimal or no therapist contact. These interventions have gained some empirical support as well. For example, a bibliotherapy treatment targeting symptoms of panic and agoraphobia was self-administered over 8 weeks (Lindren et al., 1994). Results indicated that this form of treatment was superior to a waitlist control condition and comparable to the same treatment delivered by a therapist during eight group therapy sessions. Other investigations empirically supported guided exposure treatment for panic disorder with agoraphobia in which only telephone contact with the therapist (Swinson et al., 1995; McNamee et al., 1989) or simple self-exposure instructions from a psychiatrist (Ghosh and Marks, 1987) were provided. In this latter investigation, other participants randomized to a self-administered bibliotherapy condition or to a computer program intervention condition reported substantial improvements equivalent to the psychiatrist instruction condition. Minimalist bibliotherapy interventions for panic also may prevent relapse when delivered after initial treatment. Wright and colleagues (2000) found that bibliotherapy and minimal therapist contact provided during a 6-month follow-up period resulted in greater improvements on panic and avoidance measures when compared to a waitlist control group.

Some recent self-help interventions were designed to treat an array of clinical anxiety problems instead of a specific anxiety disorder diagnosis. This transdiagnostic approach is consistent with current trends in CBT development (e.g., Barlow et al., 2004; Norton, 2008) and ultimately may be a more pragmatic and theoretically satisfying approach to anxiety treatment in primary care. Indeed, one such assisted bibliotherapy treatment for mild-to-moderate anxiety was developed for and tested in a primary care setting (Reeves and Stace, 2005). Seven weekly 20-min "coaching" sessions were provided along with six module booklets teaching several established cognitive-behavioral anxiety management strategies. Although only 9 of 19 patients referred for treatment completed, these patients reported significant improvements on symptom measures. In addition, 75% of treatment completers found the intervention "very useful" on satisfaction measures. All of these patients reported using the strategies at least "often," and over 80% reported that the strategies were a part of their daily routine. Bibliotherapy might also be useful for the parents of anxious children, although this approach was not as efficacious as a standard group treatment in a randomized trial (Rapee et al., 2006).

Computer-based delivery formats provide an alternative to written therapy materials. Such computerized minimal therapist contact interventions have received increasing attention in recent years, and a growing body of research supports the inclusion of these interventions in stepped care models. In a recent review of this literature, Titov (2007) concluded that computerized CBT for anxiety, particularly when guided by a therapist, is a promising alternative. Although this form of treatment has received more attention for depression symptoms, some Internet-based depression treatments also reduced scores on anxiety measures (e.g., Andersson et al., 2005). Newer computer-based treatments specific to anxiety have received preliminary empirical support as well. Titov identified six randomized controlled trials and two uncontrolled trials of computerized CBT for panic, all of which found significant treatment effects. In addition, one randomized controlled trial and one uncontrolled trial demonstrated effectiveness of computerized treatments specifically designed for social phobia. Computerized CBT for symptoms of posttraumatic stress was supported by two randomized controlled trials and one uncontrolled trial. Titov also identified one randomized controlled trial and one uncontrolled trial supporting a commercially available computerized treatment for panic and/or phobias known as the FearFighter program (Marks et al., 2004). Since the review by Titov, an additional investigation of the feasibility and effectiveness of FearFighter was conducted by Hayward and colleagues (2007), a research group independent of the treatment program developers. Patients in rural areas of Scotland reported few difficulties using the treatment, and both general practitioners and patients provided high ratings of treatment acceptability. Significant improvements across a range of phobia, anxiety, and depression outcome measures also were found. In most of the investigations described in this paragraph, computer-assisted treatment included some degree of therapist contact. However, this therapist contact often included telephone and/or e-mail contact.

While encouraging, results from initial computerized CBT trials should be interpreted with some degree of caution. In another review of this literature, Andersson and colleagues (2005) concluded that Internet-based self-help with minimal therapist contact is a promising treatment for panic, and they found no evidence that such treatments are harmful. However, they also emphasized the need for large-scale trials and the need to evaluate these treatments within the larger stepped care treatment delivery context. Titov (2007) noted several methodological limitations of this outcome literature, including the potential for sampling bias, lack of adequate clinical assessment, high dropout rates, and small sample sizes.

Similar limitations have been identified for bibliotherapy and other minimal therapist contact treatment research studies (Newman et al., 2003). In addition, one overarching issue involves all forms of alternative low-cost treatments: How much therapist contact is needed to achieve desired clinical outcomes? In their review of self-administered and minimal-contact anxiety treatments, Newman and colleagues found that self-administered exposure treatment for specific phobias yielded significant benefits, particularly for highly motivated patients who found the treatment materials credible. Minimal therapist contact may be important for other patients, perhaps because of the externally imposed structure provided, and these interventions benefited the majority of specific phobia patients treated. Purely self-administered treatments for panic have not been widely studied, but self-help treatments guided by brief therapist contacts consistently were superior to waitlist control conditions. Brief computer-assisted CBT appeared equivalent to traditional 12 session individual therapy, and such minimal therapist contact treatments may be sufficient for the majority of patients presenting with panic symptoms. However, patients with severe agoraphobia may need additional therapist contact. Purely self-administered treatment for OCD may not be adequate, and therapist-guided self-help treatments and other brief CBT protocols produced only modest effects. Results from a few studies examining brief CBT for GAD and for social phobia provided preliminary empirical support for this practice. Newman and colleagues concluded that purely self-administered treatment appears most effective for specific phobia, whereas some degree of therapist contact seems optimal for panic disorder. Indeed, one investigation of purely self-administered bibliotherapy treatment for panic disorder failed to produce expected treatment effects (Febbraro et al., 1999), despite the use of self-help materials with established effectiveness in previous research. Brief CBT treatments with minimal therapist contact are promising for specific phobia and panic and appear superior to no treatment for OCD, GAD, and social phobia.

Quality Improvement Outcomes

Primary care patients complaining of anxiety symptoms have a variety of choices other than the traditional treatment options of intensive psychotherapy and/or medication. Many patients who otherwise would not pursue active treatment may benefit from a stepped care approach. Less costly or invasive alternatives could be attempted first; additional treatment would only be offered if these lower cost treatments fail.

Watchful Waiting

The "watchful waiting" approach generally is not recommended for patients with full anxiety disorder diagnoses, as these conditions infrequently remit spontaneously when left untreated (e.g., Yonkers et al., 2003). Nevertheless, patients reporting only mild anxiety symptoms in the absence of a full diagnosis may prefer to begin with the watchful waiting approach. Some patients may report recent symptoms of a subclinical severity that do not seem to interfere with daily functioning or cause notable distress. These symptoms may never develop into full anxiety disorders, and some may be easily explained by current stressful life events expected to resolve in a short time. Patients who choose to monitor their condition before engaging in active treatment might benefit from general information about potential warning signs. For example, patients might agree to re-contact their provider for further treatment if anxiety symptoms increase in frequency or intensity, if fear or anxiety alters behavior or causes changes in routine, or if the symptoms begin to interfere with social/occupational functioning or cause noticeable distress. Information about dependable resources, such as a list of self-administered bibliotherapy or computerized treatment programs, also could be provided. Patients who begin with a watchful waiting approach may choose to visit the Anxiety Disorders Association of America (ADAA) website (http://www.adaa.org) to learn more about clinical warning signs and to complete self-assessment measures.

Psychoeducation

Psychoeducation interventions for anxiety typically present fundamental information about the nature of worry, anxiety, and fear. Clients learn about the adaptive nature of anxiety and the protective function of the "fight or flight" fear response. Clients identify specific anxiety-provoking thoughts, sensations, and behaviors believed to maintain anxious symptoms within a cognitive-behavioral theoretical model. As reviewed above, psychoeducation alone may be sufficient in some anxiety disorder cases. Researchers have begun to examine how to predict which patients may benefit from this form of treatment versus which patients may need therapist contact treatments. Baillie and Rapee (2004) evaluated relationships between predictive variables and rate of improvement among panic patients within a stepped care treatment investigation. The authors developed a prognostic scale based on various self-report measures of panic symptoms, other anxiety symptoms, agoraphobia, and interoceptive fear. This prognostic scale proved significantly better than chance at predicting which patients recovered from a given psychoeducation or self-help intervention and which patients required therapy involving therapist contact.

Although many psychoeducation interventions are specific to diagnosis or type of anxiety symptoms, transdiagnostic psychoeducation interventions that teach common principles underlying all anxiety disorders have emerged in the stepped care literature (e.g., Houghton and Saxon, 2007). Information about how fears develop, the role of physiology in fear maintenance, and basic principles of CBT is presented to groups of patients with a variety of anxiety disorder diagnoses. Patients learn how to conduct exposure and reduce escape/avoidance behavior on their own in addition to common cognitive therapy strategies.

Bibliotherapy

Bibliotherapy materials convey essential psychoeducation information and provide patients written instructions to guide them through self-administered therapy exercises. Motivated clients who wish to attempt behavior change on their own before resorting to therapist contact treatments are most likely to benefit from this approach. Several written patient workbooks and self-help books based on empirically supported CBT practices are commercially available to anxiety patients. For example, the self-help book *Women Who Worry Too Much* (Hazlett-Stevens, 2005) provides essential information about the nature of anxiety and worry followed by specific exercises designed to teach cognitive therapy, behavior therapy, relaxation, and mindfulness skills. Most bibliotherapy resources are specific to the type of anxiety problem, such as panic, phobias, social anxiety, and generalized anxiety or chronic worry. A list of recommended self-help bibliotherapy resources for each anxiety condition appears in Hazlett-Stevens (2009).

Another type of bibliotherapy resource for anxiety patients involves patient workbooks originally designed for therapist-guided treatments. Although not yet studied in isolation, patients are increasingly using these workbooks for self-help purposes. Many of these patient workbook materials are available from Oxford University Press (http://www.oup.com). Examples include *Mastery of Your Anxiety and Panic, 4th ed.* (MAP-4; Barlow and Craske, 2006) and *Mastering Your Fears and Phobias, 2nd ed.* (Antony et al., 2006).

Computer-Based Intervention/E-Health

This promising treatment alternative may help overcome several common barriers to traditional treatment delivery methods, such as cost, travel time for rural patients, social stigma, and a lack of available skilled clinicians within a local geographical area (Titov, 2007). Several research studies have demonstrated that administration of computer-based treatments is feasible in natural settings (Proudfoot, 2004). Computerized treatment programs for anxiety were developed from empirically supported CBT practices, often with an interactive multimedia format and a program structure containing individual modules to teach specific cognitive and behavioral techniques. Available websites for the treatment of panic and phobias include Panic Center (http://www.paniccenter.net/), Panic Online (http://www.med.monash.edu.au/mentalhealth/paniconline/), and FearFighter (http://www.fearfighter.com/index.htm). Patients complaining of more general anxiety symptoms, social anxiety, and/or comorbid depression may benefit from Beating the Blues (http://www.ultrasis.com/products/product.jsp?product_id=1) or Clinical Management and Treatment Education (CLIMATE; http://www.climategp.tv). Patients suffering from obsessive compulsive symptoms may benefit from a program entitled BT STEPS, although careful monitoring of treatment compliance and response also may be needed (Newman et al., 2003).

Group Therapy

Group therapy is most often clinically indicated for social anxiety, as the presence of other group members provides ample opportunity for in-session therapeutic exposure and role plays for the purpose of behavioral rehearsal. Group therapy formats also might provide a cost-effective way of delivering CBT for panic and GAD symptoms. The same psychoeducation information included in individual CBT protocols is presented to group therapy patients. During group sessions, group members engage in discussion and collaboration when working through a given group member's specific anxiety episode or situation. This process allows all group members to learn the cognitive and behavioral strategies as the therapist addresses individual concerns. Group therapy also provides patients with the possible additional benefit of peer social support.

Individual Therapy

Most CBT protocols for anxiety disorders originally involved outpatient individual psychotherapy sessions. Many of these treatments are tailored to a specific diagnosis, but most involve some form of psychoeducation, anxiety management strategies such as relaxation, cognitive therapy or restructuring, and systematic exposure to internal and external fear cues. As reviewed above, some abbreviated protocols are now available, particularly for the treatment of specific phobias, panic, and agoraphobia. In addition, brief outpatient CBT treatments specifically designed for use in primary care settings have been developed. In the CCAP treatment described previously (Roy-Byrne et al., 2005), primary care patients were screened for panic disorder in the waiting room. Eligible patients received six individual face-to-face CBT sessions over the first 3 months followed by six brief follow-up phone contacts spaced over the following 9 months.

The Coordinated Anxiety Learning and Management project (CALM; Sullivan et al., 2007) is another promising primary care treatment innovation. Anxiety clinical specialists conduct initial assessments of primary care patients on site. Patients then choose CBT, medication, or both. The CBT intervention allows for flexible treatment of any one of four anxiety disorders as well as any concurrent depression and/or alcohol abuse. Computer-assisted treatment delivery provides patients with an additional option. This treatment program is conducted within a stepped care framework. A large randomized controlled trial of the CALM program involving four geographical clinic locations is currently underway.

Medication

Antidepressant medications, particularly the selective serotonin reuptake inhibitors (SSRIs) and the serotonin–norepinephrine reuptake inhibitors (SNRIs), are considered first-line medications for anxiety disorders. These medications are administered in regular daily doses during the course of treatment. When effective, these medications provide general anxiety symptom relief over time. In contrast, anti-anxiety agents such as the benzodiazepines are fast acting and therefore provide more immediate anxiety symptom relief. However, this type of medication often undermines CBT procedures and objectives by providing patients a means of immediate escape from fear responses and associated bodily sensations of arousal.

Inpatient Treatment

Inpatient treatment for anxiety disorders is only indicated in the most severe cases. For example, OCD patients consumed by compulsive rituals that prevent fundamental activities of daily living may require residential treatment. Another example may involve an extremely isolated agoraphobic patient seriously contemplating suicide. In short, inpatient treatment is warranted only when symptoms severely impair patients' ability to care for themselves or when other significant clinical concerns about immediate physical safety arise. For other severe cases, intensive outpatient therapy protocols provide a promising alternative to inpatient hospitalization. These treatments are administered over several full days per week but do not require residence in the treatment facility.

Consumer Preferences and Cultural Sensitivity

Few investigations have examined relationships between cultural factors and anxiety treatment preferences in the primary care setting. In the study of primary care patient preferences among individuals reporting panic attacks mentioned above (Hazlett-Stevens et al., 2002), patients who described their ethnicity as Black/African-American or as Asian/Pacific Islander were less likely to endorse willingness to consider medication treatment for panic than White/Caucasian patients. Interestingly, reported willingness to consider meeting with a behavior specialist was not associated with any demographic, cultural, or physical health variables.

Triage Agenda

Clinicians typically consider two factors at the initial point of triage: clinical severity of the problem and patient treatment preference. As mentioned above, watchful waiting may be selected in some subclinical cases and could be augmented by providing patients a list of self-help resources. Treatment typically begins as soon as possible for patients with symptoms sufficient for DSM-IV diagnosis demonstrating clinically significant impairment or distress. Clinicians inform these patients of their diagnosis and describe empirically supported CBT treatment methods. Various treatment delivery options including psychoeducation, bibliotherapy, computer-based CBT, and outpatient CBT sessions with a therapist are described. Patients indicating a desire to learn about their condition and to attempt cognitive and behavioral changes on their own might begin with self-administered bibliotherapy or computer-assisted treatment. Once a patient has completed the treatment program, the clinician could conduct further assessment to see if more intensive treatment is warranted. Patients wanting to learn more about their symptoms from an instructor in a class setting would likely select a psychoeducation intervention instead. This intervention approach might be best for patients with only moderate levels of distress or reporting a recent onset of symptoms. Individual or group therapy sessions might be recommended afterward if symptoms persist or if patients require further assistance implementing suggested treatment strategies. For patients requiring outpatient psychotherapy, a group setting is best for socially anxious patients. Group therapy also may be a worthwhile and cost-effective CBT delivery method for patients struggling with panic and generalized anxiety. Patients with high levels of clinical severity, with a previous history of treatment failure, or who do not feel comfortable in a group therapy setting may prefer individual therapy instead.

Some patients may benefit from further medication consultation and trials of antidepressant medication independent of the approach selected for psychosocial treatment. Clinicians could describe the potential benefits of medication while emphasizing that CBT intervention can be pursued concurrently. Patients who decide to take medication should be cautioned against interpreting side effect symptoms as threatening, thereby exacerbating anxiety symptom cycles. In addition, patients who take medication and simultaneously make effortful cognitive and behavioral changes should be cautioned against mistakenly attributing all gains to the medication. In some cases, patients request or require benzodiazepine medications to eliminate anxiety or fear sensations during discrete episodes. In these cases, patients should be made aware of the counter-therapeutic and anxiety-maintaining long-term effects of this coping strategy. Patients selecting this medication approach might not be motivated at the time to invest in cognitive and behavioral change and instead are seeking short-term relief in specific situations.

Research and Development Agenda

While promising, many cost-effective treatments suitable to the primary care setting require further empirical evaluation. Brief CBT protocols, such as the CCAP and CALM interventions described above, were designed specifically for primary care and appear feasible to disseminate across many primary care settings. The brief large group psychoeducation intervention for patients with any of the anxiety disorders (Houghton and Saxon, 2007) is another promising option, and the recent proliferation of bibliotherapy and computer-assisted treatment programs is also encouraging. However, experts in this area consistently call for additional large-scale studies with improved research methodology. Furthermore, several critical questions remain regarding the implementation of stepped care models: Which patients are most likely to benefit from which treatments? How much therapist contact is needed for optimal effectiveness? What patient factors are most important when making triage decisions?

Dissemination Agenda

A final consideration involves how to disseminate effective treatments to patients who would benefit from services. Early dissemination efforts began with the development of streamlined, cost-effective versions of the full individual psychotherapy

CBT protocols with established empirical support. Clinical researchers next subjected these alternative interventions to empirical investigation and since have gathered numerous preliminary findings supporting the effectiveness of various alternatives. Researchers increasingly have collected feasibility and acceptability data in addition to effectiveness data, demonstrating that these interventions are possible to implement in settings other than traditional mental health specialty treatment settings. However, a final step remains at the level of the healthcare delivery system: development of institutional policies and practices promoting systematic assessment and triage of anxiety conditions. In an ideal future, primary care patients routinely would be assessed for anxiety (as well as other emotional disorders such as depression) and subsequently offered an array of treatment options whenever appropriate.

References

Allen LB, McHugh RK, Barlow DH. Emotional disorders: a unified protocol. In: Barlow DH, editor. Clinical handbook of psychological disorders: a step-by-step treatment manual. 4th ed. New York: Guilford; 2007. p. 216–49.

Andersson G, Bergström J, Carlbring P, Lindefors N. The use of the internet in the treatment of anxiety disorders. Curr Opin Psychiatry. 2005;18:73–7.

Antony MM, Craske MG, Barlow DH. Mastering Your Fears and Phobias: Workbook. 2nd ed. New York: Oxford University Press; 2006.

Baillie A, Rapee RM. Predicting who benefits from psychoeducation and self help for panic attacks. Behav Res Ther. 2004;42:513–27.

Barlow DH, Allen LB, Choate ML. Toward a unified treatment for emotional disorders. Behav Ther. 2004;35:205–30.

Barlow DH, Craske MG. Mastery of your anxiety and panic: client workbook. 4th ed. New York: Oxford University Press; 2006.

Brown TA, DiNardo PA, Barlow DH. Anxiety disorders interview schedule for DSM-IV (ADIS-IV). San Antonio, TX: Psychological Corporation; 1994.

Dobscha SK, Corson K, Gerrity MS. Depression treatment preferences of VA primary care patients. Psychosomatics. 2007;48:482–8.

Eisenthal S, Emery R, Lazare A, Udin H. "Adherence" and the negotiated approach to patienthood. Arch Gen Psychiatry. 1979;36:393–8.

Febbraro GA, Clum GA, Roodman AA, Wright JH. The limits of bibliotherapy: a study of the differential effectiveness of self-administered interventions in individuals with panic attacks. Behav Ther. 1999;30:209–22.

First MB, Spitzer RL, Gibbon M, Williams JBW. Structured clinical interview for DSM-IV-TR Axis I disorders. New York: Biometrics Research Department, New York State Psychiatric Institute; 2001.

Ghosh A, Marks IM. Self-treatment of agoraphobia by exposure. Behav Ther. 1987;18:3–16.

Hayward L, MacGregor AD, Peck DF, Wilkes P. The feasibility and effectiveness of computer-guided CBT (FearFighter) in a rural area. Behav Cogn Psychoth. 2007;35:409–19.

Hazlett-Stevens H. Assessment and treatment of anxiety in primary care. In: James LC, O'Donohue WT, editors. The primary care toolkit: Practical resources for the integrated behavioral care provider New York: Springer; 2009. p.169–82.

Hazlett-Stevens H. Women who worry too much: how to stop worry and anxiety from ruining relationships, work, and fun. Oakland, CA: New Harbinger; 2005.

Hazlett-Stevens H, Craske MG. Brief cognitive-behavioral therapy: definition and scientific foundations. In: Bond FW, Dryden W, editors. Handbook of brief cognitive behaviour therapy. New York: Wiley; 2002. p. 1–20.

Hazlett-Stevens H, Craske MG, Roy-Byrne PP, Sherbourne CD, Stein MB, Bystritsky A. Predictors of willingness to consider medication and psychosocial treatment for panic disorder in primary care patients. Gen Hosp Psychiatry. 2002;24:316–21.

Houghton S, Saxon D. An evaluation of large group CBT psycho-education for anxiety disorders delivered in routine practice. Patient Educ Couns. 2007;68:107–10.

Kobak KA, Taylor LH, Dottl SL, Greist JH, Jefferson JW, Burroughs D, Mantle JM, Katzelnick DJ, Norton R, Henk HJ, Serlin RC. A computer-administered telephone interview to identify mental disorders. J Am Med Assoc. 1997;278:905–10.

Lindren DM, Watkins PL, Gould RA, Clum GA, Asterino M, Tulloch HL. A comparison of bibliotherapy and group therapy in the treatment of panic disorder. J Consult Clin Psychol. 1994;62:865–9.

Marks IM, Kenwright M, McDonough M, Whittaker M, Mataix-Cols D. Saving clinicians' time by delegating routine aspects of therapy to a computer: a randomized controlled trial in phobic/panic disorder. Psychol Med. 2004;34:9–17.

McNamee G, O'Sullivan G, Lelliott P, Marks I. Telephone-guided treatment for housebound agoraphobics with panic disorder: exposure vs. relaxation. Behav Ther. 1989;20:491–7.

Newman MG, Erickson T, Przeworski A, Dzus E. Self-help and minimal-contact therapies for anxiety disorders: is human contact necessary for therapeutic efficacy? J of Clin Psychol. 2003;59:251–74.

Newman MG, Holmes M, Zuellig AR, Kachin KE, Behar E. The reliability and validity of the panic disorder self-report: a new diagnostic screening measure of panic disorder. Psychol Assessment. 2006;18:49–61.

Newman MG, Kachin KE, Zuellig AR, Constantino MJ, Cashman-McGrath L. The social phobia diagnostic questionnaire: preliminary validation of a new self-report diagnostic measure of social phobia. Psychol Med. 2003;33:623–35.

Newman MG, Zuellig AR, Kachin KE, Constantino MJ, Przeworski A, Erickson T, Cashman-McGrath L. Preliminary reliability and validity of the generalized anxiety disorder questionnaire-iv: a revised self-report diagnostic measure of generalized anxiety disorder. Behav Ther. 2002;33:215–33.

Norton PJ. An open trial of a transdiagnostic cognitive-behavioral group therapy for anxiety disorder. Behav Ther. 2008;39:242–50.

Proudfoot JG. Computer-based treatment for anxiety and depression: is it feasible? Is it effective? Neurosci and Biobehav Rev. 2004;28:353–63.

Rapee RM, Abbott MJ, Lyneham HJ. Bibliotherapy for children with anxiety disorders using written materials for parents: a randomized controlled trial. J Consul Clin Psychol. 2006;74: 436–44.

Raue P, Schulberg H.C. Psychotherapy and patient preferences for the treatment of major depression in primary care. In: Henri MJ, editor. Trends in depression research. Hauppauge, NY: Nova Science Publishers; 2007. p. 31–51.

Reeves T, Stace JM. Improving patient access and choice: assisted bibliotherapy for mild to moderate stress/anxiety in primary care. J Psychiatr Mental Health Nurs. 2005;12:341–6.

Roy-Byrne PP, Craske MG, Stein MB, Sullivan G, et al. A randomized effectiveness trial of cognitive behavior therapy and medication for primary care panic disorder. Arch Gen Psychiatry. 2005;62:290–8.

Schulberg HC, Block MR, Madonia MJ, Scott CP, et al. Treating major depression in primary care practice: eight-month clinical outcomes. Arch Gen Psychiatry. 1996;53:913–9.

Sheehan DV, Lecrubier Y. MINI International Neuropsychiatric Interview for DSM-IV (English Version 5.0.0). Tampa: University of South Florida; 2002.

Sheehan DV, Lecrubier Y, Harnett-Sheehan K, Amorim P, Janavs J, Weiller E, Hergueta T, Baker R, Dunbar GC. The Mini-International Neuropsychiatric Interview (M.I.N.I.): the development and validation of a structured diagnostic psychiatric interview for DSM-IV and ICD-10. J Clin Psychiatry. 1998;59(Suppl. 20):22–33.

Spitzer RL, Kroenke K, Williams JB. Validation and utility of a self-report version of PRIME-MD: the PHQ primary care study. Primary Care Evaluation of Mental Disorders. Patient Health Questionnaire. J Am Med Assoc. 1999;282:1737–74.

Spitzer RL, Williams JBW, Kroenke K, Linzer M, deGruy FV, Hahn SR, Brody D, Johnson JG. Utility of a new procedure for diagnosing mental disorders in primary care: The PRIME-MD 1000 study. J Am Med Assoc. 1994;272:1749–56.

Sullivan G, Craske MG, Sherbourne C, Edlund MJ, et al. Design of the Coordinated Anxiety Learning and Management (CALM) study: innovations in collaborative care for anxiety disorders. Gen Hosp Psychiatry. 2007;29:379–87.

Swinson RP, Fergus KD, Cox BJ, Wickwire K. Efficacy of telephone-administered behavioral therapy for panic disorder with agoraphobia. Behav Res Ther. 1995;33:465–9.

Titov N. Status of computerized cognitive behavioural therapy for adults. Aust N Z J Psychiatry. 2007;41:95–114.

van Schaik DJF, Klijn AFJ, van Hout HPJ, van Marwijk HWJ, et al. Patients' preferences in the treatment of depressive disorder in primary care. Gen Hosp Psychiatry. 2004;26:184–9.

Wright J, Clum GA, Roodman A, Febbraro GA. A bibliotherapy approach to relapse prevention in individuals with panic attacks. J Anxiety Disord. 2000;14:483–99.

Yonkers KA, Bruce SE, Dyck IR, Keller MB. Chronicity, relapse, and illness—Course of panic disorder, social phobia, and generalized anxiety disorder: Findings in men and women from 8 years of follow-up. Depress Anxiety. 2003;17:173–9.

Zimmerman M, Mattia JI. The reliability and validity of a screening questionnaire for 13 DSM-IV Axis I disorders (the psychiatric diagnostic screening questionnaire) in psychiatric outpatients. J Clin Psychiatry. 1999;60:677–83.

Zimmerman M, Mattia JI. The psychiatric diagnostic screening questionnaire: development, reliability, and validity. Compr Psychiatry. 2001a;42:175–89.

Zimmerman M, Mattia JI. A self-report scale to help make psychiatricdiagnoses: The psychiatric diagnostic screening questionnaire (PDSQ). Arch Gen Psychiatry. 2001b;58:787–94.

Chapter 4
Panic Disorder

Gerhard Andersson and Per Carlbring

Brief Description of the Problem

Panic disorder is an anxiety disorder that is characterized by recurrent and unexpected panic attacks. A panic attack is defined as a discrete period of intense fear or discomfort in the absence of real danger. In the diagnostic system DSM-IV a panic attack is further defined as being accompanied by at least 4 of 13 somatic or cognitive symptoms developed abruptly and reaching a peak within 10 min (APA, 2000). Attacks that have fewer than four somatic or cognitive symptoms are referred to as limited symptom attacks. Symptoms can include, for example, sweating, palpitations, trembling, feeling of choking, nausea, dizziness, depersonalization, fear of losing control, and fear of dying. Recurrent, unexpected panic attacks are required for a diagnosis of panic disorder (with or without agoraphobia; APA, 2000). Apart from this, the attacks are followed by at least 1 month of persistent concern about having another attack and/or worry about the possible implications or consequences of the attacks and/or significant behavioral change related to the attacks. The frequency and severity of the panic attacks may vary among individuals suffering from panic disorder (Taylor, 2000), but when a diagnosis can be confirmed it is highly likely that the individual suffers from a debilitating condition with marked negative consequences for quality of life (Taylor, 2006). Panic disorder is a rather common and prevalent disorder with a lifetime prevalence of 1.5–3.5% (Taylor, 2000). The age of onset for panic disorder is typically between late adolescence and the mid-thirties and a majority are females (APA, 2000). The condition may recur even after effective immediate treatment, but relapse rates may differ between different treatments (e.g., psychological versus pharmacological treatments).

Agoraphobia can develop as a consequence of full or subclinical panic disorder. The essential feature of agoraphobia is the anxiety about being in places or

G. Andersson (✉)
Department of Behavioural Sciences and Learning, Linköping University, Linköping, SE-581 83, Sweden
e-mail: gerhard.andersson@liu.se

W.T. O'Donohue, C. Draper (eds.), *Stepped Care and e-Health*,
DOI 10.1007/978-1-4419-6510-3_4, © Springer Science+Business Media, LLC 2011

situations from which escape might be difficult or in which help may not be available in the event of having an unexpected or situationally predisposed panic attack or panic-like symptoms (APA, 2000). People with agoraphobia tend to fear and avoid a range of situations or places such as being alone outside the home, crowds, traveling by car, bus, train, or plane (Taylor, 2000). Some individuals expose themselves to the feared situations, but endure these experiences with a high level of anxiety and many become increasingly dependent on significant others (as they are better off to confront a feared situation when accompanied with a companion). Approximately one-third to one-half of individuals diagnosed with panic disorder also have agoraphobia (Barlow, 2002).

Comorbidity with other anxiety disorders is common among individuals with panic disorder with or without agoraphobia (Taylor, 2000), and it is also common with panic attacks in other anxiety disorders such as social phobia sometimes making diagnostic differentiation difficult. The most common comorbid disorders are social phobia (occurring in 15–30% of people diagnosed with panic disorder), obsessive-compulsive disorder (8–10%), specific phobia (10–20%), and general anxiety disorder (25%). According to Taylor (2000), around 50–65% of people who develop panic disorder will also develop major depression at some point in their lives. Also substance abuse frequently co-occurs with panic disorder (Zvolensky et al., 2006). Axis-II disorders, such as avoidant, dependent, and histrionic personality disorders are common in clinical setting with about 40–50% of patients with panic disorder fulfilling the criteria for a personality disorder (Taylor, 2000).

Several studies have found that patients with panic disorder are among the highest users of medical services and therefore are an enormous economic burden for the healthcare system (Mitte, 2005). It is therefore important to develop cost-effective interventions including stepped care procedures. Fortunately, evidence-based treatment exists including less therapist-intensive treatments (Starcevic, 2008). Indeed, clinical trials have shown that treatment for panic disorder, based on cognitive-behavioral principles, enables 75–95% of patients to be panic free following treatment and that the improvements are maintained for at least 2 years (Taylor, 2000).

Assessment/Triage

Assessment and subsequent triage of individuals with suspected panic disorder range from brief self-screening instruments to thorough structured interviews. One increasingly used instrument is the Panic Disorder Severity Scale (PDSS), which is a commonly used clinician administered measure of PD severity (Shear et al., 1997). It measures the frequency of full panic attacks as well as limited symptom attacks. It also rates the experienced distress from attacks, worry about attacks, effect of PD on social and professional functioning, as well as degree of interoceptive- and agoraphobic avoidance. The PDSS is usually administered in an interview but can also be used as a self-report instrument.

A range of self-report measures have been used in research and in clinical practice. To give a few examples, this includes panic-specific measures like the Agoraphobic Cognitions Questionnaire and The Body Sensations Questionnaire (Chambless et al., 1984), which measure panic-specific cognitions and fear of physical symptoms, respectively. Agoraphobic avoidance can be measured by the Mobility Inventory for agoraphobia (Chambless et al., 1985). Another commonly used measure is the Anxiety Sensitivity Index (Reiss et al., 1986), which measures fear of anxiety-related sensations. It is also common to measure more general anxiety symptoms, for example, by using the Beck Anxiety Inventory (Beck et al., 1988). Questionnaire assessment of panic disorder symptoms can feasibly be administered using the Internet (Carlbring et al., 2007).

When it comes to diagnostic instruments it is common to use the Structured Clinical Interview for the DSM-IV (SCID; First et al., 1995) or the Anxiety Disorders Interview Schedule Revised (Di Nardo et al., 1994) to confirm a diagnosis of panic disorder with or without agoraphobia. As medical conditions such as vestibular deficits and asthma may occur as co-existing conditions it is often important to medically examine patients or check medical files from general practice. Some patients may seek out numerous medical tests but it is also common that they avoid medical consultations for fear of having a disease detected.

Once interview and questionnaire data have been collected a decision on further treatment should be made in collaboration with the patient. In this chapter we focus on adult patients. Panic disorder can, however, occur in children and adolescents (Taylor, 2000), but it may be that panic attacks in children more often are elicited in response to a situation (e.g., crowds) rendering a diagnosis of panic disorder less suitable. Older adults can also have panic disorder, which may require special considerations in assessment and treatment, in particular in relation to comorbid medical conditions.

Stepped Care Options

Watchful Waiting

Panic disorder tends to be chronic if not treated and shows only low spontaneous remission rates in its natural course (Kessler et al., 1994). It may, however, vary in severity and symptoms can fluctuate. When panic disorder is treated the prognosis can be good, although relapse may occur (Starcevic, 2008). However, only about 25% of the sufferers of panic disorder seek professional help for their panic problems. Instead they seek other forms of health care for somatic conditions (Lidren et al., 1994), and the demand versus available treatment gap is particularly large when it comes to evidence-based psychological treatments (Postel et al., 2008). A limited amount of qualified therapists, long waiting periods, and high costs probably restrict the opportunity to receive accurate help.

Psychoeducation

Psychoeducation is an integral part of most cognitive-behavioral (CBT) treatment protocols and is also included in pharmacological treatments, albeit to a lesser extent. Increasingly, other psychological treatment formats such as psychodynamic therapy include psychoeducation. Usually, psychoeducation consists of information about the condition and some explanatory mechanism (e.g., catastrophic misinterpretation of bodily signals) is presented. Some forms of psychoeducation also involve asking the client to register symptoms in line with a model such as the panic circle developed by Clark (1986). Psychoeducation may also include information about prognosis, treatment options and their outcomes, and also tailored information to help the client understand maintaining factors.

There may be initial effects of psychoeducation that will facilitate further progress in treatment. For example, Shear et al. (1994) found that by starting treatment with psychoeducation the subsequent treatment, which was either based on CBT or a non-prescriptive supportive therapy, did not differ. It is more questionable if psychoeducation on its own confers any benefits and in studies in which an information only control condition has been included this has generally not resulted in any improvements (e.g., Klein et al., 2006). It may be premature to exclude psychoeducation as a sole intervention. Indeed, Baillie and Rapee (2004) argued that it is important to search for predictors of outcome in briefer treatments as they can be a part of a stepped care approach to treatment.

Bibliotherapy

Bibliotherapy refers to the use of written instructional materials, often in the form of a self-help book or manual, to guide the patient through the course of treatment (Watkins and Clum, 2008). Bibliotherapy is probably not sufficient for individuals with severe panic disorder and comorbidity and can also be unsuited for individuals with limited reading abilities or lack of motivation to follow a self-directed program (Taylor, 2000). Treatment ingredients presented in self-help books are derived from face-to-face treatment manuals. A brief outline of the contents of a Swedish self-help material (Carlbring and Hanell, 2007) is presented in Table 4.1.

Several studies have shown that bibliotherapy for panic disorder is an effective treatment when it is delivered with minimal therapist contact (e.g., Gould et al., 1993; Gould and Clum, 1995; Hecker et al., 1996; Hecker et al., 2004; Lidren et al., 1994). Carlbring et al. (2000) reviewed the available self-help books at that time and their corresponding studies and found that bibliotherapy for panic disorder can be effective, with a moderate to large effect size ($d = 0.5 - 1.5$).

In the study by Gould et al. (1993) bibliotherapy was compared to individual therapy and to a waitlist control group. A total number of 33 patients diagnosed with panic disorder were allocated to one of the three groups. Participants receiving individual therapy met with a therapist for 1 h twice a week during the 4 weeks of treatment. The treatment was based on the content of the self-help book. Participants

Table 4.1 Overview of the Swedish self-help material on panic disorder

Chapters 1 and 2 cover psychoeducation and socialization to the treatment. Chapter 3 includes breathing retraining and a hyperventilation test. Chapters 4 and 5 contain information and exercises regarding cognitive restructuring, and Chapters 6 and 7 instructions on how to do interoceptive exposure. The following two chapters (Chapters 8 and 9) deal with exposure in vivo, and the material ends with a chapter on relapse prevention and assertiveness training. At the end of each chapter, the reader is presented with a quiz to test the level of knowledge gained after the completion of that particular chapter. For example, a question might be "What happens if you experience anxiety for a prolonged period and stay in the situation?" For each chapter, the reader is also given homework assignments, which usually consist of some type of practical exercise. An example is to do exposure from a list of anxiety provoking situations such as spinning a chair to experience dizziness.

in the bibliotherapy condition were asked to read the self-help book *Coping with Panic* (Clum, 1990) at their own pace and to apply the strategies described in the book. The participants in this group had telephone contact for about 10 min on two occasions (weeks 2 and 4) during the course of the treatment. The self-help book consisted of psychoeducation about panic disorder, cognitive and behavioral strategies (such as relaxation, breathing retraining, cognitive restructuring, and exposure exercises), and application of the material. The results from the study indicate that participants in the bibliotherapy group, in general, showed significantly more improvement than participants in the waitlist and were not significantly different from those in the individual therapy group. Seventy-three percent of the patients in the bibliotherapy condition, 56% in the individual therapy condition, and 36% in the waitlist condition were panic free at post-treatment assessment. The overall effect size was $d = 1.5$ for bibliotherapy compared to the waitlist.

In a replication and extension of their original study, Gould and Clum (1995) compared a 4 week self-help treatment to a waitlist control. The self-help book utilized in the study was *Coping with Panic* which the participants were encouraged to read at their own pace. Apart from this primary intervention the participants were also given an informational videotape and a relaxation audiotape. The videotape explained the etiology of panic disorder, the spiraling and circular relationship between panic symptoms and cognitions, and modeled diaphragmatic breathing. The audiotape consisted of instructions on progressive muscle relaxation. Of the 25 participants 84% met the criteria for panic disorder with agoraphobia and the remaining met the criteria for panic disorder without agoraphobia. The proportions of panic-free subjects were 46% for the self-help treatment group and 25% for the waitlist at post-treatment and 69 and 25%, respectively, at the 2-month follow-up. The study strongly supports the effectiveness of self-help relative to waitlist condition both post-treatment and at a 2-month follow-up. The study showed a medium effect size ($d = 0.5$) at post-treatment and a large effect size ($d = 0.8$) at the follow-up.

In another study Lidren et al. (1994) compared an 8-week bibliotherapy treatment and group therapy to a waitlist control. The participants in both treatment groups were given the book *Coping with Panic* and the subjects in the self-help group were contacted over the telephone at weeks 2, 5, and 8 to determine if subjects were reading, comprehending, and using the strategies described. Participants receiving group therapy met weekly for 90 min with a therapist in groups of six to process and practice material covered in the text. Results indicated that both bibliotherapy and group treatment were more effective than the waitlist condition in reducing frequency of panic attacks, severity of physical panic symptoms, catastrophic cognitions, agoraphobic avoidance, and depression and also more effective in increasing self-efficacy. Before treatment commenced 30 participants out of 36 met the criteria for panic disorder with agoraphobia and the remaining met the criteria for panic disorder without agoraphobia. The proportions of panic-free patients at post-treatment and 6-month follow-up were 83% (75%) for bibliotherapy, 83% (92%) for group therapy, and 25% for the waitlist. Both interventions maintained their effects throughout the follow-up periods at 3 and 6 months and produced clinically significant levels of change. A post-test comparison between the bibliotherapy and the waitlist conditions across all dependent measures revealed a large effect size ($d = 1.5$).

In a study by Hecker et al. (1996) self-directed and therapist-directed CBT for panic disorder were compared. All the 16 participants were provided with Barlow and Craske's (1989) *Mastery of your anxiety and panic*. Subjects in the therapist-directed groups met with a therapist for 12 weekly sessions, during which material in the book was discussed and worked through. Therapists also met with the self-directed group, but only three times over 12 weeks to assign readings and answer questions. The book used in the study consisted of material covering basic information about panic, anxiety, and panic disorder from a CBT perspective; muscle relaxation training and breathing retraining; common cognitive distortions associated with panic; and instructions for monitoring and challenging irrational thinking. Interoceptive and in vivo exposure exercises were other areas that were presented in the book. In both conditions participants improved with treatment and maintained their gains at a 6-month follow-up. There were no differences between the two treatment conditions on the outcome measures. The proportions of panic-free self-directed patients at post-treatment and at 6-month follow-up were 60% (80%) and the proportions of panic-free therapist-directed patients at post-treatment and at 6-month follow-up were 63% (71%). The average within-group effect size for the self-help condition was $d = 1.1$ at post-treatment and $d = 1.0$ at 6-month follow-up.

In another study by Hecker et al. (2004) four sessions of CBT group therapy (Group) or one meeting with a therapist plus three telephone calls (Telephone) contacts were compared. The 48 included participants worked with *Mastery of your anxiety and panic* during 10 weeks. The participants who received group therapy met at weeks 1, 3, 5, and 7 and during the group meetings the therapist assigned readings, provided an overview of the information to be covered in the readings and answered participants' questions. In the other group participants met alone with the therapist who provided them with a copy of the book and instructed them to read the first four chapters. Therapists then telephoned participants at three different occasions to assess the compliance and the comprehension with the reading. The proportions of panic-free patients at post-treatment were 16% for group and 57%

for telephone and 24% for group and 36% for telephone at the 6-month follow-up assessment. The results from the study revealed significant improvement over the course of treatment and maintenance of gains over the follow-up period and the study indicates that self-help treatment with brief therapist contact is a viable treatment for panic disorder.

One crucial question is if bibliotherapy for panic disorders requires therapist contact and if so how much? This question was directly addressed in a study by Febbraro et al. (1999) who compared bibliotherapy alone ($n = 17$); bibliotherapy plus monitoring ($n = 15$); monitoring alone ($n = 13$); or waitlist control ($n = 18$) conditions. The monitoring consisted of self-observation and rating of panic symptoms. In this study there was no contact with the researchers at pre-treatment assessment as participants assessed themselves. It was not necessary for participants to meet criteria for panic disorder to be included in the study. All participants had approximately 1 h of telephone or in-person contact during the post-treatment assessment, when a clinical interview was conducted. There were no significant differences between the groups at post-treatment, but some within-group effects. Febbraro et al. questioned the efficacy of bibliotherapy and self-monitoring interventions when practiced without contact with a clinician who conducts the assessments and monitors treatment compliance. In a later study Febbraro (2005) contrasted three conditions; bibliotherapy alone ($n = 9$), bibliotherapy plus phone contact ($n = 9$), and phone contact alone ($n = 12$). In this trial dropout rate from inclusion to completion was substantial with 18 out of 48 not completing the trial. In terms of clinically significant change there were large differences between the three groups on a measure of full panic attacks (55.6%, 100%, and 33.3% for the three conditions, respectively). Overall, the study showed superior outcome for the telephone-guided bibliotherapy when compared with the unguided self-help and phone contact alone.

A similar conclusion was reached in another study in which standard therapist contact ($n = 37$) was compared with minimal contact treatment ($n = 32$) and finally a third group ($n = 35$) who received pure bibliotherapy (Powers et al. 2000). They found a much better outcome for the standard therapist contact group and the group with minimal therapist contact. For example, using a criterion of clinically significant change on the Hamilton Anxiety Scale, 83.3% improved in the standard therapist contact group, 67.7% in the minimal contact treatment group, and only 34.5% in the pure bibliotherapy group.

In sum, most studies on bibliotherapy for panic disorder suggest that guidance is needed, but in one study by our research group we discovered that unguided biblio-therapy can work if a clear deadline is provided (Nordin et al., 2010). Participants were randomized to either unassisted bibliotherapy ($n = 20$) with a scheduled follow-up telephone interview or to a waiting list control group ($n = 19$). Following a structured psychiatric interview, participants in the treatment group were sent a self-help book consisting of 10 chapters based on cognitive-behavioral strategies for the treatment of panic disorder. No therapist contact of any kind was provided during the treatment phase which lasted for 10 weeks. Results showed that the treatment group had, in comparison to the control group, improved on all outcome measures at post-treatment and at 3-month follow-up. The tentative conclusion drawn from these results is that pure bibliotherapy with a clear deadline can be effective for people suffering from panic disorder with or without agoraphobia. It is, however, also best to regard bibliotherapy as an early intervention for less severe cases, in particular if unguided.

Computer-Assisted and Internet-Delivered Interventions

Treatment via the Internet has increasingly been investigated in research and promising findings have been observed for various conditions (Andersson, 2009). Moreover, the results for anxiety and depression have been summarized in a meta-analysis (Spek et al., 2007), and several controlled studies have been published after that review. Briefly, there are many ways in which Internet-based treatment can be delivered ranging from mostly text-based programs to interactive programs with audio files and film clips.

Panic disorder was one of the first conditions for which Internet treatment was developed and there are controlled trials in which Internet treatment has been contrasted against a waiting list, and trials in which Internet treatment has been compared with face-to-face treatment. Finally, there are now two effectiveness trials in which Internet treatment has been delivered under more clinically representative conditions. All programs to date dealing with panic disorder have been based on CBT and all have included some form of guidance with the exception of one open access trial which showed a very large dropout rate (Farvolden et al., 2005).

In Australia a research group showed promising outcomes in two small trials (Klein and Richards, 2001; Richards and Alvarenga, 2002). The later research did studies with larger samples and an extended treatment program (Klein et al., 2006; Richards et al., 2006). In most trials of Internet treatment psychologists have provided the support but in one trial the Australian group found that it worked equally well when general practitioners provided the guidance (Shandley et al., 2008). In one trial they compared their Internet treatment with a standard face-to-face treatment and found equivalent outcomes (Kiropoulos et al., 2008). The authors found that 30.4% (14/46) of their *Panic online* treatment participants reached the criteria of high end-state functioning, with the corresponding figure in the face-to-face group being 27.5% (11/40). High end-state was defined as being free of panic and having a panic disorder clinician severity rating of less than 2 (on a 0–8 scale). Finally, in one trial they examined whether frequency of therapist contact affected treatment outcomes (Klein et al., 2009). Fifty-seven people with panic disorder were randomly allocated to Internet treatment with either frequent (three emails per week) or infrequent (one email per week) support from a psychologist. Post-treatment, intention-to-treat analyses on 57 participants revealed that both treatments were effective at improving panic disorder and agoraphobia severity ratings, panic-related cognitions, negative affect, and psychological and physical quality of life domains, with no differences between conditions. High end-state functioning was achieved by 28.6 and 27.6% of the frequent and infrequent participants, respectively. The authors concluded that the results provide evidence that the effectiveness of internet-based mental health interventions may be independent of the frequency of therapist support and may therefore be more cost-effective than previously reported.

Our Swedish group has independently conducted similar research with three controlled Internet trials all showing positive outcomes (Carlbring et al., 2001, 2003, 2006) and a direct comparison between face-to-face and Internet-delivered CBT (Carlbring et al., 2005). In the Carlbring et al. (2003) study two active online treatments were compared (CBT versus applied relaxation), showing small differences in outcome. In terms of effect sizes we have generally found high standardized effect sizes, both for primary panic-related outcomes and secondary outcomes including quality of life. For example, in the trial in which we added brief weekly supportive telephone calls (Carlbring et al., 2006), the mean between-group effect size across all measures was $d = 1.00$, and outcomes were sustained at 9-month follow-up. In an open uncontrolled trial we found that the results from the efficacy trials with participants recruited via advertisement were replicated in a psychiatric setting with patients referred from general practice or psychiatry (Bergström et al., 2009). In the latest large trial group live CBT was compared with Internet treatment again showing that Internet treatment can be as effective as face-to-face treatment (Bergström et al., 2010).

A third research group has independently tested Internet-delivered CBT for panic disorder, again showing that the treatment concept appears to hold (Schneider et al., 2005).

In sum, there are now several studies suggesting that at least a significant proportion of persons with panic disorder with or without agoraphobia can be successfully treated with guided self-help over the Internet. However, as with bibliotherapy patients need to be able to read and understand text and in the case of Internet treatment they should also have access to the Internet and be able to use computers at a basic level. Security issues must be handled as well, but this is increasingly less of an issue at least in Sweden where safe solutions have been developed and integrated into health care (www.internetpsykiatri.se).

Group Therapy

In common with many forms of CBT panic treatment has also been tested as a group treatment (Telch et al., 1993), usually with 8–12 participants per group and with a similar duration as individual treatment (i.e., 10–15 weekly sessions). Typically, sessions last for 2 h with a break in the middle and one to two therapists lead the group. Overall, this format is suitable for panic treatment and is generally set up with the ingredients presented in Table 4.1 (e.g., psychoeducation, exposure, homework). However, the group format has the advantage of having the other group members to share experiences with. Moreover, group members can reinforce progress given a good group climate. While some clinicians have expressed concerns that group treatment can be a suboptimal option (Morrison, 2001), this is not confirmed by the empirical literature on panic disorder. However, few direct comparisons have been made and meta-analyses are not conclusive regarding the relative merits of individual versus group treatment. As with bibliotherapy and Internet treatment not all patients are suitable for group treatment, as the more idiosyncratic characteristics can be difficult to handle in a group. For example, in cases with comorbid social anxiety disorder, this may prevent them from being active in the group in relation to the rest of the participants and "safety behaviors" (used to prevent perceived catastrophes) can be used in the group sessions which may hinder progress. Moreover, it is not necessarily the case that group treatment saves time and costs. However, Roberge et al. (2008) conducted a randomized, controlled trial to examine the cost-effectiveness of cognitive-behavioral treatment (CBT) for panic disorder with agoraphobia. A total of 100 participants were randomly assigned to standard ($n = 33$), group ($n = 35$), and brief ($n = 32$) treatment conditions. Their results showed no significant differences between treatment conditions. Compared with standard CBT, brief and group CBT incurred lower treatment costs and had a superior cost-effectiveness ratio. Recently intensive group treatment has been tested with positive results (Bohni et al., 2009), and this could possible decrease the costs further.

As with Internet treatment there are indications that individual treatment is preferred over group treatment and that dropout is somewhat higher in group treatment (Sharp et al., 2004). However, since costs are likely reduced in group treatment and our own clinical experience of patients changing their preference once they are in group, we believe that group CBT should be presented as an option that could be followed by individual treatment or medication in a stepped care procedure.

Individual Therapy

Individual psychological treatment for panic disorder is widely regarded as an evidence-based treatment and appears in many treatment guidelines (e.g., NICE in the United Kingdom). The most established form is CBT, as attested by several meta-analyses (e.g., Mitte, 2005; Westen and Morrison, 2001), and good quality controlled trials (e.g., Clark et al., 1994).

There is one controlled trial on manualized individual psychodynamic psychotherapy (Milrod et al., 2007), but so far this is not replicated and appears to be more time consuming than other psychological treatments. However, psychodynamic therapy might be feasible in the presence of comorbid personality disorders (Milrod et al., 2007).

Other studies have found effects of applied relaxation (Öst and Westling, 1995). However, Siev and Chambless (2007) reviewed the literature and found that CBT was a specific treatment for panic disorder which performed better than relaxation.

The treatment components in individual CBT for panic disorder includes the ingredients presented in the previous sections, but the individual format allows for more tailoring. In particular with difficult and more complicated cases, individual face-to-face treatment can be indicated (Hackmann, 1998). In particular, tailoring is needed not only in cases with severe agoraphobia, but also in the presence of drug and alcohol problems and as mentioned personality disorders. While the presence of personality disorders may be predictive of a negative treatment outcome (Mennin and Heimberg, 2000), we found that a positive indication of avoidant personality disorder was predictive of better outcome (Andersson et al., 2008) in individual CBT for panic disorder. This could possibly be because we used a combined format in which text material was used as an adjunct to the treatment sessions and this gives the therapist more room for other issues such as personality dysfunction. Hackmann (1998) recommended using images when working with difficult patients when verbal techniques were not sufficient. In our own clinical experience concurrent drug use can be problematic, but not necessarily implicating worse outcome. This is in line with what some other researchers have reported (McEvoy and Shand, 2008).

Medication

Pharmacological treatment of panic disorder with or without agoraphobia is a common treatment option for the acute treatment phase (Baldwin et al., 2005), and a range of pharmacological interventions are effective. For example, tricyclic antidepressants (TCA) and selective serotonin reuptake inhibitors (SSRIs) have been proven to be effective in treating panic disorder (Baldwin et al., 2005). Moreover, high-potency benzodiazepines have been used although they appear in treatment guidelines to a lesser extent. The three main classes of medication (e.g., SSRIs, TCAs, and benzodiazepines) do not appear to differ much in terms of efficacy and attrition rates (Mitte, 2005), but overall SSRI's are often the pharmacological treatment of choice. For example, withdrawal problems with benzodiazepines favor the use of antidepressants. No differences in efficacy have been demonstrated between the two groups of antidepressants that are used most frequently (SSRI and TCAs), but the side effects of TCAs have led to a preference for SSRIs over TCAs. SSRIs plus psychological (commonly CBT) appear slightly more effective than SSRIs alone (Starcevic, 2008) in the acute phase, but this is not clear when it comes to longer follow-up periods (Foa et al., 2002). Our impression is that combined treatment can be useful in comorbid cases with, for example, major depression. We have, however, often seen cases who have stable dose of medication (SSRIs) but still fulfill the criteria for panic disorder and respond well to psychological treatment.

Inpatient Treatment

Inpatient treatment is most often in question for suspected physical problems (Barlow, 2002), but also in cases with suicide risk even if this is relatively rare. Obviously, panic attacks occur in association with a range of mental health problems such as psychosis and severe depression. Patients with severe and refractory anxiety may be in need of inpatient treatment but in our impression panic disorder is then often not the only reason.

Consumer Preferences and Cultural Sensitivity

In many settings it has been found that patients prefer psychological treatments over pharmacological (Taylor, 2000), but this is not a well-investigated area when it comes to regular clinical practice. In one study on panic disorder, we found differences in treatment credibility between live versus Internet treatment (Carlbring et al., 2005), but no differences in outcome. A later prediction study confirmed that treatment credibility did not predict outcome (Andersson et al., 2008). However, what is needed is data on treatment preferences in clinical settings. This also relates to cultural sensitivity as treatments developed in once society will not necessarily work equally well when transported to another culture. In many countries such as our own a significant proportion will not have our language as their native tongue, rendering cultural sensitivity important. Another important factor is where the research has been conducted. For example, treatment of panic disorder often occurs in primary care settings. While there are studies showing that psychological treatments alone or in conjunction with medication work well in primary care, the strongest treatment effects are often seen in treatment trials with recruited patients.

Triage Agenda

Baillie and Rapee (2004) did a study in which they investigated predictors of who was likely to improve from brief interventions and who is likely to require more intensive assistance. In their study 117 people with panic attacks received a psychoeducational booklet, a self-help workbook, and brief group CBT over a 9-month period. They found that baseline levels of social anxiety and general mental health predicted outcome, suggesting that more severe cases require intensive treatment and proposed that it is possible to identify who will benefit from psychoeducation, self-help or face-to-face therapy as the first step in stepped care.

Otto et al. (2000) analyzed different treatment options and found that CBT was at least equal to pharmacotherapy in terms of pretreatment severity and treatment outcome. They also found that CBT was more cost-effective.

Research and Development Agenda

In this chapter we concentrated on reviewing the literature on bibliotherapy and recent Internet-delivered treatments. There are several new research venues such as combined pharmacological and exposure-based strategies using D-cycloserine (Starcevic, 2008) and using computers in face-to-face treatments (e.g., Craske et al., 2009). We also expect further research activities within other forms of psychotherapy than CBT, such as psychodynamic treatment. Another possible development could involve the incorporation of acceptance-based strategies in research on panic disorder (Eifert and Heffner, 2003), and overall it may be that different conceptualizations of panic disorder could inform treatment. Diagnostic heterogeneity and predictors and moderators of treatment outcome remain a challenge to investigate. Moreover, research on the biological and psychological underpinnings of panic disorder is likely to continue and might lead to further developments of treatments.

Dissemination Agenda

It is well known that effective psychological treatments are not accessed to the extent required in relation to costs and patient preferences. Effectiveness studies suggest that treatment of panic disorder works in regular clinical settings when the provider is a trained therapist (e.g., Addis et al., 2004; Wade et al., 1998). To a much lesser extent other providers of treatment have been studied, and there are relatively few studies on less therapist-intensive treatments (e.g., guided bibliotherapy) conducted in regular clinical settings. More information is needed about the costs of panic disorder and that the suffering involved can be avoided by means of effective treatments. Finally collaborative care efforts have shown promising outcomes (Roy-Byrne et al., 2005), suggesting that a collaborative care effort with relatively untrained CBT providers can work well in a general practice setting.

References

Addis ME, Hatgis C, Krasnow AD, Jacob K, Bourne L, Mansfield A. Effectiveness of cognitive-behavioral treatment for panic disorder versus treatment as usual in a managed care setting. J Consult Clin Psychol. 2004;72:625–35.

American Psychiatric Association. Diagnostic and statistical manual of mental disorders. 4th ed., text revision ed. Washington, DC: American Psychiatric Press; 2000.

Andersson G. Using the internet to provide cognitive behaviour therapy. Behav Res Ther. 2009;47:175–80.

Andersson G, Carlbring P, Grimlund A. Predicting treatment outcome in Internet versus face to face treatment of panic disorder. Computers in Human Behavior. 2008;24:1790–1801.

Baillie AJ, Rapee RM. Predicting who benefits from psychoeducation and self help for panic attacks. Behav Res Ther. 2004;42:513–27.

Baldwin DS, Anderson IM, Nutt DJ, Bandelow B, Bond A, Davidson JR, et al. Evidence-based guidelines for the pharmacological treatment of anxiety disorders: recommendations from the British Association for Psychopharmacology. J Psychopharmacol. 2005;19: 567–96.

Barlow DH. Anxiety and its disorders. The nature and treatment of anxiety and panic (Vol. 2). New York: Guilford press; 2002.

Barlow DH, Craske MG. Mastery of your anxiety and panic. San Antonio: the Psychological Corporation; 1989.

Beck AT, Epstein N, Brown G, Steer RA. An inventory for measuring clinical anxiety: psychometric properties. J Consult Clin Psychol. 1988;56:893–7.

Bergström J, Andersson G, Karlsson A, Andreewitch S, Rück C, Carlbring P, et al. An open study of the effectiveness of internet treatment for panic disorder delivered in a psychiatric setting. Nord J Psychiatry. 2009;63:44–50.

Bergström J, Andersson G, Ljótsson B, Rück C, Andréewitch S, Karlsson A, et al. Internet-versus group-administered cognitive behavior therapy for panic disorder in a psychiatric setting: a randomized equivalence trial. BMC Psychiatry. 2010;10, 54.

Bohni MK, Spindler H, Arendt M, Hougaard E, Rosenberg NK. A randomized study of massed three-week cognitive behavioural therapy schedule for panic disorder. Acta Psychiatr Scand. 2009;120(3):187–95.

Carlbring P, Brunt S, Bohman S, Austin D, Richards JC, Öst L-G, et al. Internet vs. paper and pencil administration of questionnaires commonly used in panic/agoraphobia research. Comput Hum Behav. 2007;23:1421–34.

Carlbring P, Ekselius L, Andersson G. Treatment of panic disorder via the internet: A randomized trial of CBT vs. applied relaxation. J Behav Ther Exp Psychiatry. 2003;34:129–40.

Carlbring P, Hanell Å. Ingen panik: Fri från panik-och ångestattacker i 10 steg med kognitiv beteendeterapi. [No panic: free from panic and anxiety]. Stockholm: Natur och Kultur; 2007.

Carlbring P, Bohman S, Brunt S, Buhrman M, Westling BE, Ekselius L, Andersson G. Remote treatment of panic disorder: a randomized trial of Internet-based cognitive behavior therapy supplemented with telephone calls. Am J Psychiat. 2006;163:2119–25.

Carlbring P, Nilsson-Ihrfelt E, Waara J, Kollenstam C, Buhrman M, Kaldo V, et al. Treatment of panic disorder: live therapy vs. self-help via internet. Behav Res Ther. 2005;43:1321–33.

Carlbring P, Westling BE, Andersson G. A review of published selfhelp books for panic disorder. Scand J Behav Ther. 2000;29:5–13.

Carlbring P, Westling BE, Ljungstrand P, Ekselius L, Andersson G. Treatment of panic disorder via the Internet: a randomized trial of a self-help program. Behav Ther. 2001;32:751–64.

Chambless DL, Caputo G, Jasin S, Gracely EJ, Williams C. The mobility inventory for agoraphobia. Behav Res Ther. 1985;23:35–44.

Chambless DL, Caputo GC, Bright P, Gallagher R. Assessment of fear of fear in agoraphobics: the body sensations questionnaire and the agoraphobic cognitions questionnaire. J Consult Clin Psychol. 1984;52:1090–7.

Clark DM. A cognitive approach to panic. Behav Res Ther. 1986;24:461–70.

Clark DM, Salkovskis PM, Hackmann A, Middleton H, Anastasiades P, Gelder M. A comparison of cognitive therapy, applied relaxation and imipramine in the treatment of panic disorder. Br J Psychiatry. 1994;164:759–69.

Clum GA. Coping with panic. Pacific Grove: Brooks/Cole Publishing; 1990.

Di Nardo PA, Moras K, Barlow DH, Rapee RM. Reliability of DSM III R anxiety disorder categories: using the anxiety disorders interview schedule revised (ADIS R). Arch Gen Psychiatry. 1993;50:251–6.

Craske MG, Rose RD, Lang A, Welch SS, Campbell-Sills L, Sullivan G, et al. Computer-assisted delivery of cognitive behavioral therapy for anxiety disorders in primary-care settings. Depress Anxiety. 2009;26:235–42.

Di Nardo P, Brown TA, Barlow DH. anxiety disorders interview schedule for DSM-IV. San Antonio, TX: The Psychological Corporation; 1994.

Eifert GH, Heffner M. The effects of acceptance versus control contexts on avoidance of panic-related symptoms. J Behav Ther Exp Psychiatry. 2003;34:293–312.

Farvolden P, Denisoff E, Selby P, Bagby RM, Rudy L. Usage and longitudinal effectiveness of a Web-based self-help cognitive behavioral therapy program for panic disorder. J Med Internet Res. 2005;7(1):e7.

Febbraro GA. An investigation into the effectiveness of bibliotherapy and minimal contact interventions in the treatment of panic attacks. J Clin Psychol. 2005;61:763–79.

Febbraro GAR, Clum GA, Roodman AA, Wright JH. The limits of bibliotherapy: a study of differential effectiveness of self-administered interventions in individuals with panic attacks. Behav Ther. 1999;30:209–22.

First MB, Spitzer RL, Gibbon M, Williams JBW. Structured clinical interview for DSM-IV Axis I disorders (SCID-I). Washington, D.C: American Psychiatric Press; 1995.

Foa EB, Franklin ME, Moser J. Context in the clinic: How well do cognitive-behavioral therapies and medications work in combination? Biol Psychiatry. 2002;52:987–97.

Gould RA, Clum GA. Self-help plus minimal therapist contact in the treatment of panic disorder: a replication and extension. Behav Ther. 1995;26:533–46.

Gould RA, Clum GA, Shapiro D. The use of bibliotherapy in the treatment of panic disorder: a preliminary investigation. Behav Ther. 1993;24:241–52.

Hackmann A. (1998). Cognitive therapy panic and agoraphobia: working with complex cases. In: Tarrier N, Wells A, Haddock G, editors. Treating complex cases. The cognitive behavioural therapy approach. Chichester: Wiley; 1998. p. 27–45.

Hecker JE, Losee MC, Fritzler BK, Fink CM. Self-directed versus therapist-directed cognitive behavioural treatment for panic disorder. J Anxiety Disord. 1996;10:253–65.

Hecker JE, Losee MC, Roberson-Nay R, Maki K. Mastery of Your Anxiety and Panic and brief therapist contact in the treatment of panic disorder. Anxiety Disord. 2004;18:111–26.

Kessler RC, McGonagle KA, Zhao S, Nelson CB, Hughes M, Eskleman S, Wittchen H-U, Kendler KS. Lifetime and 12-month prevalence of DSM-III-R psychiatric disorders in the United States. Arch Gen Psychiatry. 1994;51:8–19.

Kiropoulos LA, Klein B, Austin DW, Gilson K, Pier C, Mitchell J, et al. Is internet-based CBT for panic disorder and agoraphobia as effective as face-to-face CBT? J Anxiety Disord. 2008;22:1273–84.

Klein B, Austin D, Pier C, Kiropoulos L, Shandley K, Mitchell J, et al. Internet-based treatment for panic disorder: does frequency of therapist contact make a difference? Cogn Behav Ther. 2009;38:121–31.

Klein B, Richards JC. A brief internet-based treatment for panic disorder. Behav Cogn Psychother. 2001;29:113–7.

Klein B, Richards JC, Austin DW. Efficacy of internet therapy for panic disorder. J Behav Ther Exp Psychiatry. 2006;37:213–38.

Lidren DM, Watkins PL, Gould RA, Clum GA, Asterino M, Tulloch HL. A comparison of bibliotherapy and group therapy in the treatment of panic disorder. J Consult Clin Psychol. 1994;62:865–9.

McEvoy PM, Shand F. The effect of comorbid substance use disorders on treatment outcome for anxiety disorders. J Anxiety Disord. 2008;22:1087–98.

Mennin DS, Heimberg RG. The impact of comorbid mood and personality disorders in the cognitive-behavioral treatment of panic disorder. Clin Psychol Rev. 2000;20:339–57.

Milrod BL, Leon AC, Barber JP, Markowitz JC, Graf E. Do comorbid personality disorders moderate panic-focused psychotherapy? An exploratory examination of the American psychiatric association practice guideline. J Clinl Psychiatry. 2007;68:885–91.

Milrod B, Leon AC, Busch F, Rudden M, Schwalberg M, Clarkin J, et al. A randomized controlled clinical trial of psychoanalytic psychotherapy for panic disorder. Am J Psychiatry. 2007;164:265–72.

Mitte K. A meta-analysis of the efficacy of psycho- and pharmacotherapy in panic disorder with and without agoraphobia. J Affective Disord. 2005;88:27–45.

Morrison N. Group cognitive therapy: treatment of choice or suboptimal option? Behav Cogn Psychoth. 2001;29:311–32.

Nordin S, Carlbring P, Cuijpers P, Andersson G. Expanding the limits of bibliotherapy for panic disorder. Randomized trial of self-help without support but with a clear deadline. Behav Ther. 2010;41:267–76.

Öst L-G, Westling BE. Applied relaxation vs cognitive behaviour therapy in the treatment of panic disorder. Behav Res Ther. 1995;33:145–58.

Otto MW, Pollack MH, Maki KM. Empirically supported treatments for panic disorder: costs, benefits and stepped care. J Consult Clin Psychol. 2000;68:556–63.

Postel MG, de Haan HA, De Jong CA. E-therapy for mental health problems: a systematic review. Telemed e-Health. 2008;14:707–14.

Powers MB, Sharp DM, Swanson V, Simpson RJ. Therapist contact in cognitive behaviour therapy for panic disorder and agoraphobia in primary care. Clin Psychol Psychother. 2000;7:37–46.

Reiss S, Peterson RA, Gurksy DM, McNally RJ. Anxiety sensitivity, anxiety frequency and the prediction of fearfulness. Behav Res Ther. 1986;34:1–8.

Richards JC, Alvarenga ME. Extension and replication of an Internet-based treatment program for panic disorder. Cogn Behav Ther. 2002;31:41–7.

Richards JC, Klein B, Austin DW. Internet CBT for panic disorder: does the inclusion of stress management improve end-state functioning? Clin Psychol. 2006;10:2–15.

Roberge P, Marchand A, Reinharz D, Savard P. Cognitive-behavioral treatment for panic disorder with agoraphobia: a randomized, controlled trial and cost-effectiveness analysis. Behav Modif. 2008;32:333–51.

Roy-Byrne PP, Craske MG, Stein MB, Sullivan G, Bystritsky A, Katon W, et al. A randomized effectiveness trial of cognitive-behavioral therapy and medication for primary care panic disorder. Arch Gen Psychiatry. 2005;62:290–8.

Schneider AJ, Mataix-Cols D, Marks IM, Bachofen M. Internet-guided self-help with or without exposure therapy for phobic and panic disorders. Psychother Psychosom. 2005;74: 154–64.

Sharp DM, Power KG, Swanson V. A comparison of the efficacy and acceptability of group versus individual cognitive behaviour therapy in the treatment of panic disorder and agoraphobia in primary care. Clin Psychol Psychother. 2004;11:78–82.

Shandley K, Austin DW, Klein B, Pier C, Schattner P, Pierce D, et al. Therapist-assisted, Internet-based treatment for panic disorder: can general practitioners achieve comparable patient outcomes to psychologists? J Med Internet Res. 2008;10(2):e14.

Shear MK, Brown TA, Barlow DH, Money R, Sholomskas DE, Woods SW, et al. Multicenter collaborative panic disorder severity scale. Am J Psychiatry. 1997;154:1571–5.

Shear MK, Pilkonis AA, Cloitre M, Leon AC. Cognitive behavioral treatment compared with nonprescriptive treatment of panic disorder. Arch Gen Psychiatry. 1994;51:395–401.

Siev J, Chambless DL. Specificity of treatment effects: cognitive therapy and relaxation for generalized anxiety and panic disorders. J Consult Clin Psychol. 2007;75:513–22.

Spek V, Cuijpers P, Nyklicek I, Riper H, Keyzer J, Pop V. Internet-based cognitive behaviour therapy for symptoms of depression and anxiety: a meta-analysis. Psychol Med. 2007;37: 319–28.

Starcevic V. Treatment of panic disorder: recent developments and current status. Expert Rev Neurother. 2008;8:1219–32.

Taylor CB. Panic disorder. Brit Med J. 2006;332:951–5.

Taylor S. Understanding and treating panic disorder. Cognitive-behavioral approaches. Chichester: Wiley; 2000.

Watkins PL, Clum GA. (Eds.). Handbook of self-help therapies. New York: Routledge; 2008.

Telch MJ, Lucas JA, Schmidt NB, Hanna HH, LaNae Jaimez T, Lucas RA. Group cognitive-behavioral treatment of panic disorder. Behav Res Ther. 1993;31:279–87.

Wade WA, Treat TA, Stuart GL. Transporting an empirically supported treatment for panic disorder to a service clinic setting: a benchmarking strategy. J Consult Clin Psychol. 1998;66:231–9.

Westen D, Morrison K. A multidimensional meta-analysis of treatments for depression, panic, and generalized anxiety disorder: an empirical examination of the status of empirically supported therapies. J Consult Clin Psychol. 2001;69:875–99.

Zvolensky MJ, Bernstein A, Marshall EC, Feldner MT. Panic attacks, panic disorder, and agoraphobia: associations with substance use, abuse, and dependence. Curr Psychiatry Rep. 2006;8:279–85.

Chapter 5
Post-traumatic Stress Disorder

Computer-Based Stepped Care: Practical Applications to Clinical Problems

Crissa Draper and Matthew Ghiglieri

Introduction

The implementation of stepped care model in the treatment of post-traumatic stress disorder is a much-needed innovation in the system of health-care delivery. While other disorders really only occur at the level of the individual, PTSD has the potential to affect a significant number of individuals within communities all at once, such as in the event of major traumatic events like terrorist attacks, war, or natural disasters. While the disorder can also affect people individually, such as in the case of sexual assault or car accidents, the ability to affect entire regions and large numbers of individuals at once creates a need for minimizing therapist time while maximizing outcomes for individuals. As with any disorder, it is also essential to devise a system which allows individuals to seek modes of therapy that appeal to them as consumers, and to allow them the level of care they need based on the severity of their symptom set. The stepped care model potentially allows individuals to try and treat problems in ways that are more cost-effective, less invasive, and less intensive and step away from these variables if initial treatments failed or to "fail forward."

While the majority of individuals experience a trauma at some point in their lives (Yehuda et al., 1998), the majority of these also recover in time from these incidents without further trouble. However, a relatively small but not uncommon sub-section of this population will go on to experience distress related to the event, including re-experiencing, avoidance of stimuli reminiscent of the trauma, and hyperarousal symptoms. Post-traumatic stress disorder (PTSD) ranges from 47% of rape victims to 12% of traffic accident victims, to 5–8% of natural disaster victims (Resick, 2001). Many more may experience sub-clinical symptoms that may be distressing or disrupting.

The majority of individuals with PTSD do not seek treatment, and of those who do, a substantial percentage (estimated to range as high as 82%) do not comply with treatment, and 19–27% of clients drop out (Burstein, 1986; Hembree et al., 2003;

C. Draper (✉)
Department of Psychology, University of Nevada-Reno, Mail Stop 0298, Reno, NV 89557, USA
e-mail: crissadraper@gmail.com

W.T. O'Donohue, C. Draper (eds.), *Stepped Care and e-Health*,
DOI 10.1007/978-1-4419-6510-3_5, © Springer Science+Business Media, LLC 2011

Tarrier et al., 2006). Additionally, the vast majority of licensed clinical psychologists (83%) have never used exposure therapy to treat PTSD, even though exposure therapy is widely regarded as the golden standard in individual treatment of PTSD (Becker et al., 2004). This shows a clear need for the development of additional options for individuals suffering from post-traumatic distress.

In this chapter, a stepped care model for the assessment and treatment of trauma-related distress will be discussed, as will the evidence or research agenda for each step. Consumer preferences, triage agenda, and dissemination agenda will also be discussed.

Consumer Preference

As stated earlier, the majority of individuals do not seek treatment for PTSD and those who do are likely to drop out. Those who stay in therapy are not likely to receive an evidence-based treatment. This is due at least in part to the fact that around 80% of therapists who do not use the gold standard in treating PTSD—exposure therapy—say it is because they are worried that it might upset the client (Becker et al., 2004). From this discussion, the need for assessing and considering consumer preference regarding treatment for PTSD is clear.

In one study, it was found that for undergraduate students who had imagined a sexual assault and were given brief information on different types of treatment, 87% would choose exposure therapy, 7% would choose medication, and 6% would choose no treatment (Zoellner et al., 2003). This is clearly not entirely accurate based on the high expectations of treatment seeking being so distant from the actual levels of treatment seeking, but it is interesting to note that the idea of exposure therapy far outweighs these alternatives in terms of consumer preferences from a non-clinical sample.

Another study compared 14 different treatments in terms of the acceptability and preference of a non-clinical sample (Tarrier et al., 2006). The study gave undergraduate students a brief description of what the different types of treatment entailed, including known advantages and disadvantages, approximate duration, and methods of delivery. The rankings were as follows:

1. Cognitive therapy
2. Cognitive therapy with exposure
3. Imaginal exposure
4. Psychoeducation
5. In vivo exposure
6. Stress management
7. Group therapy
8. Family therapy
9. Guided imagery and rescripting

10. Psychodynamic psychotherapy
11. Virtual reality
12. Computer-based therapy
13. Eye movement desensitization
14. e-Therapy

From these data, we can determine that in general, people prefer individual treatments in which there is interaction with a mental health-care practitioner and do not seem to endorse the newer therapies or those involving technology (Tarrier et al., 2006). It is unknown whether the idea of the therapy itself or the information regarding the research basis of the treatment was more powerful in individuals' rankings; therefore, these data may look different with an increase in research surrounding the newer technologies. Additionally, the endorsement of these treatments does not imply a lack of discomfort. The discomfort rankings from most to least are as follows:

1. Imaginal exposure
2. In vivo exposure
3. Group therapy
4. Family therapy
5. Cognitive therapy with exposure
6. Virtual reality
7. Guided imagery and rescripting
8. Cognitive therapy
9. Psychodynamic therapy
10. EMDR
11. e-Therapy
12. Computer-based therapy
13. Stress management
14. Psychoeducation

Because we have seen from the previous data that expectations about treatment seeking from individuals who are not experiencing post-traumatic distress do not seem to be an accurate representation of behavior (Zoellner et al., 2003), it may be that the distress rankings could be more accurate in terms of behaviors than acceptability. There are no data regarding the treatment-seeking behaviors of these different modalities, but it is interesting to note that the lower steps on the stepped care model are generally lower in the distress rankings, which may provide insight into what keeps distressed, non-treatment seekers out of therapy. Generally, we have very little information regarding the preferences of treatment seekers or distressed non-treatment seekers, but this does give us some insight as to what people tend to prefer, which seems to be, above all else, that which is backed by data (Tarrier et al., 2006).

Assessment

The clinician-administered PTSD Scale for DSM-IV (CAPS) is generally considered to be the gold standard for assessment of PTSD (Blake et al., 1995; Vaishnavi et al., 2006; Weathers et al., 2001; Brewin, 2005). The CAPS is a structured clinical interview based on the DSM-IV criteria for PTSD. CAPS has great psychometric properties, including high inter-rater reliability (from 0.92 to 1.00), high test–retest reliability (from 0.77 to 0.96), and high internal consistency, with alphas for the three-symptom clusters ranging from 0.85–0.87 to 0.94 for the total test score (Hovents et al., 1994; Blake et al., 1995). However, it has been criticized in that it is particularly time consuming, up to an hour to administer (Bradley et al., 2005; IOM, 2006). Because of this, it is not ideal for all clinical situations (Vaishnavi et al., 2006). The structured clinical interview is a similar instrument both in its psychometric properties and in its time consumption (First et al., 1995). Several individuals have noted the need for a more parsimonious assessment and have found several assessments to meet this challenge (Brewin, 2005; Vaishnavi et al., 2006), as detailed below.

In one study, the authors looked at civilian PTSD self-report assessments with 30 items or fewer that had been validated against structured clinical interviews and found 13 measures meeting this criteria, listed in the table below:

Measure name		References
Impact event scale	IES	Horowitz et al. (1979)
PTSD checklist	PCL-C	Weathers et al. (1991)
Post-traumatic stress diagnostic scale	PDS	Foa et al. (1997)
Post-traumatic stress symptom scale	PSS-SR	Foa et al. (1993a)
Davidson trauma scale	DTS	Davidson et al. (1997)
Self-rating scale for post-traumatic stress disorder	SRS-PTSD	Carlier et al. (1998)
The startle, physiological arousal, anger, and numbness items from the Davidson trauma scale	SPAN	Meltzer-Brody et al. (1999)
Screen for post-traumatic stress symptoms	SPTSS	Carlson (1997)
Post-traumatic stress disorder questionnaire	PTSD-Q	Cross and McCanne (2001)
Penn Inventory for post-traumatic stress disorder	Penn	Hammarberg (1992)
Trauma-screening questionnaire	TSQ	Foa et al. (1993b) and Foa et al. (1997)
Disaster-related psychological screening test	DRPST	Chou et al. (2003)
Self-rating inventory for post-traumatic stress disorder	SRIP	Hovens et al. (2002)
Brief DSM PTSD	DSMPTSD-IV	Fullerton et al. (2000)

The author found that "the performance of some currently available instruments is near to their maximal potential effectiveness, and those instruments with fewer items, simpler response scales, and simpler scoring methods perform as well if not better than longer and more complex measures" (Brewin, 2005, p. 53). For the actual and opportunity costs of both the therapists and the clients, it would be ideal to identify screening instruments with the least amount of time and effort required with the most sensitivity and specificity for the given task. Brewin found that the IES and the TSQ fared well in sensitivity (IES 0.89; TSQ 0.76–0.86), specificity (IES 0.88–0.94; TSQ 0.93–0.97), positive predictive power (IES 0.67–0.89; TSQ 0.86–0.91), negative predictive power (IES 0.88–0.89; TSQ 0.92–0.93), and efficiency (IES 0.89–0.94; TSQ 0.92–0.97) and both had been validated on independent samples (Brewin, 2005). From this account these measures should be considered a lower stepped assessment for screening individuals seeking lower stepped treatment.

The IES is a 15-item self-report scale, which asks individuals to rate symptoms specific to intrusion and avoidance on a four-point scale. Originally, the cutoff score was determined to be 19 (Horowitz et al., 1979), although it was later found to have greater specificity (0.88–0.94) while still maintaining good sensitivity (0.89) when using a cutoff score of 35 (Wohlfarth et al., 2003).

The TSQ is a 10-item self-report measure based on Foa's PSS-SR (Foa et al., 1993a), but modified to require a forced choice of whether the individual has experienced each symptom at least twice in the past week, as opposed to the original version which gave more options. When the cutoff score of 6 is used, this measure has been found to have high sensitivity (0.76–0.86) and specificity (0.93–0.97) when compared to CAPS (sensitivity 0.84; specificity 0.95) (Brewin et al., 2002).

Additionally, because these assessments are self-report measures, it is feasible that they could adequately translate to self-help treatment or treatments with minimal therapist interaction. Several studies have shown that Web-based administration of assessments are as valid via computer administration and may actually increase reporting accuracy when compared to both pen-and-paper assessments and practitioner-administered assessments due to anonymity, especially in the case of questions dealing with stigmatizing issues such as drug use and sexual behavior (Alemi et al., 1994; Hasley, 1995; Johnson et al., 2001). While no studies have been conducted regarding automated assessments for PTSD, it may follow because of these results and the stigma-surrounding PTSD that computerized self-report assessments are likely at least as accurate—and possibly more so—than more traditional methods.

Vaishnavi and colleagues compared the short PTSD rating interview (SPRINT) to the CAPS, also in the hopes of finding an assessment that would minimize the time needed to obtain an accurate diagnosis of PTSD (Vaishnavi et al., 2006). In this study, it was found that the two measures correlated highly in nearly every symptom cluster other than the SPRINT scores referring to somatic symptoms and social functioning, which were measured against the total score. According to this chapter, the CAPS took an average of 19 min to administer, whereas the SPRINT took only 8.9 min (Vaishnavi et al., 2006). It should be noted that this administration time seems to be a low average when compared to other studies reporting administration time (Brewin, 2005). Therefore, the SPRINT may be considered in the lower steps of clinician-administered assessments, such as adjunctive or individual therapies.

The SPRINT is an 8-item clinical interview that assesses the core symptoms of PTSD, as well as some other mental health difficulties that are common with this disorder, including somatic malaise, stress vulnerability, and functional impairment. The test has been shown to have good test–retest reliability (ICC of 0.778, $p < 0.0001$), internal consistency (Cronbach's 0.77 at baseline, 0.88 at endpoint), convergent validity ($p < 0.0001$ against Davidson Trauma Scale, Stress Vulnerability Scale, and Sheehan Disability Scale), and discriminate validity ($r = 0.10$ against social support) (Connor and Davidson, 2001).

While it is essential within a stepped care model to explore less invasive and costly assessments, with such high correlations to the best assessment available, it may be that these parsimonious measures may be ideal for assessing in any or all circumstances (Brewin, 2005).

Additionally, the majority of assessments assume that a diagnosis is either present or not and do not account for sub-clinical presentations. One benefit of the stepped care model is that individuals who may not be diagnosable but are suffering in some way (for example, if only one domain of diagnosis is present but is extreme, such as experiencing through nightmares, but not avoiding or experiencing hyperarousal) may still seek treatment and may do so in a way that is not pathologizing, by seeking help on a lower step in the model. Therefore, assessments in this model may be more functional, simply asking face-valid questions about what the individual may want to work on.

Watchful Waiting

While there have been several attempts at preventing the development of PTSD after the experience of a trauma, there has been little evidence to suggest that these interventions are useful, and in fact several studies have shown that these interventions may be iatrogenic. As Litz stated in 2008, "there is consensus within the academic community that any one-size-fits-all intervention for all who are exposed to trauma is not only infeasible, but for most, unnecessary, or for others, too early and intrusive, and too little (Litz, 2008, p. 503)."

PTSD is a difficult disorder in the sense of engaging in watchful waiting, because the trigger is clear, which may make people want to react and prevent possible impending pathology. As MacFarlane wrote in 1989, "There is always the danger after a disaster for mental health workers to view the victims as being psychologically damaged in a way that requires intervention. In the vast majority this is not the case (MacFarlane, 1989)."

However, experiencing difficultly after a traumatic event is normative. In the first 48 h after experiencing a trauma, the vast majority of individuals will experience post-traumatic stress symptoms and these symptoms should seem as normal; the majority of these individuals (66%; Kessler et al., 1995) have spontaneous remission of their symptoms over time. Several standards of care recommend that no treatments be offered within 2 weeks of the trauma and some studies suggest even longer (Ehlers et al., 2003). During these first weeks post-trauma, it is recommended that individuals simply wait to see if symptoms improve. As Litz noted in 2008, "there is more agreement about what not to do than what to do (Litz, 2008, p. 503)." In the event that PTSD symptoms are present at least 2 weeks after the trauma, and preferably a month or more, then it may be appropriate for that individual to seek a higher level in the stepped care model; however, as the majority of research in this area is cross-sectional, it is unclear what the natural trajectory of post-traumatic distress would be. More research would be needed to determine the optimal time period to linger in watchful waiting before seeking help (Litz, 2008).

Early Interventions

In the context of immediate trauma, or the first few hours or days after experiencing a trauma, several attempts have been made at preventing the development of PTSD. Psychological debriefing is one attempt at preventing PTSD symptoms in traumatized groups, but in 11 studies with adequate control, researchers have found that at best these treatments do not actually prevent symptoms. At worse, they may pathologize individuals who have been traumatized, which may actually increase the risk of developing PTSD symptoms (Gist and Devilly, 2002; Emmerik and Kamphuis, 2002). It is not recommended that such debriefings be offered, but instead that individuals engage in a watchful waiting process. Additionally, several psychopharmacological interventions have been tested in the prevention of PTSD symptoms and neither performed better than placebo (Forbes et al., 2007; Litz, 2008).

Psychological first aid is another intervention used immediately post-trauma. This intervention has not been tested to date, but was created on an empirical basis on the existing literature, and takes into account the risk and resilience following a trauma (Vernberg et al., 2008). Additionally, the intervention was created to be "applicable and practical in field settings," and was designed to be used in various settings in which a disaster has occurred. The intervention is based on five basic principles that have received "broad empirical support for facilitating positive adaptation following trauma" (Vernberg et al., 2008, p. 382) such as

1. Promoting sense of safety
2. Promoting calming
3. Promoting sense of self- and community efficacy
4. Promoting connectedness
5. Instilling hope
   (Hobfoll et al., 2007)

Because of its evidence-based approach, this intervention is recommended by several practice guidelines in the immediate aftermath of disasters (Litz, 2008; NIMH,

2002). The intervention should be provided by mental health practitioners and is currently delivered on the level of the individual. However, with the data outstanding, it is yet to be seen how effective this hopeful early intervention will prove.

In the acute-phase post-trauma, several empirically validated options are available. Self-monitoring and repeated assessment with no further intervention have been shown to be an effective treatment alone for a small amount of individuals in the late stages of acute stress or the early stages of acute PTSD (Ehlers et al., 2003; Foa et al., 2006). Both cognitive therapy and cognitive behavioral therapy have been shown to be effective treatments at this stage (Ehlers et al., 2003; Foa et al., 2006). Therefore, it is at this point in the time line for individuals who are experiencing post-trauma distress that individuals should engage in self-monitoring of these symptoms for a matter of several weeks before moving to another step.

Psychoeducation

Psychoeducation is an often used portion of treatment for post-traumatic stress disorder. Traditionally, psychoeducation regarding what trauma symptoms might look like and what to expect have been integrated into other steps in the stepped care model; however, psychoeducation may be used alone for individuals either in early stages after the trauma or with less severe post-traumatic distress.

There is little evidence that psychoeducation in and of itself is helpful in the treatment of post-traumatic distress. As Wesley and colleagues said in 2008, "Perhaps it could be assumed that psychoeducation, like education in general, is so obviously a 'good thing' that it requires no evidence." There is a small amount of literature supporting psychoeducation in theory, or as integrated into other treatments, but very little testing the effectiveness of psychoeducation alone. This may be due to the lack of conceptualizing treatment on a stepped care continuum that contributes to the lack of having more or stronger evidence.

The small literature on this intervention is mixed, which may seem counterintuitive. However, psychoeducation is a core component both of critical incident stress debriefing and psychological first aid; the first of course has been found to be iatrogenic, while the second has not been experimentally tested, as stated earlier, but is widely regarded as having utility (Litz, 2008; NIMH, 2002). Only one trial directly testing psychoeducation on adults was found (Turpin et al., 2005) and it concluded that psychoeducation within 1–2 weeks post-trauma provided worse outcomes. On the other hand, school-based psychoeducation for children exposed to war was found to be an effective tier in reducing PTSD symptoms (Layne et al., 2008).

Psychoeducation has also been tested several times as the control group for other therapies, consistently showing "modest therapy gains" (Wessely et al., 2008), but not comparing positively to any of the interventions against which it was tested.

It is theorized that people who have received psychoeducation regarding what they might expect in coping with the trauma may find these reactions to be "less disturbing," and may feel normalized by the experiences instead of pathologized (Wessely et al., 2008, p. 288). On the other hand, it has been theorized that by telling individuals what symptoms they may experience, it may actually increase their experience of such symptoms by increasing awareness of the possibility (Howland et al., 1990). Additionally, Wesley and colleagues noted in 2008 that it might be fragilizing the public to believe that people generally need to be informed of normative reactions to traumatic events. This belief may be in line with why the treatment for children was effective, in that they may not yet have learned to normalize these reactions, whereas adult might have (Layne et al., 2008; Wessely et al., 2008).

Another important benefit of psychoeducation is that it may improve treatment seeking. One study has shown that brief psychoeducation regarding what therapy might look like increased attitudes toward treatment seeking (Gonzalez et al., 2002). As psychological first aid posits, it may be essential to be non-directive when providing such information, and as many standards point out, it may be best to engage in at least 1 month of watchful waiting before engaging in psychoeducation. Although this suggestion has not been empirically tested, it may have been the difference leading to moderate gains when compared to other treatments for PTSD (NICE, 2007; Wessely et al., 2008).

Stress inoculation training is a specific form of intervention based on psychoeducation and has shown generally positive results in preventing PTSD when provided before the trauma occurs; however, this lacks the generalizability to the majority of types of trauma an individual may experience.

Bibliotherapy

While bibliotherapy seems to be an effective treatment for depression and many anxiety disorders (Gould et al., 1993; Scogin et al., 1990; den Boer et al., 2004; Mains and Scogin, 2003), there does not appear to be any evidence that bibliotherapy as a stand-alone treatment is effective for the treatment of post-traumatic stress symptoms.

Understanding Your Reactions to Trauma: A Booklet for Survivors of Trauma and Their Families, a workbook by Claudia Herbert, was tested as an early intervention in the prevention of PTSD symptoms. Individuals in the bibliotherapy group were found to have worse outcomes on several measures than the repeated assessment group, including the PDS self-report on post-traumatic distress, the CAPS assessments of frequency and intensity of PTSD symptoms, the Beck Anxiety Inventory, the Beck Depression Inventory, and self-report of disability (Ehlers et al., 2003). However, this may have been a timing effect in attempting to treat symptoms at the acute phase; more research would be needed to determine whether this or another form of bibliotherapy may be helpful in the treatment of post-traumatic distress during the recommended treatment phase at least 1 month after the trauma (Forbes et al., 2007; NICE, 2007).

Although there are many books on coping with trauma, there is not much in the way of scientific literature testing the efficacy of these books as bibliotherapy. One workbook that does not appear to have been tested, called *Reclaiming Your Life from a Traumatic Experience* (Rothbaum et al., 2007) was developed as an adjunctive to individual therapy and is based on empirically tested treatments. Because this book is not intended to be a stand-alone treatment, it will be discussed further in the dissemination agenda section.

Computer-Based Interventions

Computer-based interventions (CBI, also known as Internet-based interventions, computer-based cognitive behavioral therapy, or e-health) are an up and coming step in the stepped care model for many disorders. In treating anxiety and depression, effect sizes from several interventions are comparable to more traditional individual psychotherapy (Amstadter et al., 2009). It is important to note that CBIs are more than just bibliotherapy on the Web, but are instead interventions that are tailored to the individual, much like individual services.

There have been several experimental studies testing the effects of CBIs on post-traumatic distress. These treatments may be conceptualized as falling on different steps of the stepped care model, in that they involve varying levels of cost, intrusion, and anonymity.

Hirai and Clum conducted a brief CBI which included psychoeducation, several types of relaxation training, cognitive restructuring, and exposure treatment through writing about the experience (Hirai and Clum, 2005). The treatment consists of eight modules, organized to be one weekly session each. The therapist contact was made only when participants needed prompting to return to the site or when clients needed technical assistance, but instructions and all active ingredients of therapy were only delivered through the site.

The sample included individuals suffering distress due to several types of trauma, including car accidents, interpersonal violence, eyewitness, life-threatening disease, and losses due to suicide or murder. While the sample size was rather small, the intervention proved to have significant gains when controlled to wait-list on measures including depression (61% of the Internet intervention reached clinical significance vs. 14% of the wait-list on the Beck Depression Inventory), anxiety (54% vs. 7% on the State Trait Anxiety Inventory), and trauma distress (69% vs. 27% on trauma avoidance on the Impact of Event Scale Revised, and 54% vs. 0% on the Active Coping with Trauma Scale). The intervention was a stand-alone intervention that could be done completely on the computer, which may prove to increase treatment seeking for individuals high in stigma (Hirai and Clum, 2005). The intervention is not currently available to the public.

Litz and colleagues produced another brief CBT CBI, with similar ingredients to the Hirai and Clum intervention, and also including Stress Inoculation Training. The intervention called DE-STRESS (delivery of self-training and education for stressful situations) was slightly different though, in that it was therapist assisted. Individuals using this treatment were first assessed face-to-face for a 2-h intake before proceeding to the Web-based treatment. The treatment was intended to be an 8-week program, with daily logins (or several times daily when the client chose to do so). Litz and colleagues reported that clients did not end up logging in daily as would be ideal, they did were "engaged sufficiently over time and absorbing the bulk of the intervention." The program also included therapist monitoring throughout and therapists were actually monitored immediately and automatically notified in the event that the client endorsed severe depression (Litz et al., 2004, 2007).

The Litz sample was also small, as the trial was intended to be a proof-of-concept trial, and included those exposed to the September 11 Pentagon attack and service members in the Iraq war. The CBI was tested against supportive counseling and was found to be more effective in reducing PTSD symptom severity, avoidance, hyperarousal symptoms, and depression (Litz et al., 2007). The CBI group showed a higher percentage of clinically significant change and scored lower on depression ($t = 2.15, \mathrm{df} = 16, p < 0.05$), anxiety ($t = 2.06, \mathrm{df} = 16, p = 0.06$), and PTSD symptoms ($t = 2.02, \mathrm{df} = 16, p = 0.06$). The study is currently being run in several military sites, but is not yet available to the general public.

Ruggerio and his colleagues developed what might be seen as a more functional CBI for individuals who are experiencing multiple types of distress as a result of trauma. The Web site provided different modules for different problems associated with trauma, including sleep hygiene, substance abuse, generalized anxiety, smoking cessation, and of course a PTSD module. The proof-of-concept small trial showed the site to be feasible as an overall treatment package for individuals suffering from post-traumatic distress in terms of participant satisfaction, engagement, and pre/post-knowledge about the various disorders targeted. No data were discussed in this proof-of-concept trial regarding pre/post-assessments of functioning or symptoms. The intervention is not available to the public at this time (Ruggiero et al., 2006).

Lange and colleagues developed and tested a CBI as an adjunctive therapy to be used alongside individual therapy. The site included online assessments which were automated for inclusion criteria and instant feedback to clients, information about the process and procedure, informational pages, and writing exposure assignments to be done online. The treatment was intended to be completed in a 5-week period. The writing exposure assignments were reviewed by therapists during individual treatment and feedback and instruction were provided (Lange et al., 2003). Two studies on different populations (college and community samples) were found to have large effect sizes compared to a wait-list control and the community sample showed both statistically and clinically significant changes in all categories compared to wait-list (45% of the Interapy program reached clinical significance vs. 8% in the Impact of Events Scale of intrusions, 50% vs. 80% in IES of avoidance; in the SCL-90, clinical significance for depression was 55% vs. 5%; anxiety was 52% vs. 0%; somatization was 52% vs. 5%; and sleeping problems was 21% vs. 5%). The site is available to the public at www.interapy.nl, but is written in Dutch.

Individual Therapy

While individual therapy is a moderately high step in the stepped care model, it is by far the most widely used and studied step in the treatment of PTSD, as with the treatment of most other disorders. For individual treatment of PTSD, there is ample research to suggest that exposure therapy is the gold standard for treating PTSD (Foa et al., 2008; Forbes et al., 2007; IOM, 2006; NICE, 2007). Eye Movement Rapid Desensitization (EMDR) has also proven effective, especially when combined with in vivo exposure (Forbes et al., 2007; Rothbaum et al., 2005). Several modifications to these treatments, including the integration of dialectical behavior therapy-based techniques, stress inoculation, and similar skills training, are thought to be useful in treating real-life samples that may have comorbid disorders, as is so common with traumatized individuals (Becker and Zayfert, 2001; Trappler and Newville, 2007; Wagner and Linehan, 2006; Wagner et al., 2007; IOM 2006).

EMDR has often been criticized as having the same active ingredient as exposure therapy, and that it may not in fact be the eye movements acting as mediators, but instead the exposure to the stimuli (Perkins and Rouanzoin, 2002; Rogers and Silver, 2002). If assuming this criticism to be accurate and viewing this therapy in terms of a stepped care model, it may be useful to think about EMDR as a "packaging" for consumer preference. Whereas Terrier and colleagues found that EMDR was significantly lower in consumer acceptability and preference (Tarrier et al., 2006), it is important to remember that consumer preferences are at the level of the individual, and although most people would prefer direct exposure, there may be some who would find direct exposure unacceptable but EMDR preferable.

Because exposure therapy and EMDR are so widely researched elsewhere, it is outside the scope of this chapter to go into further detail about the treatments. Please see Foa et al. (2008) for further reading.

Virtual Reality

It does not appear that virtual reality has previously been conceptualized as a step in the stepped care model, but in fact this type of therapy is a clear next step in the event that imaginal exposure has failed. Some individuals may not have strong enough imaginations to engage in imaginal exposure with enough detail to be effective, and additionally because PTSD is marked by avoidance of stimuli reminding the individual of the trauma, this might be a barrier in the implementation of imaginal exposure for some (Difede and Hoffman, 2002; Jaycox et al., 1998; Rizzo et al., 2009). Several studies have shown that individuals who were left untreated after trying imaginal exposure were then successfully treated through virtual reality exposure therapy (VRET, (Difede and Hoffman, 2002; Rothbaum et al., 2001).

Virtual reality (VR) is a technology-based intervention in which individuals are immersed within a virtual environment structured to be that which they are avoiding; in the case of PTSD, the environment of the trauma. Sometimes other senses are incorporated as well, including scent-delivery technology and the use of inert guns as joysticks or vibrating controllers to emulate olfactory and tactile senses as well as the already included audiovisual stimuli. Because the startup costs can be high for this type of therapy, the treatments are generally constrained to situations that may be useful to many people. Most virtual reality therapies have therefore simulated the environment of wars including Vietnam and Iraq and have been used to treat veterans of these wars (Rizzo et al., 2009; Rothbaum et al., 2001).

When a client engages in virtual reality therapy, they generally put on a virtual reality helmet with speakers built in and navigate their environment with a joystick. A therapist walks the client through the scenario as one would thorough an imaginal exposure exercise, but also has control over the environment. The clinician has an interface through a separate monitor that will allow them to add different triggers into the environment as suitable.

As Rizzo and colleagues stated in 2007, the addition of this new medium may also increase treatment seeking, even to the high-need spectrum of those with post-traumatic distress. As he stated, "The current generation of young military personnel, having grown up with digital gaming technology, may actually be more attracted to and comfortable with participation in a VR application approach as an alternative to what is viewed as traditional 'talk therapy'" (Rizzo et al., 2009, p. 22). Additionally several studies show efficacy and effectiveness data in using virtual reality exposure therapy (VRE) for several other anxiety disorders that regularly find success with exposure therapy, including panic disorder and specific phobia with effect sizes ranging from 0.92 to 1.79 according to a meta-analysis by Parsons and Rizzo; however, PTSD data so far tends to be smaller in scale (Botella et al., 2007; Emmelkamp, 2005; Parsons and Rizzo, 2008; Rizzo et al., 2007).

A case study found that virtual reality was helpful in reducing PTSD symptoms based on significantly lower CAPS scores for Vietnam veterans suffering from the disorder. Although the original sample size was a mere eight, each one showed a reduction in symptoms (ranging from 15 to 65%; Rothbaum et al., 1999). A follow-up study with 16 subjects also proved significant reduction in symptoms, again showing no iatrogenic effects for any subjects (Rothbaum et al., 2001).

VRE has also been developed for civilians from the events of 9/11, showing both a powerful change in depression (83% reduction) and PTSD symptoms (90% reduction) as a proof-of-concept trial and a large effect size (1.54) against a wait-list control (Difede and Hoffman, 2002; Difede et al., 2007). Effects were maintained at 6-month follow-up. Additionally, this study presented interesting data in that 5 of the 13 participants in the RCT had previously not responded to imaginal exposure in the past, providing preliminary evidence for the importance of including virtual reality in a stepped care model where individual therapy has previously failed (Difede et al., 2007).

Another major project in the VRE for PTSD literature is Virtual Iraq. This project was designed to evaluate the value of treatment of VRE for soldiers returning from Iraq with PTSD, and specifically to target a population with low treatment-seeking tendencies, with the idea that a generation raised on technology would feel more comfortable seeking therapy when it was more technologically based. This platform has run a handful of studies, all with promising results (Gerardi et al., 2008; Reger and Gahm, 2008; Mclay et al., under review; Rizzo et al., 2009; Yeh et al., 2009). The most impressive data came from a sample of 20 individuals, 16 of whom no longer met criteria after completing VRE treatment (Rizzo et al., 2009).

Medication

There is minimal evidence to suggest the use of drug treatment in minimizing post-traumatic distress. Many studies have been done and the few that found drugs to be more effective than placebo have low effect sizes. These effects are also offset by side effects of psychopharmacological treatments. The United States Institute of Medicine has stated that medication should not be considered as an evidence-based treatment for PTSD and the Australian and the UK standards of care both state that it should be the last option considered (Forbes et al., 2007; IOM, 2006; NICE, 2007). In the event that psychopharmacology must be implemented, these standards suggest using SSRIs (such as paroxetine and venlafaxine), and stepping down off the medication after 1 year in the event that the medication is successful (Forbes et al., 2007; NICE, 2007). According to the American Psychological Association, SSRIs are the only medications with evidence allowing the organization to "recommend with substantial clinical confidence" (especially in the case of females who are suffering from PTSD due to sexual assault), while TCAs and MAOIs were recommended with moderate confidence, and benzodiazepines, anticonvulsants, antipsychotics, and adrenergic inhibitors were under the "may be recommended" category and were recommended to be used only for symptoms such as improving sleep, but not as an entire treatment for PTSD (APA, 2004).

Inpatient Treatment

In general, it is rare that individuals with PTSD need or are given inpatient treatments. However, there is a subset of trauma survivors with PTSD symptoms that far exceed the traditional presentation of PTSD distress. This presentation has been titled Disorder of Extreme Stress Not Otherwise Specified (DESNOS) or complex PTSD and it is not uncommon for clients with this presentation to fail forward into inpatient treatment centers (Trappler and Newville, 2007).

Additionally, comorbidities with PTSD tend to be the rule instead of the exception. Some comorbidities, such as severe depression and borderline personality disorder, may necessitate the use of inpatient treatment (Ruggiero et al., 2006; Trappler and Newville, 2007). In fact, it has been considered whether BPD is actually just complicated PTSD, due to the similar symptoms and the high likelihood that individuals with BPD also suffer from PTSD (Driessen et al., 2002).

In the cases of complex PTSD and borderline personality disorder, individuals who suffer severe traumatic abuse early in their development may benefit from skills training, specifically DBT skills including emotion regulation, distress tolerance, interpersonal effectiveness, and mindfulness (Wagner and Linehan, 2006; Wagner et al., 2007), or Skill Training in Affect Regulation (STAIR), which also focuses on emotion regulation and mindfulness skills (Trappler and Newville, 2007). While these interventions do not have substantial evidence, several case studies substantiate the utility of DBT (Wagner et al., 2007), and STAIR showed positive results compared to supportive therapy in a small randomized controlled trial in an inpatient facility (Trappler and Newville, 2007).

Triage Agenda

When considering triage for an individual seeking treatment for trauma-related distress, one may want to consider the severity of symptoms, timing, cost barriers (including insurance coverage), physical barriers (including time, transportation, living in a rural area), and consumer preference.

In the event that no other barriers exist for a client, it would be ideal to determine treatment based on treatment severity. In this case, it might be beneficial to determine how distressed an individual is and how much the distress is impairing the rest of their life, and choose the lowest step likely to benefit that individual, allowing the fail-forward aspect of stepped care to allow the client to move upward when needed. More research is needed to determine the best way to assess severity and to triage based on severity with an empirical basis.

Timing may be an important step in determining appropriate care. For example, individuals experiencing post-trauma distress within hours or days of the trauma are within the normative range and should clearly be triaged to the watchful waiting condition. While psychological first aid looks like a promising early intervention, currently the data are not there to triage individuals to this intervention in the early stages after trauma. After 1 month, low steps in the model, including self-monitoring and e-health, may be all that is needed to halt the progress of symptoms. Three months or more after the trauma, it may be appropriate to refer to the treatment severity triage agenda.

Cost and physical barriers may limit an individual's access to services to treatments like psychoeducation, bibliotherapy, and e-health. Until further research is produced regarding the efficacy of the first two, e-health should be the treatment of choice to accommodate these barriers.

More data are needed regarding consumer preferences in most steps in the model. While it appears that non-clinical individuals tend to endorse treatments with contact with therapists more highly, these treatments are also ranked as more distressing, so it is unclear what preferences would actually go into making decisions to seek treatment (Tarrier et al., 2006). More information is needed regarding treatment preferences in general, and in triage for specific patients, individual preferences should be used to assess the best placement for that individual.

Research Agenda

While ample research has been done on individual therapy for PTSD and adequate research has been done on e-health interventions and virtual reality, the rest of the stepped care model needs significantly more information.

As was mentioned in the Triage Agenda section, the model is desperate for clear guidelines regarding timing-related triage issues. When is it too early to start screening for distress, to start treatment, and of what kind? Is there a trajectory of post-traumatic distress that could map on to the stepped care model?

Additionally, triage would be well met by measures better defining severity. Currently, most measures have been tested in terms of PTSD as a binary diagnosis—either you have it or you do not. However, research shows that PTSD exists on a continuum (Ruscio et al., 2002; Palm et al., 2009) and the nuances of the stepped care model allow for individuals with varying levels of distress and symptoms to receive treatment matched in this way. More research would be needed to assess for what severity measured in what way would best be treated by what step.

Consumer preferences are also lacking in terms of opinions of treatment seekers, or how that maps on to behaviors, and should be examined to determine both the development of new treatments and the marketing of current and new treatments to consumers.

Lastly, more information needs to be obtained regarding how the important differences between types of trauma may inform triage into the stepped care system. For example, whereas individual therapy can account for different types of therapy and adjust accordingly, there may be forms of psychoeducation that would be more effective for individuals who have survived a physical injury, such as a car accident, vs. those who have experienced personal violence, such as a rape (Litz, 2008).

Dissemination Agenda

While there are many questions remaining in how to best implement the stepped care model for post-traumatic distress, it appears that even when important research questions are answered, they might not make their way to the distressed clients in need of successful treatment. As stated previously, it has been well researched that exposure is the gold standard for the treatment of PTSD. This treatment has been around for decades, but has not yet made its way into many practices around the United States (Becker et al., 2004).

In a survey of 852 licensed psychologists in several locations in the United States, only 17% of those surveyed reported ever using exposure to treat PTSD (Becker et al., 2004). A lack of training was the most cited barrier to providing this treatment, but it appears that training does not actually account for the whole problem. Of those both trained in exposure, and those who are experienced PTSD therapists, fewer than half of these therapists used exposure more than 50% of the time and around 33% of these therapists reported not using exposure at all (Becker et al., 2004). Further, in one e-health study for generally distress (The Therapeutic Learning Program, Gould 1989), those in the computer group showed similar scores to those in the individual treatment group in all measures except the therapist subjective rating of patient functioning, which the study stated "was due in part to a pretreatment difference in favor of individual therapy versus TLP" (Jacobs et al., 2001, p. 94).

This proves the importance of dissemination in the expansion of this treatment to a stepped care model. Further work needs to be done on getting individuals' treatments that are likely to work, both from the side of increasing treatment seeking from individuals and from the side of increasing the use of evidence-based practice and evidence-based triage. From the Becker Survey, it is obvious that training is not enough. Quality improvement, accountability, and consumer preferences (which in a perfect world would be guided by consumer information) need to provide a contingency management plan on providing treatments that are likely to work, so that individuals may start to get the help that they need. In developing future treatments, disseminability ease and modes should be considered. For example, the book *Reclaiming Your Life From a Traumatic Experience* by Barbara Rothbaum and colleagues provides practitioners with the opportunity to learn exposure therapy through an adjunctive workbook that can be done with clients and guides practitioners through the empirically supported treatment week-by-week. Again, while training is not a sufficient step in dissemination, it is a necessary one; this and issues of natural contingencies should be considered when developing new treatments.

References

Alemi F, Stephens R, Parran T, Llorens S, Bhatt P, Ghadiri A, et al. Automated monitoring of outcomes: application to treatment of drug abuse. Med Decis Making. 1994;14(2):180–7. doi:10.1177/0272989X9401400211.

Amstadter AB, Broman-Fulks J, Zinzow H, Ruggiero KJ, Cercone J. Internet-based interventions for traumatic stress-related mental health problems: a review and suggestion for future research. Clin Psychol Rev. 2009. doi:10.1016/j.cpr.2009.04.001.

Becker CB, Zayfert C. Integrating DBT-based techniques and concepts to facilitate exposure treatment for PTSD. Cogn Behav Pract. 2001;8(2):107–22. doi:10.1016/S1077-7229(01)80017-1.

Becker CB, Zayfert C, Anderson E. A survey of psychologists' attitudes towards and utilization of exposure therapy for PTSD. Behav Res Ther. 2004;42(3):277–92. doi:10.1016/S0005-7967(03)00138-4.

Blake DD, Weathers FW, Nagy LM, Kaloupek DG, Gusman FD, Charney D S, et al. The development of a clinician-administered PTSD scale. J Trauma Stress. 1995;8(1):75–90.

Botella C, García-Palacios A, Villa H, Baños R, Quero S, Alcañiz M, et al. Virtual reality exposure in the treatment of panic disorder and agoraphobia: a controlled study. Clin Psychol Psychother. 2007;14(3):164–75.

Bradley R, Russ E, Dutra L, Westen D. A multidimensional meta-analysis of psychotherapy for PTSD. Am J Psychiatry. 2005;162(2):214–27.

Brewin CR, Rose S, Andrews B, Green J, Tata P, McEvedy C, et al. Brief screening instrument for post-traumatic stress disorder. Br J Psychiatry. 2002;181(2):158–62. doi:10.1192/bjp.181.2.158.

Brewin CR. Systematic review of screening instruments for adults at risk of PTSD. J Traum Stress. 2005;18(1):53–62. doi:10.1002/jts.20007.

Burstein A. Treatment noncompliance in patients with posttraumatic stress disorder. Psychosomatics. 1986;27:37–40.

Carlier I, Lamberts R, Van Uchelen A, Gersons B. Clinical utility of a brief diagnostic test for posttraumatic stress disorder. Psychosom Med. 1998;60(1):42–7.

Carlson EB. Trauma assessments: a clinician's guide. 1st ed. New York: The Guilford Press; 1997.

Chou FH, Su TT, Ou-Yang W, Chien I, Lu M, Chou P. Establishment of a disaster-related psychological screening test. Aust N Z J Psychiatry. 2003;37(1):97–103.

Connor KM, Davidson JR. SPRINT: a brief global assessment of post-traumatic stress disorder. Int Clin Psychopharmacol. 2001;16(5):279–84.

Cross MR, McCanne TR. Validation of a self-report measure of posttraumatic stress disorder in a sample of college-age women. J Traum Stress. 2001;14(1):135–47. doi:10.1023/A:1007843800664.

Davidson JRT, Book SW, Colket JT, Tupler LA, Roth S, David D, et al. Assessment of a new self-rating scale for post-traumatic stress disorder. Psychol Med. 1997;27(01):153–60.

den Boer PCAM, Wiersma D, Van Den Bosch RJ. Why is self-help neglected in the treatment of emotional disorders? A meta-analysis. Psychological Medicine: A Journal of Research in Psychiatry and the Allied Sciences. 2004;34(6):959–71.

Difede J, Hoffman HG. Virtual reality exposure therapy for world trade center post-traumatic stress disorder: a case report. CyberPsychol. Behav. 2002;5(6):529–35.

Difede J, Cukor J, Jayasinghe N, Patt I, Jedel S, Spielman L, et al. Virtual reality exposure therapy for the treatment of posttraumatic stress disorder following September 11, 2001. J Clin Psychiatry. 2007;68(11):1639–47.

Driessen M, Beblo T, Reddemann L, Rau H, Lange W, Silva A, et al. [Is the borderline personality disorder a complex post-traumatic stress disorder?—The state of research]. Der Nervenarzt. 2002;73(9):820–9. doi:10.1007/s00115-002-1296-1.

Ehlers A, Clark DM, Hackmann A, McManus F, Fennell M, Herbert C, et al. A randomized controlled trial of cognitive therapy, a self-help booklet, and repeated assessments as early interventions for posttraumatic stress disorder. Arch Gen Psychiatry. 2003;60(10):1024–32. doi:10.1001/archpsyc.60.10.1024.

Emmelkamp PMG, Krijn M, Hulsbosch AM, de Vries S, Schuemie MJ, van der Mast CAPG. Virtual reality treatment versus exposure in vivo: a comparative evaluation in acrophobia. Behav Res Ther. 2002;40:509–11, 516.

Emmelkamp PM. Technological innovations in clinical assessment and psychotherapy. Psychotherapy and Psychosomatics. 2005;74(6):336–43.

Emmerik A, Kamphuis J. Single session debriefing after psychological trauma: a meta analysis. Lancet. 2002;360:736–41.

First M, Spitzer RL, Gibbon M, Williams JB. Structured clinical Interview for DSM-IV axis i disorders. New York: New York State Psychiatric Institute; 1995.

Foa EB, Cashman L, Jaycox L, Perry K. The validation of a self-report measure of post-traumatic stress disorder: the posttraumatic diagnostic scale. Psychol Assessment. 1997;9: 445–51.

Foa EB, Zoellner LA, Feeny NC. An evaluation of three brief programs for facilitating recovery after assault. J Trauma Stress. 2006;19(1):29–43. doi:10.1002/jts.20096.

Foa EB, Keane TM, Friedman MJ, Cohen JA. Effective Treatments for PTSD, Second Edition: practice guidelines from the international society for traumatic stress studies. 2nd ed. The Guilford Press.

Foa EB, Riggs DS, Dancu CV, Rothbaum BO. Reliability and validity of a brief instrument for assessing post-traumatic stress disorder. J Trauma Stress. 1993a;6(4):459–73. doi:10.1007/BF00974317.

Foa EB, Riggs DS, Dancu CV, Rothbaum BO. Reliability and validity of a brief instrument for assessing post-traumatic stress disorder. J Trauma Stress. 1993b;6(4):459–73. doi:10.1007/BF00974317.

Forbes D, Creamer M, Phelps A, Bryant R, McFarlane A, Devilly GJ, et al. The Australian guidelines for the treatment of adults with acute stress disorder and posttraumatic stress disorder. Aust N Z J Psychiatry. 2007;41(8):637–48.

Fullerton CS, Ursano RJ, Epstein RS, Crowley B, Vance KL, Craig KJ. Measurement of posttraumatic stress disorder in community samples. Nord J Psychiatry. 2000;54:5–12.

Gist R, Devilly GJ. Post-trauma debriefing: the road too frequently travelled. Lancet. 2002;360(9335):741–2. doi:10.1016/S0140-6736(02)09947-6.

Gonzalez JM, Tinsley HEA, Kreuder KR. Effects of psychoeducational interventions on opinions of mental illness, attitudes toward help seeking, and expectations about psychotherapy in college students. J Coll Student Dev. 2002;43(1):51–63.

Gould RA, Clum GA, Shapiro D. The use of bibliotherapy in the treatment of panic: A preliminary investigation. Behavior Therapy. 1993;24(2):241–52.

Hammarberg M. Penn inventory for posttraumatic stress disorder: psychometric properties. Psychol Assessment. 1992;4:67–76.

Hasley S. A comparison of computer-based and personal interviews for the gynecologic history update. Obstet Gynecol. 1995;85(4):494–8. doi:10.1016/0029-7844(95)00012-G.

Hembree EA, Foa EB, Dorfan NM, Street GP, Kowalski J, Tu X. Do patients drop out prematurely from exposure therapy for PTSD? J Trauma Stress. 2003;16(6):555–62. doi:10.1023/B:JOTS.0000004078.93012.7d.

Hirai M, Clum GA. An Internet-based self-change program for traumatic event related fear, distress, and maladaptive coping. J Trauma Stress. 2005;18(6):631–6. doi:10.1002/jts.20071.

Hobfoll SE, Watson P, Bell CC, Bryant RA, Brymer MJ, Friedman MJ, et al. Five essential elements of immediate and mid-term mass trauma intervention: empirical evidence. Psychiatry. 2007;70(4):283–315; discussion 316–69. doi:10.1521/psyc.2007.70.4.283.

Horowitz M, Wilner N, Alvarez W. Impact of event scale: a measure of subjective stress. Psychosom Med. 1979;41(3):209–18.

Hovens JE, Bramsen I, van der Ploeg HM. Self-rating inventory for posttraumatic stress disorder: review of the psychometric properties of a new brief Dutch screening instrument. Percept Mot Skills. 2002;94(3 Pt 1):996–1008.

Hovens JEJM, Van der Ploeg HM, Bramsen I, Klaarenbeek MTA, Schreuder BJN, Rivero VV. The development of the self-rating inventory for posttraumatic stress disorder. Acta Psychiatr Scand. 1994;90:172–83.

Howland JS, Baker MG, Poe T. Does patient education cause side effects? A controlled trial. J Fam Pract. 1990;31(1):62–4.

IOM. Posttraumatic stress disorer: diagnosis and assessment. Washington, DC: Institute of Medicine; 2006. p. 87.

Jacobs MK, Christensen A, Snibbe JR, Dolezal-Wood S, Huber A, Polterok A. (2001). A comparison of computer-based versus traditional individual psychotherapy. Prof Psychol-Res Pract. 2001;32(1):92–6.

Jaycox LH, Foa EB, Morral AR. Influence of emotional engagement and habituation on exposure therapy for PTSD. J Consult Clin Psychol. 1998;66(1):185–92.

Johnson AM, Copas AJ, Erens B, Mandalia S, Fenton K, Korovessis C, et al. Effect of computer-assisted self-interviews on reporting of sexual HIV risk behaviours in a general population sample: a methodological experiment. AIDS (London, England). 2001;15(1):111–15.

Kessler RC, Sonnega A, Bromet E, Hughes M, Nelson CB. Posttraumatic stress disorder in the national comorbidity survey. Arch Gen Psychiatry. 1995;52(12):1048–60.

Lange A, Rietdijk D, Hudcovicova M, van de Ven J, Schrieken B, Emmelkamp PMG. Interapy: a controlled randomized trial of the standardized treatment of posttraumatic stress through the internet. J Consult Clin Psychol. 2003;71(5):901–9. doi:10.1037/0022-006X.71.5.901.

Layne CM, Saltzman WR, Poppleton L, Burlingame GM, Pasalić A, Duraković E, et al. Effectiveness of a school-based group psychotherapy program for war-exposed adolescents: a randomized controlled trial. J Am Acad Child Adolesc Psychiatry. 2008;47(9):1048–62. doi:10.1097/CHI.0b013e31817eecae.

Litz BT. Early intervention for trauma: where are we and where do we need to go? A commentary. J Trauma Stress. 2008;21(6):503–6. doi:10.1002/jts.20373.

Litz BT, Williams L, Wang J, Bryant R, Engel Jr, CC. A therapist-assisted internet self-help program for traumatic stress. Prof Psychol-Res Pr. 2004;35(6):628–34.

Litz BT, Engel CC, Bryant RA, Papa A. A Randomized, Controlled Proof-of-Concept Trial of an Internet-Based, Therapist-Assisted Self-Management Treatment for Posttraumatic Stress Disorder. Am J Psychiatry. 2007;164(11):1676–84. doi:10.1176/appi.ajp.2007.06122057.

MacFarlane A. (1989). Treatment of PTSD. Br J Med Psychol. 1989;62:81–90.

Mains JA, Scogin FR. The effectiveness of self-administered treatments: a practice-friendly review of the research. J Clin Psychol. 2003;59(2):237–46.

Meltzer-Brody S, Churchill E, Davidson JRT. Derivation of the SPAN, a brief diagnostic screening test for post-traumatic stress disorder. Psychiat Res. 1999;88(1):63–70. doi:10.1016/S0165-1781(99)00070-0.

NICE. Management of post-traumatic stress disorder in adults and children. London: National Institute of Clinical Excellence; 2007.

NIMH. Mental health and mass violence: Evidence-based early psychological intervention for victims/survivors of massviolence. A workshop to reach consensus on best practices. Washington, DC: National Institute of Mental Health; 2002.

Parsons TD, Rizzo AA. Affective outcomes of virtual reality exposure therapy for anxiety and specific phobias: a meta-analysis. J Behav Ther Exp Psychiatry. 2008;39(3):250–61.

Palm KM, Strong DR, MacPherson L. Evaluating symptom expression as a function of a posttraumatic stress disorder severity. J Anxiety Disorders. 2009;23(1):27–37.

Perkins BR, Rouanzoin CC. A critical evaluation of current views regarding eye movement desensitization and reprocessing (EMDR): clarifying points of confusion. J Clin Psychol. 2002;58(1):77–97. doi:10.1002/jclp.1130.

Resick PA. Stress and trauma. Hove, England: Psychology Press; 2001.

Rizzo A, Reger G, Gahm G, Difede J, Rothbaum BO. Virtual reality exposure therapy for combat-related PTSD. In Post-Traumatic Stress Disorder, Retrieved 5 May 2009, from http://dx.doi.org/10.1007/978-1-60327-329-9_18 (2009). p. 1–25.

Rizzo A, Rothbaum B, Graap K. (2007). Virtual reality applications for the treatment of combat-related PTSD. Combat stress injury: Theory, research, and management (pp. 183–204). New York, NY US: Routledge/Taylor & Francis Group.

Rogers S, Silver SM. Is EMDR an exposure therapy? A review of trauma protocols. J Clin Psychol. 2002;58(1):43–59. doi:10.1002/jclp.1128.

Rothbaum BO, Hodges LF, Ready D, Graap K, Alarcon RD. Virtual reality exposure therapy for Vietnam veterans with posttraumatic stress disorder. J Clin Psychiatry. 2001;62(8):617–22.

Rothbaum B, Foa E, Hembree E. (2007). Reclaiming your life from a traumatic experience: a prolonged exposure treatment program workbook. 1st ed. New York: Oxford University Press, USA; 2007.

Rothbaum BO, Astin MC, Marsteller F. Prolonged exposure versus eye movement desensitization and reprocessing (EMDR) for PTSD rape victims. J Trauma Stress. 2005;18(6):607–16. doi:10.1002/jts.20069.

Rothbaum BO, Hodges LF, Ready D, Graap K, Alarcon RD. Virtual reality exposure therapy for Vietnam veterans with posttraumatic stress disorder. J Clin Psychiatry. 2001;62(8):617–22.

Rothbaum BO, Hodges L, Alarcon R, Ready D, Shahar F, Graap K, et al. Virtual reality exposure therapy for PTSD Vietnam veterans: a case study. J Trauma Stress. 1999;12(2):263–71.

Ruggiero KJ, Resnick HS, Acierno R, Coffey SF, Carpenter MJ, Ruscio AM, et al. Internet-based intervention for mental health and substance use problems in disaster-affected populations: a pilot feasibility study. Behav Ther. 2006;37(2):190–205. doi:10.1016/j.beth.2005.12.001.

Ruscio AM, Ruscio J, Keane, TM. The latent structure of Posttraumtic Stress Disorder: A taxometric investigation of reactions to extreme stress. Journal of Abnormal Psychology. 2002;111:290–301.

Scogin F, Jamison C, Davis N. Two-year follow-up of bibliotherapy for depression in older adults. Journal of Consulting and Clinical Psychology. 1990;58:665–67.

Tarrier N, Liversidge T, Gregg L. The acceptability and preference for the psychological treatment of PTSD. Behav Res Ther. 2006;44(11):1643–56. doi:10.1016/j.brat.2005.11.012.

Trappler B, Newville H. Trauma healing via cognitive behavior therapy in chronically hospitalized patients. Psychiatr Q. 2007;78(4):317–25. doi:10.1007/s11126-007-9049-8.

Turpin G, Downs M, Mason S. Effectiveness of providing self-help information following acute traumatic injury: randomised controlled trial. Br J Psychiatry. 2005;187(1):76–82. doi:10.1192/bjp.187.1.76.

Vaishnavi S, Payne V, Connor K, Davidson JR. A comparison of the SPRINT and CAPS assessment scales for posttraumatic stress disorder. Depress Anxiety. 2006;23(7):437–40. doi:10.1002/da.20202.

Vernberg EM, Steinberg AM, Jacobs AK, Brymer MJ, Watson PJ, Osofsky JD, et al. Innovations in disaster mental health: psychological first aid. Prof Psychol-Res Pr., 2008;39(4):381–8.

Wagner AW, Linehan MM. Applications of dialectical behavior therapy to posttraumatic stress disorder and related problems. In: Follette VM, Ruzek JI, editors. Cognitive-behavioral therapies for trauma. 2nd ed. New York: Guilford Press; 2006; p. 117–45.

Wagner AW, Rizvi SL, Harned MS. Applications of dialectical behavior therapy to the treatment of complex trauma-related problems: when one case formulation does not fit all. J Trauma Stress. 2007;20(4):391–400. doi:10.1002/jts.20268.

Weathers FW, Huska JA, Keane TM. The PTSD Checklist—Civilian Version (PCL-C). Boston veterans affairs medical center: national center for PTSD; 1991.

Weathers FW, Keane TM, Davidson JR. Clinician-administered PTSD scale: a review of the first ten years of research. Depress Anxiety, 2001;13(3):132–56.

Wessely S, Bryant RA, Greenberg N, Earnshaw M, Sharpley J, Hughes JH. Does psychoeducation help prevent post traumatic psychological distress? Psychiatry. 2008;71(4):287–302. doi:10.1521/psyc.2008.71.4.287.

Wohlfarth TD, van den Brink W, Winkel FW, ter Smitten M. Screening for posttraumatic stress disorder: an evaluation of two self-report scales among crime victims. Psychol Assessment. 2003;15(1):101–9.

Yehuda R, McFarlane A, Shalev AY. Predicting the development of posttraumatic stress disorder from the acute response to a traumatic event. Biological Psychiatry. 1998;44(12):1205–1313.

Zoellner LA, Feeny NC, Cochran B, Pruitt L. Treatment choice for PTSD. Behav Res Ther. 2003;41(8):879–86.

Chapter 6
Social Phobia (Social Anxiety Disorder)

Gerhard Andersson and Per Carlbring

Brief Description of the Problem

Social phobia, or social anxiety disorder (SAD), is defined in the DSM-IV as a marked and persistent fear of one or more social performance situations in which embarrassment may occur (APA, 2000). Exposure to unfamiliar people or possible scrutiny of others typically evokes anxiety and tends to be avoided or endured under great distress. SAD is argued to exist on a continuum varying in severity and number of symptoms. SAD is associated with substantial impairment in quality of life (Safren et al., 1997) and is highly prevalent with prevalence rates well above 10% (Furmark, 2002). A recent large study estimated lifetime and 12-month prevalence of social phobia of 12.1 and 7.1%, respectively (Ruscio et al., 2008). SAD may vary in severity, and most researchers distinguish between more limited specific (e.g., speaking in front of an audience) versus generalized social phobia (Hofmann, 2007), in which problems occur in several social situations. As evidenced by controlled trials and meta-analyses there are effective psychosocial treatments for SAD (Acarturk et al., 2009; Rodebaugh et al., 2004). However, far from all sufferers seek treatment (Baldwin and Buis, 2004), and there is a gap between help seeking and the number of people who have SAD. The high prevalence of SAD is also a problem for health care, and barriers to accessing expert assistance include shortage of skilled therapists, long waiting lists, and costs. These barriers particularly disadvantage geographically isolated people, such as those in regional and rural areas where traveling time is an added burden. Another problem is that those with generalized social phobia may not seek therapy due to the fear of embarrassment associated with help seeking (Postel et al., 2008). Therefore, a major challenge is to increase the accessibility and affordability of evidence-based psychological treatments for social phobia and to consider stepped care approaches.

G. Andersson (✉)
Department of Behavioural Sciences and Learning, Linköping University, Linköping, SE 581 83, Sweden
e-mail: gerhard.andersson@liu.se

W.T. O'Donohue, C. Draper (eds.), *Stepped Care and e-Health*, 99
DOI 10.1007/978-1-4419-6510-3_6, © Springer Science+Business Media, LLC 2011

Assessment/Triage

Assessment and subsequent triage of individuals may contain several steps. The first option is self-screening. Increasingly, persons with SAD may recognize that they have SAD by means of resources on the World Wide Web (Erwina et al., 2004; Shepherd and Edelmann, 2005). The Internet and publicity on SAD may also influence help seeking. In addition, screening of SAD can be done via the Internet and reliable screening instruments have been developed (Furmark et al., 1999).

While screening can be a useful first step, self-reported problems cannot replace a structured diagnostic interview conducted by a clinician. There is a gap between research and clinic. In research it is common to use the Structured Clinical Interview for the DSM-IV (SCID; First et al., 1995) or the Anxiety Disorders Interview Schedule Revised (Di Nardo et al., 1993) to confirm a diagnosis of SAD. Moreover, diagnoses of comorbid problems may be needed such as other anxiety disorders, mood disorders, and addictions. Since the overlap between the anxiety disorders and the mood disorders is substantial, it is feasible to assess the presence of major depression. In clinical settings it may not be possible to conduct lengthy structured interviews, and in those cases triage may be informed by the clinical impression and self-report. There are several useful self-report inventories for the measurement of symptoms of SAD, such as the Liebowitz Social Anxiety Scale self-report version (LSAS-SR; Baker et al., 2002), the Social Phobia Scale (SPS), and Social Interaction Anxiety Scale (SIAS; Mattick and Clarke, 1998).

Once interview and questionnaire data have been collected a decision on further treatment should be made in collaboration with the patient. In this chapter we focus on adult patients, as the situation differs with children and adolescents.

Stepped Care Options

Watchful Waiting

Depending on the level of severity watchful waiting is probably a self-selected option as many patients with SAD wait for many years until they seek help. We could not locate any studies on consumer preferences for this option, but it is unlikely that SAD of a more severe kind will remit on itself. Indeed, the mean age of onset of SAD is commonly in adolescence (Tillfors, 2004). It is not necessarily the case that early identification of SAD will prevent further development of the condition, and in particular among adolescents the stability of SAD symptoms may vary (Gren-Landell et al., 2009). However, overall the recovery rate is poor and Ruscio et al. (2008) found that only 20–40% of SAD cases recover within 20 years of onset and only 40–60% recover within 40 years.

Psychoeducation

Psychoeducation is an integral part of most psychological treatments and in particular in CBT. It usually includes presenting a model for the condition at hand and discussions with the patient if the model fits the experienced problems (see box for additional information). While there may be initial effects from "pure" psychoeducation for anxiety disorders (e.g., Shear et al., 1994), we have not located studies in which the effects of psychoeducation only have been tested in patients with SAD. One possible exception is a study by Heimberg et al. (1998) who in their study had an educational-supportive group therapy condition. This was, however, a control condition and not strictly psychoeducation as a stand-alone treatment. There is no firm line between psychoeducation and other treatment formats, but one distinction would be that psychoeducation mainly involves information about the condition and rationale for further treatments such as medication and psychological treatments. It is important to mention that psychoeducation also can occur via other sources than therapists and health care systems. There are, for example, information on the World Wide Web (Khazaal et al., 2008), and it is likely that at least some persons with social anxiety problems read only parts of self-help books and do not follow a full self-help program.

Bibliotherapy

There is a growing literature on self-help for SAD. Bibliotherapy is a heterogeneous treatment format ranging from pure self-help to guided self-help. Self-help books can also be used in live treatments as a complement (Keeley et al., 2002), but have been studied as treatment on its own. While books on SAD may differ, they often follow the structure in face-to-face therapy, which means that psychoeducation, cognitive components, exposure exercises, and relapse prevention are included (see box for overview). Overall, research on bibliotherapy suggests that it can be as effective as face-to-face therapies under the condition that some kind of therapist guidance is given (den Boer et al., 2004; Hirai and Clum, 2006). While the literature on bibliotherapy for SAD is still limited there are independent trials suggesting that it can be effective. Rapee et al.,(2007) conducted a large trial in which they contrasted pure self-help and therapist-augmented self-help for SAD. The authors clearly showed that therapist-guided self-help was superior to self-guided treatment. Interestingly, they also added a live group treatment comparison group which did not do better than the therapist-guided bibliotherapy group. The authors concluded that pure self-help was not an effective treatment for SAD. However, in another recent trial conducted in Sweden (Furmark et al., 2009) pure bibliotherapy was better than waiting list on measures of social anxiety, general anxiety, depression, and quality of life. It may be that procedural differences and the self-help materials used explain this difference between the two studies. Another smaller study conducted by a third research group also found that guided self-help can be effective for SAD

(Abramowitz et al., 2009). In terms of consumer preferences bibliotherapy including telephone support has many advantages but we could not locate any preference studies. The improvement rates following bibliotherapy appears to be promising, but not as large as in face-to-face therapies.

Computer-Assisted and Internet-Delivered Interventions

There is an emerging database on the effects of guided Internet-delivered treatments for various conditions (Andersson, 2009), and systematic reviews and meta-analyses show promising findings (Spek et al., 2007). Internet-based treatments can be regarded as an extension of bibliotherapy, as the World Wide Web is used to present text materials often downloadable text files for the client to read and register. However, with web administration elements can be made more visually attractive and e-mail is often used to keep in contact with the client during the treatment period. At least three independent research groups have conducted controlled trials on Internet treatment. Programs are based on CBT and do not differ from CBT in what they cover (e.g., exposure). The first trials were conducted in Sweden, and in the first trials two live group exposure sessions were added (Anderssonet al., 2006). The treatment consisted of a 9-week program and support was provided through e-mail. Relatively large effects were observed with overall within- and between-groups Cohen's d effect sizes being 0.87 and 0.70, respectively. Treatment gains were maintained at 1-year follow-up. It is important to note that all participants in that trial ($N = 64$) were diagnosed with social phobia and 70% were of the generalized subtype. A brief description of the treatment is provided in the Box. The treatment follows face-to-face treatments in terms of contents.

Description of the Internet and Bibliotherapy Treatment Used in the Swedish Studies

The text, consisting of 186 pages, is divided into nine modules. The first module, which introduces the program, portrays social phobia and its symptoms, proposes possibleetiological factors, and describes facts about cognitive behavior therapy. The second module outlines a model for social phobia (by Clark and Wells, 1995) and the relationship between thoughts, feelings, behavior, and cognitive symptoms. It also defines automatic thoughts and explains how to register them. The third module provides a basic outline of thinking errors/cognitive distortions, the registration of automatic thoughts, and information about how to challenge these. Work with automatic thoughts continues in the fourth module and behavioral experiments are introduced. Formulation of specific therapeutic goals is also included in this module. The fifth module covers the principles behind exposure and reality testing, while the sixth module concerns self-focus, shifting of focus, attention training, and safety behaviors. The seventh module continues the previous work with exposure. It focuses on problems that are commonly encountered during exposure and suggests behavioral experiments. The eighth module concerns the art of listening and conversing, non-verbal communication, the ability to say no, and assertiveness (social skills). The final module informs the reader about the role of perfectionism, procrastination, and self-confidence as well as relapse prevention. The entire program is then summarized.

Each module includes information and exercises and ends with three to eight essay questions. Participants are asked to explain, in their own words, the most important sections of the module they have just completed, provide thought records, and describe their experience with and outcome of their exposure exercises. The questions are intended to promote learning and to enable the online therapists to assess whether the participants have assimilated the material and completed their homework. Also included in each module is a multiple choice quiz that the participants need to get 95% correct in order to proceed. Finally, in each module the participants are required to post a message in a discussion forum about a specific topic.

Personal feedback on the homework is usually given within 24 hours after participants have sent their answers via e-mail. On the basis of these e-mails, an assessment is made of whether the participant is ready to continue; if so, the password to the next module is sent. If not, the participant receives instructions on what needs to be completed before proceeding to the next module.

Following the first trial which included two live exposure sessions a trial was conducted in which brief weekly telephone calls were added to the Internet treatment and no live group exposure sessions. That trial showed equally good outcomes, with an average between group effect size across measures of $d = 0.95$ (Carlbring et al., 2007). In a third study the Swedish group tested if adding five live group sessions would result in better outcome than pure Internet treatment with e-mail guidance. This small study found no differences in outcome suggesting that group sessions may not be required (Tillfors et al., 2008). In terms of long-term outcomes a 30-month follow-up suggests that Internet treatment of SAD has sustainable effects (Carlbring et al., 2009).

Studies conducted in Australia have replicated and extended the findings from the Swedish studies. Titov and coworkers in Australia reported two trials (Titov et al. 2008b, c), with between group effect sizes above $d = 0.80$. They have also found that contact via e-mail fosters better compliance and results in better outcome (Titov et al. 2008a) and that effects are sustainable (Titov et al., 2009).

A third research group has independently developed a treatment program for SAD. Berger et al. (2009) in Switzerland also replicated the findings from the Swedish and Australian studies. In common with the two other groups Berger et al. had a structured program based on CBT, and guidance is provided via e-mail.

In addition to the mainly text-based online treatments there are also applications of virtual reality treatments which may become a treatment complement in the future (Botella et al., 2000; Klinger et al., 2005).

Overall, there are now strong indications that Internet treatment can work for SAD. There are no direct comparisons with live treatment and no effectiveness study. The latter refers to studies that are conducted in regular clinical settings under representative conditions (high external validity). It is highly likely that persons with SAD will find Internet treatment attractive (Erwina et al., 2005), but it is important to note that Internet treatment involves the same procedure as in live CBT, with homework assignments and live exposures. Given that the client works with the program our impression is that it can work. Combined treatments may, however, be more preferable for clinicians and for some clients. An additional challenge is to investigate the cost-effectiveness of Internet treatment for SAD. We estimate that at least half of the costs can be cut when it comes to the delivery of treatment. Initial costs for programming and preparation of material add to the initial costs. However, the indirect costs for patients may be more rapidly reduced as the patient can access treatment after work hours and costs for traveling to the therapist office are minimized.

Group Therapy

Group therapy is often the treatment of choice as it provides the facilities for group exposure and has been regarded as more cost-effective than individual treatment (Heimberg and Becker, 2002; Rodebaugh et al., 2004). The most well-researched group treatment is the one developed by Heimberg and colleagues (Heimberg and Becker, 2002). This involves not only group exposure but also other CBT components such as cognitive therapy techniques derived from the work by Beck et al. (1985). Role plays are used to integrate the cognitive components and in vivo homework assignments are an integral part. While group therapy for SAD may include different components, some clients may need social skills training. As a single treatment this is rarely sufficient (Ponniah and Hollon, 2008). Moreover, exposure in the group setting has also been used as a main component in the treatment of SAD (Ponniah and Hollon, 2008). The format of the group treatments may also vary and intensive treatments over a few weeks have been tested with promising results (Mörtberg et al., 2005; Mörtberg et al., 2007). While there is a predominance of CBT in the treatment literature (if we include behavioral and cognitive treatments under the CBT heading) there are a few studies on psychodynamic treatment (Knijnik et al., 2004) and interpersonal treatments (Borge et al., 2008). None of these have generated better outcomes than CBT, but may broaden the treatment options for SAD. They may hence expand the number of clinicians with treatment orientations other than CBT who can deliver effective treatments for SAD.

In terms of outcome data there are several meta-analyses and systematic reviews showing that group CBT is effective (Fedoroff and Taylor, 2001; Taylor, 1996).

A more recent meta-analysis only included controlled studies and found a relatively large treatment effect (Cohen's $d = 0.70$) on measures of social anxiety (Acarturk et al., 2009). Studies have also documented long-term effects (e.g., Heimberg et al., 1993). Since social contacts and in particular public speaking is a problem for many persons with SAD, it is likely that some refrain from seeking group treatment and prefer either pharmacological treatment or individual treatment. On the other hand the group setting can be instrumental for some persons with SAD as it automatically generates opportunities for exposure. In terms of quality improvements there are many studies in which treatment components have been altered, but fewer direct comparisons of different approaches to group treatment.

Individual Therapy

Recent theoretical and empirical developments in SAD research have led to the discovery that the group setting may not be optimal for persons with SAD. Clark and Wells (1995) developed a model of SAD in which they highlighted the role of self-focused attention and the use of "safety behaviors," the latter being a term used to describe strategies used by patients with SAD to avoid an imagined social catastrophe. They also targeted anticipatory anxiety and post-event processing. In other words they proposed that persons with SAD engage in many behaviors that are not visible during a group exposure which may require individual treatment. However, some clinicians have used the developments by Clark in group work and there is no robust evidence that SAD should be better treated in the individual format although it may be more suitable in more severe SAD of the generalized subtype. Indeed, the work by Clark is probably the treatment protocol that has generated the largest effects in controlled trials (Clark et al., 2003, 2006; Mörtberg et al., 2007). In one trial individual treatment was found superior to group treatment (Stangier et al., 2003), but as mentioned it was not found to be more effective than group treatment in the meta-analysis by Acarturk et al. (2009).

Regarding consumer preferences we are not aware of any preference studies, but it is likely that many individuals with SAD would prefer individual treatment over group treatment if given a choice. Not the least we have noticed this in our own Internet trials as many persons with SAD report interest in our trials. There is an intensive research on the mechanisms behind SAD (e.g., Clark and McManus, 2002; Hofmann and Otto, 2008) and there are continuous improvements of the treatments and the work by Clark and coworkers suggests that new knowledge can have an impact on how treatment is implemented, for example, by adding video feedback (e.g., Kim et al., 2002).

Medication

Several medications for SAD have been tested and serotonin reuptake inhibitors (SSRIs) are regarded as first-line treatment by many researchers and clinicians (Stein et al. 2004). While the evidence is not clear in a clinical situation it may be needed to combine medication with psychological treatments. Comorbid conditions such as major depression may respond to medication and it is possible to conceptualize SAD as a condition involving both a psychobiological and a psychological disturbance and that there are different routes to effective treatment (Furmark et al., 2002). In contrast to the field of major depression (Cuijpers et al., 2008), there are no clear indications in the literature that more severe forms of SAD would respond better to medication than to psychological treatment (Baldwin et al., 2005). However, given the role of comorbid depression it cannot be excluded that a combination might be helpful for at least some patients. On the other hand the long-term effects of psychological treatments are probably better than for medication unless the medication is continued (Clark et al., 2003; Davidson et al., 2004; Haug et al., 2003).

A recent development in the field of combining medication with psychological treatments comes from the work by Hofmann and coworkers. In a controlled trial they found that exposure therapy for SAD may be enhanced with D-cycloserine, an agonist at the glutamatergic N-methyl-D-aspartate receptor (Hofmann et al., 2006).

While consumers may prefer psychological treatment (Baldwin et al., 2005; Huppert et al., 2003) it is not always the case. There are both advantages and disadvantages to medication and/or psychological treatments. While medications may have unwanted side effects psychological treatments may be too time consuming and for patients who know about the procedures in CBT (e.g., exposure) it may be frightening to enter psychological treatments.

Inpatient Treatment

How health care is structured will determine if individuals with SAD are treated as inpatients. There may be severe cases, often with substantial comorbidity, for which inpatient treatment is required. In addition, some persons with SAD can develop agoraphobic avoidance and become house bound. In addition to avoidance, persons with more severe generalized social anxiety may benefit from social skills training (Davidson et al., 2004). However, a study on the economic consequences of SAD showed that very few with pure social phobia had consumed any inpatient services during the last year (1.8%), but when comorbidity was present this increased substantially to 20.6% (Patel et al., 2002).

Research on persons with severe SAD is needed as consumer preferences and outcome of regular services offered are not well investigated.

Consumer Preferences and Cultural Sensitivity

We have already commented on consumer preferences for each of the treatment options. To our knowledge, there are few if any comparative studies on treatment preferences regarding SAD. However, in other fields such as major depression it is often observed that psychological treatments are preferred over pharmacological (van Schaik et al., 2004). In comparative trials of treatment options preferences are often asked for, but in spite of differences in preference they rarely affect outcome (e.g., Leykin et al., 2007). One way to investigate this matter is to ask the study participants how credible they view the treatment options. In one study on panic disorder we found differences in treatment credibility between live versus Internet treatment (Carlbring et al., 2005), but no differences in outcome. A later prediction study confirmed that treatment credibility did not predict outcome (Andersson et al., 2008). However, what is needed are data on treatment preferences in clinical settings. We are not aware of any such studies on SAD, and it cannot be inferred from research on depression that psychological treatments are preferred over medical treatment although it is likely. Another aspect is the emerging literature on different psychological treatment alternatives. To our knowledge patient preferences regarding different forms of psychological treatment (e.g., cognitive behavioral versus psychodynamic) have not been studied.

Another issue of importance when treatment options are evaluated is the role of culture. For example, shyness is commonly associated with SAD, but may be differently valued in different countries and there may be sex differences as well. Both psychological treatments and different medications may be valued differently in different cultures and subcultures. In fact, the mere diagnosis of SAD is arguably influenced by culture (Wakefield, 1992).

Triage Agenda

How to handle triage may become even more important as different treatment options emerge. There are different levels of assessment, ranging from self-report screening instruments (that can be presented online), structured clinical interviews by one clinician, and team-based diagnostic approaches. In an ideal world all patients should be properly assessed and diagnostic information should be obtained before any intervention is presented. However, our impression is that treatment is often presented without careful diagnostic information behind (for example, lack of information on comorbid conditions). We believe that it can be a mistake to do minimal assessment (e.g., very brief screening online) and then low-intensity interventions as cases who may need careful assessment and a more comprehensive treatment immediately might be missed. Indeed, the results of guided self-help suggest that a proper diagnostic procedure very well may lead to a mainly self-administered treatment. But on the other hand it is crucial to identify individuals in need of more intensive treatments and combined treatments. The triage also should take into account prior treatment experiences as they may influence the uptake of the treatment. Moreover, clinicians need to consider the potential of combined treatments, for example, group treatment and individual treatment. Clinicians should also ask clients about other treatment activities as parallel treatments might be implemented without the clinician knowing it.

Finally, stepped care approaches should be considered in the triage process. This does not necessarily mean going from simpler to more advanced treatments. Costs of treatments and the need for booster treatment can also be part of a stepped care decision-making process. Access to health care is another issue which may make distance technologies such as Internet treatment more attractive in some settings. Overall, there is a need to develop and empirically validate stepped care models of health care delivery for SAD.

Research and Development Agenda

There are several interesting research activities that may alter the way we view and treat SAD. In this chapter we have presented the recently developed treatment approach which utilizes the Internet. We have not commented on recent research activities dealing with attention modification programs for which preliminary data show very promising result for SAD (e.g., Amir et al., 2008). It is not yet clear if this new treatment which is based on information processing theory should be a stand-alone treatment or if it should be combined with other evidence-based treatments such as group CBT. We believe this new way of treating SAD represents a truly innovative approach as is does not rely on the traditional way of delivering treatments (i.e., via communication in either a therapy setting or through text).

Another interesting new research development concerns the augmentation of exposure treatment by means of medication. This also represent a truly innovative approach in which medication and psychological treatment are assumed to work in synergy rather than in parallel as is the most common assumption when SSRIs and psychological treatments are combined.

An important challenge for research is to investigate how well evidence-based treatments can be applied for different age groups. While there are numerous controlled trials on SAD for adults there are far fewer on children and adolescents. Older adults are another group for which very little treatment research on SAD exists.

A fourth challenge concerns not only with the comorbidity between different anxiety and mood disorders, but also with other conditions such as stuttering (Kraaimaat et al., 2003) and problems such as attention deficit disorders.

Overall, research activities on SAD over the last years have showed a dramatic broadening of treatment options and ways to deliver treatment. It is now important to find predictors of treatment outcome for different treatments and further develop and potentially combine existing treatments. For example, Internet treatments for SAD have so far mainly been text based, whereas virtual reality treatments rely on visual and auditory input. Computerized-assisted assessment and treatment procedures have been developed that can aid clinicians and patients in the treatment setting (Craske et al., 2009) and this represents a whole new field of investigation.

Dissemination Agenda

It is well known that evidence-based treatments for SAD often never reach the patients who need them the most. The treatment versus demand gap may be greater for psychological treatments but with the advent of guided self-help approaches that may be cost-effective it is possible that psychological treatments can become a viable treatment alternative in addition to SSRIs. Cost-effectiveness of treatments must be considered before large-scale dissemination and is not only restricted to the costs of treatment but also involves secondary costs such as reduced sick leave, less absence from work, and increased quality of life as an effect of treatment.

Dissemination of evidence treatments also involves health care and referral routes and stepped care models are inevitable when different treatments are possible. We have mentioned guided self-help as a promising early and low-cost intervention that could be included in a stepped care model, but there are other possibilities such as group education.

A final challenge is to do dissemination research. Increasingly, guidelines are put forward on how to treat SAD with evidence-based treatments but less is known about the effects of guidelines. Overall, how well a treatment works under naturalistic conditions, so-called effectiveness studies, is an integral part of dissemination as it cannot be studied before the treatment is implemented. Lincoln et al. (2003) presented data showing that CBT approaches tended to work when the treatment was transferred to four outpatient clinics in Germany. More studies are needed in this field showing that evidence-based treatments for SAD work in the clinic and not only in research studies with recruited and selected patients.

In conclusion, we are now in a position when it is timely to focus on way to disseminate evidence-based treatments for SAD is a carefully planned stepped care format and with special considerations regarding group differences and patient preferences.

References

Abramowitz JS, Moore EL, Braddock AE, Harrington DL. Self-help cognitive-behavioral therapy with minimal therapist contact for social phobia: a controlled trial. J Behav Ther Exp Psychiat. 2009;40:98–105.

Acarturk C, Cuijpers P, van Straten A, de Graaf, R. Psychological treatment of social anxiety disorder: a meta-analysis. Psychol Med. 2009;39:241–54.

American Psychiatric Association. Diagnostic and statistical manual of mental disorders. 4th ed., text revision ed. Washington, DC: American Psychiatric Press; 2000.

Amir N, Weber G, Beard C, Bomyea J, Taylor CT. The effect of a single-session attention modification program on response to a public-speaking challenge in socially anxious individuals. J Abnorm Psychol. 2008;117:860–8.

Andersson G. Using the internet to provide cognitive behaviour therapy. Behav Res Therapy. 2009;47:175–80.

Andersson G, Carlbring P, Grimlund A. Predicting treatment outcome in Internet versus face to face treatment of panic disorder. Comput Hum Behav. 2008;24:1790–801.

Andersson G, Carlbring P, Holmström A, Sparthan E, Furmark T, Nilsson-Ihrfelt E, Buhrman M, Ekselius L. Internet-based self-help with therapist feedback and in-vivo group exposure for social phobia: a randomized controlled trial. J Consult Clin Psychol. 2006;74:677–86.

Baker SL, Heinrich N, Kim H-J, Hofmann SG. The Liebowitz social anxiety scale as a self-report instrument: a preliminary psychometric analysis. Behav Res Ther. 2002;40:701–15.

Baldwin DS, Buis C. Burden of social anxiety disorder. In: Bandelow DS, Stein DJ, editors. Social anxiety disorder. New York: Marcel Dekker; 2004. p. 65–74.

Baldwin DS, Anderson IM, Nutt DJ, Bandelow B, Bond A, Davidson JR, et al. Evidence-based guidelines for the pharmacological treatment of anxiety disorders: recommendations from the British association for psychopharmacology. J Psychopharmacol. 2005;19:567–96.

Beck AT, Emery G, Greenberg RL. Anxiety disorders and phobias. A cognitive perspective. New York: Basic Books, 2009.

Berger T, Hohl E, Caspar F. Internet-based treatment for social phobia: a randomized controlled trial. J Clin Psychol. 2009;65:1021–35.

Borge FM, Hoffart A, Sexton H, Clark DM, Markowitz JC, McManus F. Residential cognitive therapy versus residential interpersonal therapy for social phobia: a randomized clinical trial. J Anxiety Disord. 2008;22:991–1010.

Botella C, Banos R, Guillén V, Perpina C, Alcaniz M, Pons A. Telepsychology: public speaking fear treatment on the internet. Cyberpsychol Behav. 2000;3:959–68.

Carlbring P, Bergman Nordgren L, Furmark T, Andersson G. Long term outcome of Internet delivered cognitive-behavioural therapy for social anxiety disorder: a 30-month follow-up. Behav Res Ther. 2009;47:848–50.

Carlbring P, Gunnarsdóttir M, Hedensjö L, Andersson G, Ekselius L, Furmark T. Treatment of social phobia: randomized trial of internet delivered cognitive behaviour therapy and telephone support. Br J Psychiatry.2007; 190:123–28.

Carlbring P, Nilsson-Ihrfelt E, Waara J, Kollenstam C, Buhrman M, Kaldo V, et al. Treatment of panic disorder: live therapy vs. self-help via internet. Behav Res Ther. 2005;43:1321–33.

Clark DM, Ehlers A, Hackmann A, McManus F, Fennell M, Grey N, et al. Cognitive therapy versus exposure and applied relaxation in social phobia: a randomized controlled trial. J Consult Clin Psychology. 2006;74:568–78.

Clark DM, Ehlers A, McManus F, Hackmann A, Fennell M, Campbell H, et al. Cognitive therapy versus fluoxetine in generalized social phobia: a randomized placebo-controlled trial. J Consult Clin Psychol. 2003;71:1058–67.

Clark DM, McManus F. Information processing in social phobia. Biol Psychiatry. 2002;51:92–100.

Clark DM, Wells A. A cognitive model of social phobia. In: Heimberg RG, Leibowitz M, Hope DA, Schneider FR, editors. Social phobia: diagnosis, assessment and treatment. New York: Guilford press; 1995. p. 63–93.

Craske MG, Rose RD, Lang A, Welch SS, Campbell-Sills L, Sullivan G, et al. Computer-assisted delivery of cognitive behavioral therapy for anxiety disorders in primary-care settings. Depress Anxiety. 2009;26:235–42.

Cuijpers P, van Straten A, van Oppen P, Andersson G. Are psychological and pharmacological interventions equally effective in the treatment of adult depressive disorders? A meta-analysis of comparative studies. J Clin Psychiatry. 2008;69:1675–85.

Davidson JR, Foa EB, Huppert JD, Keefe FJ, Franklin ME, Compton JS, et al. Fluoxetine, comprehensive cognitive behavioral therapy, and placebo in generalized social phobia. Arch of Gen Psychiatry. 2004;61:1005–13.

den Boer PC, Wiersma D, Van den Bosch RJ. Why is self-help neglected in the treatment of emotional disorders? A meta-analysis. Psychol Med. 2004;34: 959–71.

Di Nardo PA, Moras K, Barlow DH, Rapee RM. Reliability of DSM III R anxiety disorder categories: using the anxiety disorders interview schedule revised (ADIS R). Arch Gen Psychiatry. 1993;50:251–6.

Erwina BA, Turk CL, Heimberg RG, Frescoa DM, Hantula DA. The Internet: home to a severe population of individuals with social anxiety disorder? J Anxiety Disord. 2004;18:629–46.

Fedoroff IC, Taylor, S. Psychological and pharmacological treatments of social phobia: a meta-analysis. J Clin Psychopharmacol. 2001;21:311–24.

First MB, Spitzer RL, Gibbon M, Williams JBW. Structured clinical interview for DSM-IV Axis I Disorders (SCID-I). Washington, D.C: American Psychiatric Press; 1995.

Furmark T. Social phobia: overview of community surveys. Acta Psychiat Scand. 2002;105:84–93.

Furmark T, Carlbring P, Hedman E, Sonnenstein A, Clevberger P, Bohman B, Eriksson A, Hållén A, Frykman M, Holmström A, Sparthan E, Tillfors M, Nilsson-Ihrfelt E, Spak M, Eriksson A, Ekselius L, Andersson G. Bibliotherapy and internet delivered cognitive behaviour therapy with additional guidance for social anxiety disorder: randomised controlled trial. Br J Psychiatry. 2009;195:440–47.

Furmark T, Tillfors M, Everz P, Marteinsdottir I, Gefvert O, Fredrikson M. Social phobia in the general population: prevalence and sociodemographic profile. Soc psychiatry Psychiatr Epidemiol. 1999;34:416–24.

Furmark T, Tillfors M, Marteinsdottir I, Fischer H, Pissiota A, Langstrom B, et al. Common changes in cerebral blood flow in patients with social phobia treated with citalopram or cognitive-behavioral therapy. Arch Gen Psychiatry. 2002;59(5):425–33.

Gren-Landell M, Tillfors M, Furmark T, Bohlin G, Andersson G, Svedin C-G. Social phobia in Swedish adolescents: prevalence and gender differences. Soc Psychiatry Psychiatr Epidemiol. 2009;44:1–7.

Haug TT, Blomhoff S, Hellstrom K, Holme I, Humble M, Madsbu HP, et al. Exposure therapy and sertraline in social phobia: I-year follow-up of a randomised controlled trial. Br J Psychiatry. 2003;182:312–18.

Heimberg RG, Becker RE. Cognitive-behavioral group therapy for social phobia. Basic mechanisms and clinical strategies. New York: Guilford Press; 2002.

Heimberg RG, Liebowitz MR, Hope DA, Schneier FR, Holt CS, Welkowitz LA, et al. Cognitive behavioral group therapy vs phenelzine therapy for social phobia: 12-week outcome. Arch Gen Psychiatry. 1998;55:1133–41.

Heimberg RG, Salzman DG, Holt CS, Blendell KA. Cognitive-behavioral group treatment for social phobia: effectiveness at five-year follow-up. Cogn Ther Res. 1993;17:325–39.

Hirai M, Clum GA. A meta-analytic study of self-help interventions for anxiety problems. Behav Ther. 2006;37:99–111.

Hofmann SG, Heinrichs N, Moscovitch DA. The nature and expression of social phobia: toward a new classification. Clin Psychol Rev. 2004;24:769–97.

Hofmann SG, Meuret AE, Smits JA, Simon NM, Pollack MH, Eisenmenger K, et al. Augmentation of exposure therapy with D-cycloserine for social anxiety disorder. Arch Gen Psychiatry. 2006;63:298–304.

Hofmann SG, Otto MH. Cognitive behavioral therapy for social anxiety disorder. New York: Routledge; 2008.

Huppert JD, Franklin ME, Foa EB, Davidson JR. Study refusal ¨and exclusion from a randomized treatment study of generalized social phobia. J Anxiety Disord. 2003;17: 683–93.

Keeley H, Williams C, Shapiro DA. A United Kingdom survey of accredited cognitive behaviour therapists' attitudes towards and use of structured self-help materials. Behav Cogn Psychoth. 2002;30:193–203.

Khazaal Y, Fernandez S, Cochand S, Reboh I, Zullino D. Quality of web-based information on social phobia: a cross-sectional study. Depress Anxiety. 2008;25:461–5.

Kim HY, Lundh LG, Harvey A. The enhancement of video feedback by cognitive preparation in the treatment of social anxiety. A single-session experiment. J Behav Ther Exp Psychiatry. 2002;33:19–37.

Klinger E, Bouchard S, Legeron P, Roy S, Chemin I, Nugues P. Virtual reality therapy versus cognitive behavior therapy for social phobia: a preliminary controlled study. Cyberpsychol Behav. 2005;8:76–88.

Knijnik DZ, Kapczinski F, Chachamovich E, Margis R, Eizirik CL. Psychodynamic group treatment for generalized social phobia. Rev Bras Psiquiatria. 2004;26:77–81.

Kraaimaat FW, Vanryckeghem M, Van Dam-Baggen R. Stuttering and social anxiety. J Fluency Disord. 2003;27:319–31.

Leykin Y, Derubeis RJ, Gallop R, Amsterdam JD, Shelton RC, Hollon SD. The relation of patients' treatment preferences to outcome in a randomized clinical trial. Behav Ther. 2007;38: 209–17.

Lincoln TM, Rief W, Hahlweg K, Frank M, von Witzleben I, Schroeder B, et al. Effectiveness of an empirically supported treatment for social phobia in the field. Behav Res Ther. 2003;41: 1251–69.

Mattick RP, Clarke JC. Development and validation of measures of social phobia scrutiny fear and social interaction anxiety. Behav Res Ther. 1998;36:455–70.

Mörtberg E, Berglund G, Sundin Ö. Intensive cognitive behavioural group treatment for social phobia: a pilot study. Cogn Behav Ther. 2005;36:455–70.

Mörtberg E, Clark DM, Sundin Ö, Åberg-Wisted, A. Intensive group cognitive treatment and individual cognitive therapy versus treatment as usual in social phobia: A randomized controlled study. Acta Psychiatr Scand. 2007;115:142–54.

Patel A, Knapp M, Henderson J, Baldwin D. The economic consequences of social phobia. J Affect Disord. 2002;68:221–33.

Ponniah K, Hollon SD. Empirically supported psychological interventions for social phobia in adults: a qualitative review of randomized controlled trials. Psychol Med. 2008;38:3–14.

Postel MG, de Haan HA, De Jong CA. E-therapy for mental health problems: a systematic review. Telemed e-Health. 2008;14:707–14.

Rapee RM, Abbott MJ, Baillie AJ, Gaston JE. Treatment of social phobia through pure self-help and therapist-augmented self-help. Br J Psychiatry. 2007;191:246–52.

Rodebaugh TL, Holaway RM, Heimberg RG. The treatment of social anxiety disorder. Clin Psychol Rev. 2004;24:883–908.

Ruscio AM, Brown TA, Chiu WT, Sareen J, Stein MB, Kessler RC. Social fears and social phobia in the USA: results from the national comorbidity survey replication. Psychol Med. 2008;38:15–28.

Safren SA, Heimberg RG, Brown EJ, Holle C. Quality of life in social phobia. Depress Anxiety. 1997;4:126–33.

Shear MK, Pilkonis AA, Cloitre M, Leon AC. Cognitive behavioral treatment compared with nonprescriptive treatment of panic disorder. Arch Gen Psychiatry. 1994;51: 395–401.

Shepherd R-M, Edelmann RJ. Reasons for internet use and social anxiety. Pers Indiv Differ. 2005;39:949–58.

Spek V, Cuijpers P, Nyklicek I, Riper H, Keyzer J, Pop, V. Internet-based cognitive behaviour therapy for symptoms of depression and anxiety: a meta-analysis. Psychol Med. 2007;37: 319–28.

Stangier U, Heidenreich T, Peitz M, Lauterbach W, Clark DM. Cognitive therapy for social phobia: individual versus group treatment. Behav Res Ther. 2003;41:991–1007.

Stein DJ, Ipser JC, Balkom AJ. Pharmacotherapy for social phobia. Cochrane database of systematic reviews (Online)(4), CD001206; 2004.

Taylor S. Meta-analysis of cognitive-behavioral treatments for social phobia. J Behav Ther Exp Psychiatry. 1996;27:1–9.

Tillfors M. Why do some individuals develop social phobia? A review with emphasis on the neurobiological influences. Nord J Psychiatry. 2004;58:267–76.

Tillfors M, Carlbring P, Furmark T, Lewenhaupt S, Spak M, Eriksson A, Ekselius L, Westling B, Andersson G. Treating university students with social phobia and public speaking fears: internet delivered self-help with or without live group exposure sessions. Depress Anxiety. 2008;25:708–17.

Titov N, Andrews G, Choi I, Schwencke G, Mahoney A. Shyness 3: randomized controlled trial of guided versus unguided Internet-based CBT for social phobia. Aust N Z J Psychiatry. 2008a;42:1030–40.

Titov N, Andrews G, Johnston L, Schwencke G, Choi I. Shyness programme: longer term benefits, cost-effectiveness, and acceptability. Aust N Z J Psychiatry. 2009;43:36–44.

Titov N, Andrews G, Schwencke G. Shyness 2: treating social phobia online: replication and extension. Aust N Z J Psychiatry. 2008b;42:595–605.

Titov N, Andrews G, Schwencke G, Drobny J, Einstein D. Shyness 1: distance treatment of social phobia over the Internet. Aust N Z J Psychiatry. 2008c;42:585–94.

Wakefield JC. The concept of mental disorder. On the boundary between biological facts and social values. Am Psychol. 1992;47:373–88.

van Schaik D, Klijn A, van Hout H, van Marwijk H, Beekman A, de Haan M, et al. Patients' preferences in the treatment of depressive disorder in primary care. General Hosp Psychiatry. 2004;26:184–9.

Chapter 7
Substance Abuse

Michael E. Levin and Jason Lillis

The field of substance abuse treatment includes a broad range of problems from nicotine-dependent smokers and problem drinkers to polysubstance abusing individuals with co-occurring mental health problems. Intervention needs vary across such a broad scope of clinical presentations. For example, those with mild alcohol problems are not likely to progress to more severe alcoholism (Schuckit et al., 2001) and may recover without any intervention (Cunningham, 1999). Similarly, nicotine dependence does not pose the same types of challenges involved in treating more severe problems, such as managing intense withdrawal symptoms for opiate addiction. There is a tendency to overuse more invasive and costly interventions, such as individual outpatient therapy and inpatient/residential programs, even when less intense treatments, including brief therapies, bibliotherapy, and e-health, may be successful. Considering the relatively high prevalence of substance abuse problems (SAMSHA, 2008) and the treatment needs of all these individuals, expense alone might necessitate using more cost-effective approaches. Also, treatment-seeking rates are typically low (SAMSHA, 2008) while dropout rates are high (Chappel, 1994; Pulford and Wheeler, 2007), suggesting non-traditional treatment modalities could provide benefits.

A stepped care approach could match well to the range of problems and interventions indicated in substance abuse treatment as well as provide a model for integrating lower intensity, cost-effective interventions into regular treatment procedures. The current chapter will discuss stepped care for substance abuse treatment, focusing on nicotine, drug, and alcohol abuse and dependence specifically, with an emphasis on lower step options.

Stepped Care Models in Substance Abuse Treatment

There are currently no guidelines on how to implement a comprehensive stepped care program for substance abuse. However, the available research does provide starting points regarding possible treatment options and important client

M.E. Levin (✉)
Department of Psychology, University of Nevada-Reno, Mail Stop 0298, Reno, NV 89557, USA
e-mail: levinm2@gmail.com

W.T. O'Donohue, C. Draper (eds.), *Stepped Care and e-Health*,
DOI 10.1007/978-1-4419-6510-3_7, © Springer Science+Business Media, LLC 2011

Table 7.1 Outline of
treatment steps

Watchful waiting
Brief intervention
Bibliotherapy
E-Health
Mutual help groups
Outpatient therapy
Medication
Integrated care
Inpatient and residential treatment
Combined treatments

characteristics. A proposed outline of treatment steps organized by degree of invasiveness, cost of treatment, time, and reliance on trained professionals is presented in Table 7.1. There is overlap in degree of intensity across treatment steps and micro-steps are indicated within each larger treatment category when appropriate. These treatment options can be organized in a different manner, though it is recommended that models be based on a similar set of principles and orientation to available research.

Assessment and Triage

Initial assessment should take a stepped approach, with individuals presenting with more minor problems calling for briefer assessment methods than more complex presentations. Evidence-based assessment procedures for substance abuse should be followed when possible (Allen and Wilson, 2003; Donovan and Marlatt, 2005). There are a number of factors to consider when assessing for appropriateness of stepped care options that are listed in Table 7.2.

The substance abuse treatment literature suggests that more intense treatment steps are not always more effective (e.g, Moyer et al., 2002) and expected client matching variables often do not lead to more effective treatment selection (e.g,

Table 7.2 Assessment factors

Assessment Area	Examples
Presenting problem	Substance(s) being abused/dependence, co-occurring mental and/or physical health problems
Problem severity	Degree of abuse/dependence, number of substances being abused, history of substance use and relapse
Motivation	Treatment goals, whether treatment is voluntary, motivation for change
Social environment	Availability of social support, quality of social support, degree of social support for continued substance use
Personal resources	Employment, housing, education, financial resources, insurance
Personal preferences	Preferences for treatment approach and intervention modality

Project MATCH Research Group, 1997). Based on these issues, the triage protocol emphasizes using the most pragmatic and efficient approach, with a preference toward lower levels of intervention, and consideration of consumer preferences.

Watchful Waiting

Depending on the specific problem area, there may be a significant number of individuals who naturally recover from substance abuse problems without any formal treatment. The least intensive intervention level in a stepped care model is watchful waiting, where clients continue to monitor their substance use, generally with a clinician in contact. Clients are encouraged to monitor use and check-in with a treatment provider if there is increased use, further problems, or lack of improvement.

Research shows that a significant proportion of individuals achieve or maintain low levels of use without any treatment for alcohol use problems (Cunningham, 1999), cocaine use (Cohen and Sas, 1994), and cigarette smoking (Sussman, 2002), typically with lower severity problems (Cunningham, 1999). This effect may be due in part to a regression to the mean (Finney, 2007), in which individuals seeking treatment or meeting criteria for a study are more likely to be above their average severity and thus are likely to improve naturally over time. However, it does appear that self-monitoring alone can reduce substance use (Clifford and Maisto, 2000).

Watchful waiting would only be suggested for very minor substance use problems. Clients who have more personal and social resources are more appropriate for watchful waiting (Moos and Moos, 2006). It is also important to establish a client's willingness to return for treatment if the problem worsens, as some clients may need additional intervention.

Brief Intervention

Brief interventions have been proposed as an important early step, particularly for alcohol use problems (Sobell and Sobell, 2000). Length of treatment can range from a single 5-min intervention to multiple 1-h sessions, although typically no more than four total contacts. Interventions focus on early treatment targets, such as problem perception, readiness to change, and basic behavior change strategies. Treatment goals are generally client directed and tend to focus on reduction of use rather than abstinence.

Psychoeducation is a commonly used brief intervention in which clients are provided basic information about the harmful effects of substance abuse, identifying substance use problems, how to seek help, and the effectiveness of treatment options. Assessing substance use and providing personalized feedback such as potential risks of current use and relation to social norms is another technique often used in brief interventions. Self-monitoring of substance use is routinely integrated into these interventions as well.

Motivational interviewing (MI) is commonly used and well researched. MI involves a "collaborative, person-centered form of guiding to elicit and strengthen motivation for change" (Miller and Rollnick, 2009, p. 137). A core goal of MI is to reduce ambiguity and provide a catalyst for change. Guided self-change (GSC; Sobell and Sobell, 2005) is another early, brief intervention approach for substance use problems. This treatment typically includes a combination of MI techniques, self-monitoring, personalized feedback, brief skills training, and relapse prevention.

Brief interventions have focused primarily on problematic alcohol use, though promising findings suggest efficacy for drug use and smoking cessation. A meta-analysis of studies evaluating brief interventions for alcohol problems found small to medium effect sizes compared to non-active control groups, with equivalent effect sizes compared to extended intervention approaches (Moyer et al, 2002), although effects deteriorated over time. Another meta-analysis found that very brief physician advice to quit increases smoking cessation rates at 6-month follow-up compared to standard care, with slightly higher effects for more intensive brief interventions (Stead et al., 2008). Research has also supported the application of brief interventions to drug use problems, particularly using MI (Hettema et al., 2005) and GSC (Sobell and Sobell, 2005). These findings suggest that brief interventions could be effective early step treatments.

Brief interventions can be considered the next step after watchful waiting. These interventions focus on early treatment targets, particularly problem perception and barriers to change, and can be used in conjunction with initial assessment/triage protocols. They can be implemented in a variety of contexts and often do not require a highly trained specialist. Thus the cost and expertise required for this step is relatively low. Treatment is less invasive as it is generally client directed and involves a small time commitment. Brief interventions can also be conducted through bibliotherapy, e-health, and telephone calls, which further reduce intensity.

Clients may be appropriate for brief interventions when presenting with low motivation and/or commitment to engage in change efforts or when otherwise appearing resistant. Often clients drop out relatively quickly in substance abuse treatment (Pulford and Wheeler, 2007); thus, targeting barriers to treatment early may be particularly important prior to more intensive treatment steps. Brief interventions may also be indicated for less severe presentations or individuals with substantial personal and social resources, in which minimal intervention may be sufficient to enable self-directed change. Clients may step down to watchful waiting if they successfully respond to a brief intervention. Stepping up may be indicated if the client does not have the relevant skills to initiate self-directed change, the problem is relatively severe, or if the client's social context is somehow likely to not support such improvements.

Bibliotherapy

Bibliotherapy refers to the use of any self-guided written intervention ranging from a brief brochure to a comprehensive book. There are a number of bibliotherapy resources available for substance abuse problems; however, most have little or no empirical support (Rosen et al., 2002). The majority of empirically based bibliotherapy resources are based on cognitive behavioral therapy (CBT) and typically include components such as psychoeducation, identifying and avoiding triggers, goal setting, skills training, problem solving, cognitive strategies, and relapse prevention techniques. For example, Miller and Munoz developed a bibliotherapy version of behavioral self-control training in the book *Controlling Your Drinking* (2004). The American Lung Association's *Freedom from smoking self-help manual* (1999) similarly uses a number of cognitive and behavioral technologies such as stimulus control and skills training.

Meta-analyses of bibliotherapy for alcohol problems and smoking cessation have found positive, though small, effects on reductions of problematic use and abstinence when compared to no treatment control groups (Apodaca and Miller, 2003; Lancaster and Stead, 2005a). These studies also showed that bibliotherapy may be more effective for self-referred participants and specifically tailored materials. There is currently no evidence supporting the efficacy of bibliotherapy for illicit drug use problems.

Bibliotherapy represents one of the least intensive treatments as there are minimal costs, treatment is flexible and convenient, and a trained professional is not required. As bibliotherapy includes any written intervention, there is a vast range of intensity, leaving room for multiple treatment steps to be applied within this larger category.

A client may be particularly appropriate for bibliotherapy when he or she demonstrates motivation to change substance use behavior and to engage in self-guided treatment. Also, clients with a positive social support network are likely to benefit from this step. Individuals who are unlikely to enter face-to-face treatment for substance use problems due to issues including stigma, costs, time constraints, or limited access may also be appropriate for bibliotherapy.

Bibliotherapy can also be used in later treatment phases as a step down from more intensive interventions. In cases with more complex problem presentations such as co-occurring mental health problems, bibliotherapy may be contraindicated as more flexible and intense interventions are often needed. Also, this step is not suggested for illicit drug use problems due to the lack of evidence supporting its application in this area.

E-Health

E-health interventions—treatments provided over the Internet—represent a particularly important and innovative component in stepped care. Many individuals with substance use problems do not seek or receive treatment (SAMHSA, 2008), in part due to barriers such as stigma and lack of access, suggesting that current efforts are not sufficient to meet treatment need. With e-health, evidence-based interventions can be implemented in novel formats and modalities to reach and engage a broader population of individuals with substance use problems without relying on costly training of clinicians.

There are a number of Internet sites for treating substance abuse problems; however, few have any empirical support and many are not based on empirically supported intervention components or methods. E-health programs vary substantially in intervention intensity depending on the treatment model and problem being targeted. At the lowest level of intervention, web sites are available that provide psychoeducation and treatment referral information such as the WebMD alcohol abuse center (http://www.webmd.com/mental-health/alcohol-abuse/) and the American Lung Association (http://www.lungusa.org/). Mutual help programs are also available online and can be found through web sites such as Nicotine Anonymous' site (http://www.nicotine-anonymous.org/). Similar professionally moderated online peer groups have been developed such as Alcohol Help Center (Cunningham et al., 2008; http://www.alcoholhelpcenter.net/).

More intense programs can be sub-divided into brief or extended intervention models. There have been several brief intervention programs developed to screen and provide feedback on alcohol use such as the Drinker's Check-Up (DCU; http://www.drinkerscheckup.com) and the e-Check Up to Go (E-CHUG, http://www.e-chug.com). These interventions are relatively short and of low intensity, designed to provide an initial starting point for changing patterns of alcohol use. Similarly, a program for reducing drug use with postpartum women implements a brief motivational intervention called the Motivational Enhancement System (MES; Ondersma et al., 2005) that includes feedback regarding use, discussing pros and cons of change, and optional goal setting.

E-health developers have also focused on transferring more intensive, evidence-based CBT packages to a web-based format, called computerized CBT (CCBT). For example, Committed Quitters stop-smoking plan (CQ PLAN; Strecher et al., 2005) uses a range of CBT techniques to assist with smoking cessation including relapse prevention, stimulus control, and coping skills training as well as follow-up newsletters and support messages. Drinking Less (Riper et al., 2008) is a multi-component e-health intervention combining CBT and self-control technologies as well as peer interaction features. Computer-Based Training in CBT (CBT4CBT; Carroll et al., 2008) is a recently developed program for substance dependence disorders. The program includes modules targeting maladaptive cognitions related to substance use, psychoeducation, and skills training. E-health has even be used to implement a monitored contingency management program for smoking, in which clients are provided vouchers that can be redeemed for gifts by passing CO_2 screenings conducted from home with a concurrent web camera to ensure fidelity (Dallery and Glenn, 2005).

The outcome evidence is largely supportive of e-health approaches for substance abuse problems. Brief computerized interventions for problematic alcohol use have been found to reduce problem drinking in several studies (Hester et al., 2005; Doumas et al., 2009; Saitz et al., 2007). For example, a study by Hester and colleagues (2005) found that DCU led to an approximate 50% reduction in the quantity and frequency of alcohol use by 12-month follow-up, partially due to the high rate of treatment seeking after completion of DCU (approximately 40%).

Another study with mandated college students found that a brief web-based intervention involving assessment and personalized feedback led to significant effects on perceived drinking norms and alcohol use compared to a psychoeducational web site comparison group (Doumas et al., 2009). Similarly, brief e-health interventions for smoking have been found to increase cessation rates. A study by Swartz and colleagues (2006) randomized participants to a brief one-session e-health intervention tailored to user characteristics or to a waitlist control group, with those completing the intervention demonstrating significantly higher abstinence rates (12.3 vs. 5%) at 3-month follow-up. Fewer studies have evaluated the impact of brief interventions for drug use, though one series of studies found that MES for postpartum women reporting illicit drug use significantly increased state motivation (Ondersma et al., 2005) and reduced frequency of drug use (Ondersma et al., 2007).

Research has also found significant support for the impact of more intensive, multi-session e-health interventions for substance use problems. For example, a study by Riper and colleagues (2008) tested the impact of an online CCBT for alcohol use with no therapist contact in a randomized trial with 261 adult problem drinkers, finding that those randomized to the intervention reported significantly lower alcohol use at 6-month follow-up compared to a psychoeducational control group. CCBT programs for smoking cessation have generally been found to produce increased abstinence rates, particularly when tailored to user characteristics, though research has not compared interventions to active control conditions (McDaniel and Stratton, 2006). For example, a study by Strecher et al. (2005) found significantly higher user satisfaction ratings and continuous abstinence rates (23 vs. 19% at 12-week follow-up) with an intervention tailored to user characteristics compared to a non-tailored design. There have been few CCBT programs developed and tested for drug problems and substance dependence. However, a series of studies (Carroll et al., 2008, 2009) found that a CCBT program for substance dependence, in combination with standard care, increased the number of clean drug screenings, duration of abstinence from use, and engagement in treatment following the 8-week intervention compared to standard care alone, with similar findings at up to 6-month follow-up. It is important to note that the efficacy of e-health approaches vary depending on the specific population, treatment approach, and design features of the site.

Treatment dropout is a general concern with self-guided approaches and including some degree of personal contact can reduce the potential for attrition. A stepped approach applies here as well since individuals vary in their need for personal contact, with many only requiring brief contact such as through emails and phone calls and some requiring nothing at all. For example, a study by Bischof and colleagues (2008) examined the impact of providing brief telephone intervention sessions added as a step-up for treatment non-responders with an e-health intervention targeting alcohol use. The study found that at-risk alcohol users in the stepped care program reported similar outcomes, while reducing staff time in half, compared to a group where participants all received the full intervention (e-health and all three phone sessions). In fact, a significant proportion of participants only required the brief screening and feedback component to achieve treatment gains and did not require any subsequent personal contact.

E-health has a unique place in a stepped care model. Based on factors such as cost and need for professional contact, e-health is a relatively early step. E-health programs using psychoeducation and brief interventions can be placed particularly low in a stepped care model and can even be used at a community level to identify and engage potential clients into treatment. However, e-health can also be used to implement relatively intense and time-consuming treatments for clients. Thus, one may consider steps within the e-health modality including, psychoeducation, brief interventions, online support groups, and more intense treatment.

E-health is appropriate for individuals with similar characteristics as those indicated for bibliotherapy. One may consider client preferences and available treatment resources when deciding between these two modalities. E-health may be more beneficial than bibliotherapy in some cases, such as with clients reporting lower motivation or more severe and complex problem presentations due to the ability to include treatment tailoring and interactive, engaging content.

Similar to bibliotherapy, e-health may be particularly indicated for individuals with problematic drinking and nicotine dependence. There is limited, albeit promising evidence supporting the use of e-health with illicit drug use and substance dependence problems.

The anonymity, ease and convenience of accessibility, and low cost provided with e-health makes it especially helpful in treating individuals with substance abuse problems who are unlikely to seek or continue with more traditional approaches. These interventions can be easily scaled to a public health level for these reasons as well as the fact that the number of users generally has minimal impact on service delivery. E-health is thus an important factor to consider in solving the current problems in the substance abuse treatment delivery system.

Mutual Help Groups

Community-based, peer-led groups have been a mainstay of substance abuse treatment. The most well-known mutual help groups are 12-step groups such as Alcoholics Anonymous (AA) and Narcotics Anonymous (NA). Important features of these groups include a focus on abstinence as opposed to harm reduction and an appeal to a greater power for strength. Clinical psychologists have also developed evidence-based mutual help groups such as Self-Management and Recovery Training, which is adapted from CBT.

There is limited conclusive data regarding the efficacy of mutual help groups, in large part due to the methodological problems in many of the available outcome studies (Fiorentine, 1999). Several naturalistic studies have found that attending 12-step groups is associated with decreases in alcohol and drug use, particularly if participation is regular and enduring (Moos et al., 2001; Moos and Moos, 2004; Fiorentine, 1999; Gossop et al., 2007), and that these effects do not appear to be attributable to motivational confounds or simultaneous activities (Fiorentine,

1999). Unfortunately, roughly 50% of participants drop out within the first 3 months (Chappel, 1994). Overall, the current evidence suggests mutual help groups can be beneficial for some clients, but one should be cautious and continue to monitor client substance use and ongoing participation when possible.

Mutual help groups require a significant time commitment from clients and can be relatively intense treatment at times. However, this approach does not place a burden on treatment providers and incurs minimal costs. Thus, the approach is considered to be one of the lower steps. Mutual help often functions as an adjunctive component to outpatient care or as a later phase of treatment to help maintain gains and prevent relapse.

Due to the lack of clear evidence for mutual help groups, other low-step intervention options are generally suggested. Clients who appear particularly in need of direct social support and otherwise seem to be a good fit for lower step intervention may be indicated for mutual help groups. Client motivation and likelihood of continued and regular meeting attendance is important to assess based on the available outcome data. Twelve-step groups in particular may be contraindicated for clients who are uncomfortable with a spiritual emphasis.

Outpatient Therapy

Outpatient treatment represents a relatively broad set of intervention approaches and modalities. Treatment may include group, individual, and couples/family interventions. Evidence-based treatments are primarily a form of CBT, which focuses on targeting the antecedents and consequences controlling substance use behaviors, as well as skill deficits related to use such as coping and social skills. Specific treatment approaches and components include stimulus control, cue exposure, skills training, cognitive restructuring, problem solving, behavioral contracting, relapse prevention, and couples and family techniques. Contingency management has been successfully used in outpatient treatment programs as well, which involves the provision of positive reinforcing consequences, typically monetary or other material incentives, contingent upon abstinence or reduced use.

Recent meta-analysis have found strong support for the efficacy of contingency management (Griffith et al., 2000; Plebani Lussier et al., 2006), group and individual CBT (Dutra et al., 2008; Stead and Lancaster, 2005; Lancaster and Stead, 2005b), family therapy techniques (Powers et al., 2008; Stanton and Shadish, 1997), and relapse prevention (Irvin et al., 1999) for substance abuse problems. Medium effect sizes are generally observed compared to active and inactive control conditions across meta-analysis on outcomes including abstinence, reduced use, psychological distress, and general life functioning, with some variations depending on specific problem area. Polysubstance use is especially difficult to treat with outpatient therapy, with many meta-analyses finding lower or insignificant effect sizes. Relapse is a significant problem in substance abuse treatment as well. For example, long-term abstinence rates for smoking cessation interventions typically range from 10 to 30%, with a significant percent not responding to treatment or relapsing after treatment (Fiore et al., 2000).

The degree of intensity, cost, and time required for outpatient, face-to-face treatment places it at one of the higher steps within a stepped care model. One of the goals of reviewing stepped care for substance abuse problems is to heighten awareness of the range of potential lower intensity interventions that can be implemented prior to these more traditional modalities.

Clients presenting with more severe and/or complex substance abuse problems are indicated for this step. Outpatient therapy, especially CBT, can be for a broad range of problem presentations including those resistant to less intense forms of treatment, such as drug and alcohol dependence. Problems related to a client's social environment, such as marital or family conflicts, may indicate the need for couples/family care. When the treatment resources are available, contingency management is suggested. Clients lacking coping, problem solving, or social skills may be indicated for CBT due to its focus on skills training.

Medication

Pharmacotherapy is a primary treatment modality for many substance use problems. Smoking cessation medications include bupropion and nicotine replacement therapies such as nicotine patches and gums, which serve to reduce craving and withdrawal effects. Alcohol medication treatments include opiate antagonists such as naltrexone to reduce cravings, medications that produce adverse reactions to alcohol such as disulfiram (Antabuse), and acamprosate, which may reduce withdrawal symptoms. Medications for opiate dependence include methadone and buprenorphine, which primarily serve to block craving and withdrawal symptoms.

Meta-analysis of outcome trials for alcohol dependence has found substantially higher rates of abstinence with acamprosate and lower relapse rates with naltrexone compared to placebo conditions (Bouza et al., 2004; Mann et al., 2004). Research has generally found that disulfiram can decrease frequency of alcohol use if it is adhered to correctly, though it is unclear whether the medication enhances long-term abstinence rates (Rosenthal, 2006). Research has also supported the efficacy of methadone and buprenorphine in the treatment of opiate addiction, with a recent meta-analysis finding substantially lower use and attrition rates than placebo medications (Mattick et al., 2008). Differences in efficacy between methadone and buprenorphine varied depending on medication dosages, with slightly better effects with methadone on attrition and reductions in heroin use when dosage levels were matched. According to recent reviews, there are no empirically supported safe and effective pharmacological interventions for psychostimulant dependence (Preti, 2007).

A meta-analysis of interventions for smoking cessation found approximately twice the rate of smoking abstinence for those receiving medications such as bupropion and nicotine replacement compared to those receiving placebo (Fiore et al.,

2000). However, the meta-analysis consisted of tightly controlled research studies, which employ methods to ensure proper adherence to medication and sometimes include adjunctive behavioral interventions. Individuals in "real-world" settings often report high levels of non-adherence with treatment recommendations, which can substantially decrease efficacy (Shaw et al., 1998; Orleans et al., 1994)

A stepped care approach may be used within medication treatments in some cases. For example, the increased risk for mortality posed by methadone treatment has led some providers to prescribe buprenorphine, a safer, yet potentially less effective treatment. A randomized trial by Kakko and colleagues (2007) implemented a stepped care program where individuals were first treated with the lower step buprenorphine, with doses being increased and treatment eventually moving to methadone if clients did not demonstrate sufficient improvements. The study found equivalent outcomes with the stepped care approach compared to individuals who were all treated with methadone maintenance, despite the fact that only half of the clients in the stepped care condition were eventually treated with methadone.

Medications are placed fairly high in a stepped care model due to the degree of invasiveness, cost, and potential for side effects. Methadone can be fatal if misused and some medications, such as antabuse, even have intended adverse effects on clients. Nicotine replacement treatment is one of the few exceptions as it can be self-administered and used as an early step in treatment.

Medications for alcohol problems such as acamprosate and naltrexone are generally indicated for alcohol dependency. In the case of opiate dependence, providing methadone or buprenorphine is recommended. Medications for smoking are also generally recommended due to their empirical support and low intensity. Pharmacotherapy is usually not recommended without adjunctive counseling, particularly if the client appears unlikely to adhere to the medication treatment plan.

Integrated Care

Many individuals with substance abuse problems also have co-occurring physical and mental health problems. Adjunctive care for these problems is insufficient in some cases given the limitations of ensuring compliance. Integrated care provides another solution. Integrated care involves the collaboration of a multidisciplinary team including medical staff and clinicians specializing in substance abuse and mental health problems. Co-occurring problems can be treated in this framework either sequentially, concurrently, or even simultaneously at the client level. Treatment for each problem area is provided through services located within the same organization or through a network of care, enhancing communication between treatment components and ensuring consistent, effective treatment.

Research to date has generally shown that providing integrative treatments for co-occurring mental disorders can lead to improved outcomes on substance use, mental health, and general functioning compared to targeted treatment for substance abuse or mental health alone (Drake et al., 2004). There has been less research examining the efficacy of integrated care in treating co-occurring physical problems, but available research suggests it may be beneficial in increasing treatment adherence/retention with difficult-to-treat populations (O'Toole et al., 2005) and producing higher abstinence rates (Weisner et al., 2001).

Integrated care falls into one of the highest treatment steps due to the costs, professional time, and intensity involved in such treatment. Clients with serious physical health problems are likely to fit within this step, particularly if the problem is chronic and requires ongoing medical attention. Similarly, clients with more severe co-occurring mental health problems, which are unlikely to be effectively treated with adjunct care, may be indicated for this step.

Residential and Inpatient Treatment

Residential and inpatient programs are used in the treatment of more severe substance abuse problems and typically provide 24-h care/staff monitoring lasting for several weeks. Residential/inpatient programs are designed to remove clients from ineffective environments that support substance abuse and establish a healthier environment that supports clinical change.

Studies have found positive effects with residential/inpatient programs for substance abuse problems. For example, Greenfield and colleagues (2004) examined three national studies, finding between 68 and 71% of women who completed 6 months or more of long-term residential treatment achieved abstinence and that longer stays correlated with increased probability of abstinence at post-treatment. Comparisons between outpatient and residential/inpatient programs suggest generally equivalent outcomes, with more severe cases sometimes demonstrating higher post-treatment abstinence rates in residential/inpatient care (Harrison and Asche, 1999).

Clients may be appropriate for this level of care if they demonstrate high problem severity, lack resources such as housing, or have a particularly negative social environment. Practical factors, including whether the client can miss work and how treatment will be paid for, should also be considered when deciding to use this highly intensive step.

Clients typically step down to outpatient treatment or mutual help programs after residential/inpatient programs to support and consolidate treatment gains. However, many clients do not attend recommended programs once residential treatment is completed, which is important to address with clients during discharge planning.

Combined Treatment Components

Intervention steps may be combined in some cases to enhance treatment effects. Research has found that combining e-health and bibliotherapy modalities with either extended or brief interventions is an effective approach for treating substance abuse problems (Apodaca and Miller, 2003; Carroll et al., 2008, 2009; Cunningham et al., 2001). Studies have also suggested that combining 12-step groups and individual care may be more effective in achieving and maintaining abstinence than either treatment alone, particularly when outpatient therapy has a 12-step orientation (Fiorentine and Hillhouse, 2000; Humphreys et al., 1999).

Medications are often combined with outpatient treatment for substance abuse problems. At a minimum, brief counseling should accompany pharmacotherapy, particularly for opiate dependence problems. Research supports the efficacy of stepped care approaches, such as motivated stepped care (MSC; Brooner et al., 2004), which combines individual and group counseling with methadone maintenance to provide flexible treatment targets and interventions, including the use of behavioral contingencies to enhance treatment adherence (Brooner et al., 2004, 2007).

Combined treatments generally represent more intense treatment steps, although they vary depending on the specific combination. Clients may be particularly indicated for combining self-help programs with outpatient therapy when they are unlikely to engage in treatment without social support, present with severe co-occurring problems, or when treatment resources are limited. Combined pharmacological and outpatient treatment is often indicated when medical interventions are provided, particularly when there are concerns about adherence to medications. More severe problems such as alcohol dependence and opiate dependence also often require a combination of medical interventions targeting craving and withdrawal symptoms and behavioral intervention.

Adjunctive Therapy Components

Individuals with substance abuse problems often experience additional problems such as unemployment, homelessness, and health problems. Adjunctive treatments include the range of intervention components and outside resources that can be implemented such as detoxification, case management, basic health care, and mental health treatment. These treatments are not listed in a specific place within a stepped care model as they may be implemented throughout treatment and vary on level of intensity.

Detoxification is an initial treatment for current intoxication and withdrawal symptoms and can be conducted on an inpatient or outpatient basis, depending on severity of symptoms (Center for Substance Abuse Treatment, 2006). The goals of treatment are to help the client reach a stable physiological state by establishing short-term sobriety and reducing or eliminating withdrawal symptoms as well as connecting patients to further treatment. Frequent monitoring is important, as symptom intensity cannot necessarily be predicted. For outpatient detoxification, family members or friends should be involved. Patients without reliable social resources or housing should be monitored on an inpatient basis by trained clinical staff.

Some individuals with substance abuse problems may have further barriers to treatment, such as being homeless or unemployed. Adjunctive case management may be indicated to help identify and establish linkages to necessary community resources. Case management has been shown to increase successful treatment link-ages for individuals who struggle with additional factors such as being involved in the criminal justice system (Rhodes and Gross, 1997) and low-income mothers receiving welfare (Morgenstern et al., 2006). Research has found that case manage-ment can produce higher treatment linkage rates than other active interventions such as MI (Rapp et al., 2008). Case management and detoxification are often provided in combination.

Treatment for co-occurring physical and/or mental health problems may also be included as an adjunctive component. This differs from integrative care as interven-tion is implemented by a separate treatment provider. Individuals may be provided with adjunctive care rather than integrated care if the problem is less severe, if the client is likely to adhere to recommended adjunctive services, or if integrated care is simply unavailable.

Consumer Preferences

Client preference is an important factor to consider when making stepped care deci-sions. Although differences in treatment efficacy are sometimes observed depending on problem and treatment comparison, there are also many cases where there are no clinically significant differences in outcomes across treatment steps. In these cases, ensuring retention and adherence to treatment is more important and can be enhanced by matching client preferences.

There is little data on consumer preferences for substance abuse treatments and one should assess a client's preferences whenever possible. Examining treatment usage patterns provides some insight. Self- and mutual help approaches, particularly 12-step programs, appear to be popular treatment modalities. One study estimated that approximately 25 million American adults participate in a non-professional-led mutual help group in their lifetime, with substance abuse groups accounting for one-third of individuals and 70% of total participation (Kessler et al., 1997). A survey of over 1,100 smokers, not necessarily seeking treatment, found that 3% were currently using self-help materials and 28% reported using them in the past (Curry et al., 1995). Individuals often use the Internet for receiving health-related information and it has been estimated that approximately 7% (around 10.1 million) searched for information related to smoking cessation in 2004 alone (Fox, 2005). Medications for smoking cessation appear to be frequently used as well with one study estimating that in the United States over 8 million attempts to quit smok-ing included the use of medication in 1998, many of which were self-administered (Centers for Disease Control and Prevention, 2000). Thus, self- and mutual help groups are frequently used by consumers and appear to be an acceptable, if not preferred, form of treatment, particularly for smoking cessation.

Based on characteristics of treatment steps, some general inferences can be made about consumer preferences for particular interventions. The popularity of self- and mutual-guided approaches may be attributable in part to features including anonymity, flexibility and convenience, and the potential to modulate the intensity of intervention. Client characteristics such as comfort participating in groups, experience/access to a computer, and reading ability may further impact specific preferences. Brief interventions are likely to be met with a higher degree of consumer satisfaction for individuals who are more resistant or unsure about treatment, due to the client-centered approach.

We would caution, however, against basing treatment decisions solely on consumer preferences. Clients may be in treatment involuntarily or ambivalent about change, and decisions may be affected by factors such as intoxication or withdrawal symptoms. The purpose of clients' stated preferences could be unclear. To account for this, consumer preference should be balanced with evidence-based treatment decisions, particularly with clients who are more likely to state a preference for ineffective treatments.

Triage Agenda

The triage agenda consists of two phases. The first involves initial treatment matching to level of care. We have reviewed a range of potential characteristics that may indicate optimal level of care, problem area and severity, client motivational factors, social environment, personal resources, and personal preferences.

The second phase involves deciding when to move a client to an increased or decreased level of care. Criterion for moving clients differs depending on the presenting problem and may include non-response or increase in problem severity, non-adherence to treatment, or increase in relevant risk factors. Non-adherence to treatment is particularly problematic in substance abuse treatment (Brooner et al., 2004) and is critical to address in order to ensure adequate treatment as well as client safety. Criterion based on risk factors can be identified through prospective studies. For example, Breslin and colleagues (1997) found that alcohol use during treatment predicted negative outcomes, and thus these patients could be identified for more intense treatment steps earlier on in a stepped model (Breslin et al., 1999). Early response to treatment may be a particularly useful criterion for further stepped care decisions.

Treatment changes can be made by either modifying the quantity of treatment or the treatment modality. Changes in quantity can include increasing the number of sessions, frequency of sessions, or moving to a more intense intervention within the same treatment step. One may weigh factors such as client's preference, the effects from current treatment, and the availability of treatment options in deciding between potential changes (Sobell and Sobell, 2000).

An important consideration for triage protocols is that there can be significant costs for matching a client at too low on a stepped care model. Failure to make treatment gains due to insufficient treatment may frustrate clients, reduce self-efficacy and motivation, and increase likelihood of dropout. For example, Berner and colleagues (2008) found very high dropout rates in a stepped care program for alcohol dependence, which they attributed in part to a low-intensity intervention and waiting too long to move to a more intensive step.

Considering stage of treatment, such as screening/detoxification, acute treatment, and maintenance/relapse prevention, is important as well. Substance abuse problems are often chronic and recurring, demanding a particular emphasis on relapse prevention and ongoing monitoring in treatment, which can also be implemented in a stepped fashion. Using less intensive treatments that can be extended over long periods of time such as extended monitoring, phone counseling, mutual help, or self-help programs are highly effective. Clients more likely to relapse and those reporting "slips" or high urges to use may be treated with more intensive steps such as in-person relapse prevention or booster sessions.

Research Agenda

The current evidence supporting the use of stepped care models, and lower step interventions in general, suggests this is a viable approach. Yet, substantial research is needed in order to reach clear, evidence-based guidelines. Research to date has not adequately answered the larger questions of stepped care including what treatments should be included, how treatments should be sequenced, who would benefit from which step, when and how someone should change steps in treatment, and the effectiveness of stepped care models in general. However, in large part these questions represent part of a struggle within clinical psychology to answer a question that was best put forward by Gordon Paul: "What treatment, by whom, is most effective for this individual with that specific problem under which set of circumstances, and how does this come about?" (Paul, 1969, p. 44). The research needed to study the vast number of potential combinations of assessment factors, decision points, specific presenting problems, and treatment approaches is staggering, particularly when one considers that each of these points is a moving target that continues to include more and more points of interest. Many promising approaches have produced inconclusive results (i.e., Project MATCH Research Group, 1997), and the currently available literature suggests that treatment matching based on client characteristics does not enhance efficacy. Some researchers have stated that this is a problem of scientific strategy and that a new approach is needed (Morgenstern and McKay, 2007).

We believe that what is missing is a functional understanding of the critical processes underlying substance abuse problems and treatment. Without a functional understanding of problems and treatments, researchers and practitioners alike are left basing treatment matching decisions on topographical features such as number of sessions and in-person vs. self-guided approaches. The alternative avoids testing every possible combination of problem presentation and intervention, instead taking a strategic approach to theoretical and technological development. Increasing our understanding of basic, functional processes can provide a means to answering the essential questions put forth for stepped care by reducing empirical tests and clinicians' decisions to a small set of important processes and characteristics. This can then be used to develop a limited set of flexible, evidence-based principles to inform stepped care decision making. The substance abuse field continues to make substantial steps in this direction, such as the increasing focus on mechanisms of change and translational research.

Innovative developments within e-health may also greatly enhance researchers' ability to study the complex interaction of factors within stepped care models. The ability to implement highly complex treatment tailoring through computerized interventions allows for the use of cutting edge research methodologies from other fields such as Multiphase Optimization Strategy (MOST) and Sequential Multiple Assignment Randomized Trial (SMART) (Collins et al., 2007). These methodologies allow an efficient means of testing multiple components and treatment decision factors and have recently been applied to substance abuse treatment programs with great success (Stretcher et al., 2008).

Finally, the emphasis on continuous assessment within stepped care models can be used to significantly improve the research base. The focus on assessment not only supports treatment providers, but can enhance our understanding of how best to implement stepped care decisions if shared with the larger community. This data can also be used to establish quality improvement benchmarks, a feature largely missing from the current literature on substance abuse treatment. Models for integrating comprehensive and research-oriented assessment into practice guidelines for substance abuse treatment programs have been implemented in some places (Schippers et al., 2002).

Dissemination Agenda

Substance abuse is a public health problem and requires public health solutions. To date, few treatment providers use evidence-based practices (Garner, 2009), suggesting significant deficits in dissemination and training. In addition, treatment-seeking rates are low. Self-help and mutual help programs provide the potential for scalable interventions, yet systems of care are needed that can support those for whom such interventions are not sufficient. A stepped care model can integrate these approaches representing an efficient, ethical, and cost-effective method for impacting substance abuse at a public health level.

The inherent logic in stepped care models as well as the potential promise to enhance outcomes, both clinically and in terms of healthcare costs, will make their acceptance over time likely. However, beyond the mere acceptance of stepped care models there are complex and challenging barriers to actual implementation that must be overcome. One consideration is how to maintain fidelity with practice guidelines and triage protocols. The lack of clear direction in the research literature results in a heavy reliance on clinical decision making. There is thus a need for the development of training strategies and implementation programs for making effective stepped care decisions. For example, whenever possible, decision-making principles should be developed that are relatively simple in order to ensure adherence.

Another issue is developing ways for healthcare providers and systems of care to actually implement a complete stepped care model given the broad range of treatment services it entails and the need for close patient monitoring. One method that has been proposed for stepped care treatment with substance abuse problems is the core-shell model (Schippers et al., 2002), in which there is a primary provider who monitors and guides patients to relevant treatment services. Another potential option is to educate the public directly so that consumers match themselves to the available stepped care treatments.

Stepped care models offer the promise for a system of treatment that can better respond to the public health problem of substance abuse. Further research is needed to develop effective practice guidelines and there are significant barriers to dissemination that still must be overcome. Ultimately the dissemination of stepped care treatment for substance abuse will require the cooperation and drive from a number of sources including consumers, treatment providers, healthcare systems, insurers, and governing bodies.

References

Allen JP, Wilson VB. Assessing alcohol problems: a guide for clinicians and researchers. 2nd ed. U.S. department of health and human services; 2003.

American Lung Association. Freedom from smoking self-help manual. New York: American Lung Association; 1999.

Apodaca TR, Miller WR. A meta-analysis of the effectiveness of bibliotherapy for alcohol problems. J Clin Psychol. 2003;59(3):289–304.

Berner M, Gunzler C, Frick K, Kriston L, Loessl B, Bruck R, et al, Finding the ideal place for a psychotherapeutic intervention in a stepped care approach—a brief overview of the literature and preliminary results from the Project PREDICT. Int J MethodPsych. 2008;17(S1): S60–4.

Bischof G, Grothues JM, Reinhardt S, Meyer C, John U, Rumpf HJ. Evaluation of a telephone-based stepped care intervention for alcohol-related disorders: a randomized controlled trial. Drug Alcohol Depen. 2008;93:244–51.

Breslin FC, Sobell MB, Sobell LC, Buchan G, Cunningham JA. Toward a stepped-care approach to treating problem drinkers: the predictive utility of within treatment variables and therapist prognosis ratings. Addiction, 1997;92:1479–85.

Breslin FC, Sobell MB, Sobell LC, Cunningham JA, Sdao-Jarvie K, Borsoi, D. Problem drinkers: evaluation of a stepped-care approach. J Subst Abuse. 1999;10(3):217–32.

Brooner RK, Kidorf MS, King VL, Stoller KB, Neufeld KJ, Kolodner K. (2007). Comparing adaptive stepped care and monetary-based voucher interventions for opioid dependence. Drug Alcohol Depen. 2007;88S:S14–23.

Brooner RK, Kidorf MS, King VL, Peirce JM, Bigelow GE, Kolodner K, A modified "stepped care" approach to improve attendance behavior in treatment seeking opioid abusers. J Subst Abuse Treat. 2004;27:223–32.

Bouza C, Angeles M, Muñoz A, Amate JM. Efficacy and safety of naltrexone and acamprosate in the treatment of alcohol dependence: a systematic review. Addiction. 2004;99:811–28.

Carroll KM, Ball SA, Martino S, Nich C, Babuscio TA, Nuro KF, et al. Computer-assisted delivery of cognitive-behavioral therapy for addiction: a randomized trial of CBT4CBT. Am J Psychiatry. 2008;165:881–8.

Carroll KM, Ball SA, Martino S, Nich C, Babuscio BJ, Rounsaville BJ. Enduring effects of a computer-assisted training program for cognitive behavioral therapy: a 6-month follow-up of CBT4CBT. Drug Alcohol Depen. 2009;100:178–81.

Centers for Disease Control and Prevention. Use of FDA-approved pharmacological treatments for tobacco dependence—United States, 1984–1998. Morbid Mortal Week Rep. 2000;49: 665–8.

Center for Substance Abuse Treatment. Detoxification and substance abuse treatment. treatment improvement protocol (TIP) Series 45. DHHS Publication No. (SMA) 06-4131. Rockville, MD: Substance Abuse and Mental Health Services Administration; 2006.

Chappel JN. Working a program of recovery in alcoholics anonymous, J Subst Abuse Treat. 1994;11:99–104.

Clifford PR, Maisto SA. Subject reactivity effects and alcohol treatment outcome research. J Stud Alcohol. 2000;61(6):787–93.

Cohen P, Sas A. Cocaine use in Amsterdam in non-deviant subcultures. Addict Res. 1994;2:71–94.

Collins LM, Murphy SA, Strecher V. The multiphase optimizing strategy (MOST) and the sequential multiple assignment randomized trial (SMART): new methods for more potent eHealth interventions. Am J Prev Med. 2007;32:S112–8.

Cunningham JA, Sdao-Jarvie K, Koski-Jannes A, Breslin FC. Using self-help materials to motivate change at assessment for alcohol treatment. J Subst Abuse Treat. 2001;20:301–4.

Cunningham JA. Resolving alcohol-related problems with and without treatment: the effects of different problem criteria. J Stud Alcohol. 1999;60:463–6.

Cunningham JA, Mierlo TV, Fournier R. An online support group for problem drinkers: AlcoholHelpCenter.net. Patient Educ Couns. 2008;70:193–8.

Curry SJ, McBride C, Grothaus LC, Louie D, Wagner E. A randomized trial of self-help materials, personalized feedback and telephone counseling with nonvolunteer smokers. J Consult Clin Psychol. 1995;63:1005–14.

Dallery J, Glenn IM. Effects of an Internet-based voucher reinforcement program for smoking abstinence: a feasibility study. J Appl Behav Anal. 2005;38:349–57.

Donovan DM, Marlatt GA. Assessment of addictive behaviors. 2nd ed. The Guilford Press; 2005.

Doumas DM, McKinley LL, Book P. Evaluation of two web-based alcohol interventions for mandated college students. J Subst Abuse Treat. 2009;36:65–74.

Drake RE, Mueser KT, Brunette M, McHugo GJ. A review of treatments for people with severe mental illness and co-occurring substance use disorder. Psychiatr Rehabil J. 2004;27:360–74.

Dutra L, Stathopoulou G, Basden SL, Leyro TM, Powers MB, Otto MW. A meta-analytic review of psychosocial interventions for substance use disorders. Am J Psychiatry. 2008;165(2): 179–87.

Finney JW. Regression to the mean in substance use disorder treatment research. Addiction. 2007;103:42–52.

Fiore MC, Bailey WC, Cohen SJ, Dorfman SF, Goldstein MG, Gritz ER, et al. (2000). Treating tobacco use and dependence. clinical practice guideline. Rockville, MD: U.S. Department of Health and Humans Services, Public Health Service; 2000.

Fiorentine R. After drug treatment: are 12-step programs effective in maintaining abstinence? Am J Drug Alcohol Abuse. 1999;25:93–116.

Fiorentine R, Hillhouse M.P. Drug treatment and 12-step program participation: the additive effects of integrated recovery activities. J Subst Abuse Treat. 2000;18(1):65–74.

Fox S. (2005). The online health care revolution: how the web helps Americans take better care of themselves. Retrieved 2005, 2005, from URL: http://www.pewinternet.org/reports/pdfs/PIP_Health_Report.pdf

Garner BR. Research on the diffusion of evidence-based treatments within substance abuse treatment: a systematic review. J Subst Abuse Treat. 2009;36(4):376–99.

Gossop M, Stewart D, Marsden J. Attendance at narcotics anonymous and alcoholics anonymous meetings, frequency of attendance and substance use outcomes after residential treatment for drug dependence: a 5-year follow-up study. Addiction. 2007;103:119–25.

Greenfield L, Burgdorf K, Chen X, Porowski A, Roberts T, Herrell J. Effectiveness of long-term residential substance abuse treatment for women: findings from three national studies. Am J Drug Alcohol Abuse. 2004;30(3):537–50.

Griffith JD, Rowan-Szal GA, Roark RR, Simpson DD. Contingency management in outpatient methadone treatment: a meta-analysis. Drug Alcohol Depen. 2000;58:55–66.

Harrison PA, Asche SE. Comparison of substance abuse treatment outcomes for inpatients and outpatients. J Subst Abuse Treat. 1999;17(3):207–20.

Hester RK, Squires DD, Delaney HD. The drinker's check-up: 12-month outcomes of a controlled clinical trial of a stand-alone software program for problem drinkers. J Subst Abuse Treat. 2205;28(2):159–69.

Hettema J, Steele J, Miller WR. Motivational interviewing. Ann Rev Clin Psychol. 2005;1:91–111.

Humphreys K, Huebsch P, Finney J, Moos R. A comparative evaluation of substance abuse treatment: V. Substance abuse treatment can enhance the effectiveness of self-help groups. Alcohol Clin Exp Res. 1999;23:558–63.

Irvin JE, Bowers CA, Dunn ME, Wong MC. Efficacy of relapse prevention: a meta-analytic review. J Consult Clin Psychol. 1999;67:563–70.

Kakko J, Gronbladh L, Svanborg KD, Wachenfeldt JV, Ruck C, Rawlings B, et al. A stepped care strategy using buprenorphine and methadone versus conventional methadone maintenance in heroin dependence: a randomized controlled trial. Am J Psychiatry. 2007;164:797–803.

Kessler RC, Mickelson RD, Zhao S. Patterns and correlates of self-help group membership in the United States. Soc Policy. 1997;27:27–46.

Lancaster T, Stead LF. Self-help interventions for smoking cessation. Cochrane Database Syst Rev. 2005a;3.

Lancaster T, Stead L. Individual Behavioural Counselling for Smoking Cessation. Cochrane Database of Syst Rev. 2005b;2.

Mann K, Lehert P, Morgan MY. The efficacy of acamprosate in the maintenance of abstinence in alcohol-dependent individuals: results of a meta-analysis. Alcohol Clin Exp Res. 2004;28:51–63.

Mattick RP, Kimber J, Breen C, Davoli M. Buprenorphine maintenance versus placebo or methadone maintenance for opioid dependence. Cochrane Database of Systematic Reviews. 2008;2.

McDaniel AM, Stratton RM. Internet-based smoking cessation initiatives: availability, varieties, and likely effects on outcomes. Dis Manag Health Out. 2006;14(5):275–85.

Miller WR, Munoz RF. Controlling your drinking: tools to make moderation work for you. The Guilford Press; 2004.

Miller WR, Rollnick S. Ten things that motivational interviewing is not. Behav Cogn Psychoth. 2009;37:129–40.

Moos RH, Moos BS. Rates and predictors of relapse after natural and treated remission from alcohol use disorders. Addiction. 2006;101:212–22.

Moos R, Moos B. Long-term influence of duration and frequency of participation in alcoholics anonymous on individuals with alcohol use disorders. J Consult Clin Psychol. 2004;72:81–90.

Moos R, Schaefer J, Andrassy J, Moos B. Outpatient mental health care, self-help groups, and patients' 1-year treatment outcomes. J Clin Psychol. 2001;57:1–15.

Morgenstern J, Blanchard KA, McCrady BS, McVeigh KH, Morgan TJ, Pandina RJ. Effectiveness of intensive case management for substance-dependent women receiving temporary assistance for needy families. Am J Public Health. 2006;96(11):2016–23.

Morgenstern J, McKay JR. Rethinking the paradigms that inform behavioral treatment research for substance use disorders. Addiction. 2007;102:1377–89.

Moyer A, Finney JW, Swearingen CE, Vergun P. Brief interventions for alcohol problems: a meta-analytic review of controlled investigations in treatment-seeking and non-treatment-seeking populations. Addiction. 2002;97:279–92.

Ondersma SJ, Chase SK, Svikis DS, Schuster CR. Computer-based brief motivational intervention for perinatal drug use. J Subst Abuse Treat. 2005;28:305–12.

Ondersma SJ, Svikis DC, Schuster CR. Computer-based brief intervention: a randomized trial with postpartum women. Am J Prev Med. 2007;32(3):231–38.

Orleans CT, Resch N, Noll E, Keintz MK, Rimer BK, Brown TV, Snedden TM. Use of transdermal nicotine in a state-level prescription plan for the elderly. A first look at "real-world" patch users. JAMA. 1994;271:601–7.

O'Toole TP, Conde-Martel A, Young JH, Price J, Bigelow G, Ford DE. Managing acutely ill substance-abusing patients in an integrated day hospital outpatient program. J Gen Intern Med. 2005;21:570–6.

Paul GL. Behavior modification research: design and tactics. In: Franks CM, editor. Behavior therapy: appraisal and status. New York: McGraw-Hill; 1969. p. 29–62.

Plebani Lussier J, Heil S, Mongeon J, Badger G, Higgins S. A meta-analysis of voucher-based reinforcement therapy for substance use disorders. Addiction. 2006;101:192–203.

Powers MB, Vedel E, Emmelkamp PMG. Behavioral couples therapy (BCT) for alcohol and drug use disorders: a meta-analysis. Clin Psychol Rev. 2008;28:952–62.

Preti A. New developments in the pharmacotherapy of cocaine abuse. Addict Biol. 2007;12:133–51.

Project MATCH Research Group. Matching alcohol treatments to client heterogeneity: project MATCH posttreatment drinking outcomes. J Stud Alcohol. 1997;58:7–29.

Pulford J. Wheeler A. Documenting client attendance norms: raw data and implications for treatment practice. J Subst Use. 2007;12(2):95–102.

Rapp RC, Otto AL, Lane DT, Redko C, McGatha S, Carlson RG. Improving linkage with substance abuse treatment using brief case management and motivational interviewing. Drug Alcohol Depen. 2008;94(1–3):172–82.

Rhodes W, Gross M. Case management reduces drug use and criminality among drug-involved arrestees: an experimental study of an HIV prevention intervention. In: Final Summary Report Presented to the National Institute of Justice and the National Institute on Drug Abuse. U.S. Department of Health and Human Services, Rockville, MD; 1997.

Riper H, Kramer J, Smit F, Conijn B, Schippers G. Cuijpers P. Web-based self-help for problem drinkers: a pragmatic randomized trial. Addiction. 2008;103(2):218–27.

Rosen GM, Glasgow RE, Moore TE. Self-help therapy: the science and business of giving psychology away. In: Lilienfield SO, Lohr JM, Lynn LJ, edtors. Science and pseudoscience in contemporary clinical psychology. New York: Guilford Press; 2002. p. 399–424.

Rosenthal RN. Current and future drug therapies for alcohol dependence. J Clin Psychopharma. 2006;26(S1):S20–9.

Saitz R, Palfai TP, Freedner N, Winter MR, Macdonald A, Lu J, et al. Screening and brief intervention online for college students: the ihealth study. Alcohol Alcohol. 2007;42(1):28–36.

Schippers GM, Schramade M, Walburg JA. Reforming dutch substance abuse treatment services. Addict Behav. 2002;27:995–1007.

Schuckit MA, Smith TL, Danko GP, Bucholz KK, Reich T. Five-year clinical course associated with DSM-IV alcohol abuse or dependence in a large group of men and women. Am J Psychiatry. 2001;158(7):1084–90.

Swartz LH, Noell JW, Schroeder SW, Ary DV. A randomised control study of a fully automated Internet based smoking cessation programme. Tob Control. 2006;15(1): 7–12.

Shaw JP, Ferry DG, Pethica D, Brenner D, Tucker IG. Usage patterns of transdermal nicotine when purchased as a nonprescription medicine from pharmacies. Tob Control. 1998;7:161–7.

Sobell MB, Sobell LC. Guided self-change model of treatment for substance use disorders. J Cogn Psychoth Inter Q. 2005;19(3):199–210.

Sobell MB, Sobell LC. Stepped care as a heuristic approach to the treatment of alcohol problems. J Consult Clin Psychol. 2000;68(4):573–9.

Stanton MD, Shadish WR. Outcome, attrition, and family-couples treatment for drug abuse: a meta-analysis and review of the controlled, comparative studies. Psychol Bull. 1997;122: 170–91.

Stead LF, Bergson G, Lancaster T. Physician advice for smoking cessation. Cochrane Database Syst Rev. 2008;2.

Stead L, Lancaster T. Group Behaviour Therapy Programmes for Smoking Cessation. Cochrane Database Syst Rev. 2005;2.

Strecher VJ, Shiffman S, West R. Randomized controlled trial of a Web-based computer-tailored smoking cessation program as a supplement to nicotine patch therapy. Addiction. 2005;100:682–8.

Strecher VJ, McClure JB, Alexander GL, Chakraborty B, Nair VN, Konkel JM, et al. Web-based smoking-cessation programs: results of a randomized trial. Am J Prevent Med. 2008;34(5):373–81.

Substance Abuse and Mental Health Services Administration. Results from the 2007 national survey on drug use and health: national findings (Office of Applied Studies, NSDUH Series H-34, DHHS Publication No. SMA 08-4343). Rockville: MD; 2008.

Sussman S. Effects of sixty six adolescent tobacco use cessation trials and seventeen prospective studies of self-initiated quitting. Tob Induced Dis. 2002;1:35–81.

Weisner C, Mertens J, Parthasarathy S, Moore C, Lu Y. Integrating primary medical care with addiction treatment: a randomized controlled trail. JAMA. 2001;286:1715–23.

Chapter 8
Evaluating a Web-Based Cognitive Behavioral Intervention for the Prevention and Treatment of Pediatric Obesity

Brie A. Moore and William T. O'Donohue

Introduction

The prevalence of childhood obesity is increasing at an alarming rate. In the past 30 years, the percentage of overweight children has more than tripled (National Center for Health Statistics, 2002). This increase is seen in both sexes and in children of all ages, with Mexican-, African-, and Native-American children disproportionately affected (Dietz, 2004). Effective weight control treatments are needed to address this national health-care priority and serious public health concern (American Academy of Pediatrics, 2003; Healthy People, 2010).

Researchers have identified childhood obesity as one of the most challenging diseases to treat (Barlow and Dietz, 1998). Multicomponent, family-based behavioral treatments promoting calorie reduction, increased physical activity, and behavior modification (e.g., self-monitoring, stimulus control, preplanning, and positive reinforcement) repeatedly have demonstrated positive outcomes (e.g., Epstein et al., 2000). Despite these findings, much of the empirically supported treatment of pediatric obesity is characterized by high service attrition (Cote et al., 2004), modest outcomes (Jelalian and Saelens, 1999), high relapse rates (Wadden et al., 1999), and a prohibitive cost structure (Dietz, 1998; Perri, 1998). Consequently, existing approaches have had little impact on rising prevalence rates. In order to improve retention and promote long-term maintenance of treatment gains, the comprehensive treatment of pediatric obesity has recently integrated motivational interviewing and relapse prevention skills training to enhance the empirically supported treatment of pediatric obesity (Kirk et al., 2005). To address the issue of cost, researchers (Goldfield et al., 2001) have evaluated the cost-effectiveness of mixed (group and individualized) treatment as compared to group-only treatment for pediatric obesity. The group-only intervention was found to be significantly more cost-effective than the mixed treatment. Although these enhanced treatments are promising, they provide limited attention to cost, scalability, and access.

B.A. Moore (✉)
University of Nevada, Reno Pinecrest Children's Behavioral Health, 6490 S. McCarran Blvd. Ste. D1-28, Reno, NV 89509
e-mail: drmoore@pinecresthealth.com

W.T. O'Donohue, C. Draper (eds.), *Stepped Care and e-Health*,
DOI 10.1007/978-1-4419-6510-3_8, © Springer Science+Business Media, LLC 2011

To explore the feasibility of a web-based application of family-based behavioral treatment, we conducted a randomized clinical trial with 30 at-risk and overweight children and systematically measured health outcomes and parent appraisals. After a brief overview of obesity, its definition, epidemiology, and a review of the literature, this study is outlined below. We present this study in order to highlight empirically supported techniques for the assessment and web-based treatment of pediatric obesity. Furthermore, this study underscores the unique challenges present in this stepped-care approach to pediatric obesity. Namely, we highlight the importance of reducing participant burden and enhancing treatment satisfaction to facilitate retention in web-based treatment. We present this study to encourage readers to consider the benefits of adopting a stepped-care approach as a cost-effective means of addressing the serious pubic health crisis of pediatric obesity.

Overview

Decreasing the rates of obesity in children has been identified as a national healthcare priority (Healthy People, 2010). To this end, the American Academy of Pediatrics Committee on Nutrition (2003) has called for the development of effective treatments for reducing body weight, increasing fitness, and improving the long-term health of overweight children.

Epidemiology

As recently as a few decades ago, childhood obesity was a rare condition. In the 1960s, one in every 24 children aged 6- to 11-years-old was overweight (National Center for Health Statistics, 2002). With the exception of a few researchers (e.g., Bacon and Lowrey, 1967), the treatment of pediatric obesity also received little professional attention. Largely because of availability of energy-dense foods and increasingly sedentary lifestyles, the prevalence of childhood overweight in the United States is rising at an alarming rate. Over the last 30 years, the percentage of children who are overweight has more than tripled (National Center for Health Statistics, 2002). Childhood obesity affects both sexes and in children of all ages, with Mexican-American, African-American, and Native-American children particularly at risk (Dietz, 2004). Obesity is the most prevalent nutritional disease of children in this country (Dietz, 1998).

Assessment

Assessment of overweight in children requires consideration of the child's age, height, weight, pubertal status, and growth patterns. Overweight children are commonly defined as those aged 2- to 20-years-old with body mass index (BMI) greater than the 95th percentile for age and sex (American Academy of Pediatrics, 2003;

Centers for Disease Control, 2004). In addition to BMI, pediatric obesity can also be assessed via tricep and subscapular skinfold thickness and cardiovascular risk factors including elevated blood pressure, total cholesterol, and serum lipoprotein ratios. However, BMI is frequently used clinically as a cost-effective and efficient tool. Yearly tracking of BMI is recommended for all children aged two and older.

Before treatment commences, the comprehensive evaluation of pediatric obesity also involves completion of a thorough history. This practice involves exploration of family history, including a history of the weight status of the child's biological relatives, exploration of other relevant medical and psychiatric history, including the child's current academic, family, and social functioning, as well as investigation of current eating and physical activity patterns. The frequency, type, and duration of current physical and sedentary activity should be explored. It should be noted to what degree the family participates in physical pursuits and the number of hours each day and week that the child spends engaged in television watching, using the computer, or playing sedentary video games. Additionally, assessment of eating habits is paramount. This assessment should entail an investigation of the number of sweetened beverages consumed, how often the family engages in family meals or eats out, and an assessment of the number of servings of fruits and vegetables eaten on a daily basis.

Physical Comorbidities

Childhood obesity is associated with significant health problems and is an important early risk factor for both child and adult morbidity and mortality. Children who are inactive and overweight are more likely to have high blood pressure, abnormal insulin and cholesterol concentrations, and more abnormal lipid profiles. In some populations, children with obesity now account for as much as 50% of type 2 diabetes mellitus, a metabolic disorder related to obesity and sedentary lifestyles and historically rare in children (Fagot-Campagna et al., 2000). These changes increase the risk of early disability and death from heart disease, kidney disease, and other organ damage (Young-Hyman et al., 2001). Other important complications include asthma and sleep apnea, skeletal and joint problems, liver disease, and gastrointestinal complications.

Psychological Comorbidities

The psychological stress of the social stigmatization imposed on overweight children may be as damaging as the medical morbidities. Comorbidities may include poor self-esteem, body image disturbances, depression, social isolation, difficulty with peer relationships, and poor academic achievement (Ebbeling et al., 2002). Childhood obesity poses an unprecedented burden in terms of children's physical and psychological health and future health-care costs.

Review of the Literature

Researchers have concluded that family-based behavioral interventions are the standard of care for the evidence-based treatment of childhood obesity (Kazdin and Weisz, 1998). Given that these programs have adopted the most rigorous research methodology (i.e., randomized-controlled trials) and have produced the best outcomes, we have chosen to concentrate this review on family-based behavioral treatment programs targeting child weight loss (i.e., reductions in percentage overweight or body mass index). This distinction allows the review to be of manageable size. Additionally, most extant treatment outcome studies have adopted this distinction. Epstein et al. (1998), Haddock et al. (1994), Jelalian and Saelens (1999), and Cambell et al. (2001) provide reviews of a broader scope.

Behavior Modification

A number of studies have documented the short-term efficacy of comprehensive behavioral weight loss programs for children aged 12 and under. The early work of Epstein and colleagues, as well as Israel and colleagues, demonstrated that using behavior modification techniques to target exercise and dietary behavior is more effective than providing children and families with only education and more effective than no intervention. Behavior modification techniques typically adopted include self-monitoring of diet and activity, stimulus control strategies, and contingency management. Data are mixed regarding the efficacy of these components either individually or as part of a comprehensive program.

In these studies of short-term weight loss, decreases of approximately 5–20% in percent overweight were found. To examine the long-term efficacy of treatment, Epstein and colleagues have followed children and families for 5- and 10-year follow-up periods. According to Epstein et al. (1994), at 10-year follow-up 30% of children had achieved non-obese status. Consistent across studies, family-based programs targeting both parent and child weight loss and programs that target changes in both physical activity (either lifestyle activity or aerobic activity) and nutrition were more effective than others. Ten-year-follow-up data were superior for children who received diet and lifestyle activity intervention (Epstein et al., 1990; Epstein et al., 1994). More recently, studies have examined a variety of treatment modalities to determine the most efficacious components of treatment.

Parent Involvement

The degree to which parents have been actively involved in treatment has also been systematically investigated. Specifically, studies have manipulated whether parents are disengaged entirely from behavior modification or if parents are assigned a facilitator role. Similarly, studies have also examined the role of parent training versus child self-control training (Epstein, Wing, Koeske, and Valoski, 1986). Whereas short-term results do not provide sufficient evidence for recommending one strategy over another, long-term findings suggest parent participation as an integral part of treatment. At 5- and 10-year follow-up, Epstein and colleagues found that when parents were involved in actively losing weight as part of a family-based program, families that targeted both child and parent weight loss experienced superior results than families who were assigned a nonspecific target (Epstein et al., 1990, 1994).

Physical Activity

Studies have indicated that in the short term, children see equivalent results from exercise alone, whether it be aerobic (programmed) or lifestyle activity, and diet and exercise interventions (Epstein et al., 1990). However, at 11-month follow-up, lifestyle activity alone produced superior results to programmed exercise alone or with dietary modifications. Even at 5- and 10-year follow-up, children who participated in diet plus lifestyle exercise attained greater results than children who engaged in dietary changes with programmed activity such as calisthenics (Epstein et al., 1994). Studies also provide evidence to suggest that limiting access to sedentary activities and reinforcing decreases in sedentary behavior, such as reducing television, computer, game, or "screen time," is more effective than directly targeting physical activity (this strategy may also have the desirable effect of limiting caloric intake). Together, these findings suggest that lifestyle physical activity and dietary modification are essential components in long-term weight control.

In summary, multicomponent behavioral weight loss is an efficacious strategy for decreasing children's weight. This treatment approach is superior relative to both placebo and education-only conditions. However, the clinical effectiveness of these studies is limited as most children do not achieve non-obese status. There is minimal research examining the cost-effectiveness of treatment, particularly as it relates to reducing barriers to access and improving adherence and retention. Additionally, other factors besides weight alone, including knowledge acquisition, behavioral change, and health status, should be considered.

Stepped-Care Treatment Recommendations: The Application of Evidence-Based Practices

A stepped-care model is recommended by the American Academy of Pediatrics in the AAP Policy Statement titled: Prevention of Pediatric Overweight and Obesity and the AAP endorsed Expert Committee Recommendations Regarding the Prevention, Assessment, and Treatment of Child and Adolescent Overweight and Obesity. The AAP outlines the following steps in this model: (1) prevention; (2) prevention plus; (3) structured weight management; (4) comprehensive multidisciplinary intervention; and (5) tertiary care intervention.

Prevention and early intervention are relevant to all children and should involve the promotion and support for breastfeeding, encouraging family meals, limiting screen time, regular physical activity, and yearly BMI monitoring for all children aged two and older. It is of note that watchful waiting (WW) is a commonly practiced, yet not recommended course of action. Barlow and Deitz (2002) found that pediatricians are likely to conclude that watchful waiting appears the most prudent course of action due to a lack of associated comorbidities, uncertainty regarding the effectiveness of intervention, and resistance or low motivation for treatment on the part of the child or family. Motivation should be carefully considered in relation to the age of the child. Motivated parents are sufficient for changing the behaviors of a young child. However, in adolescence, low motivation may foreshadow resistance to treatment recommendations and warrants clinical intervention. However, a lack of comorbidities does not preclude action. Early and effective prevention and treatment may prevent future complications. Furthermore, because more severely overweight children are more difficult to treat, a delayed treatment will likely reduce the effectiveness of therapy (Barlow and Deitz, 2002; Nader et al., 2006). Thus, prevention strategies should be applied to all patients.

For children whose BMI values fall in the "at-risk" range (i.e., BMI between the 85th and 94th percentiles) prevention plus psychoeducation is recommended. This level of care involves psychoeducation regarding evidence-based behavioral changes that facilitate maintenance of a health weight. For example, children are encouraged to consume five servings of fruits and vegetables per day, to engage in 2 h or less of "screen time," to engage in 1 h or more of physical activity, and to consume no sugared drinks. Other family-based behavioral strategies are also encouraged, including eating regular family meals, limiting eating out, consuming a health breakfast, and preparing your own foods.

For many families, prevention and prevention plus psychoeducation are not sufficient. Children who are "at risk" for overweight and for whom prevention plus psychoeducation has not been effective, the AAP recommends structured weight management. At this level of care, the child and family receive written diet and exercise plans and engage in more frequent follow-up. After 3–6 months of structured weight management, if the child does not achieve weight and behavioral targets, the child and family are then referred to a comprehensive multidisciplinary intervention.

Comprehensive multidisciplinary intervention is recommended not only for children who have not attained significant gains at lower levels of care but also for children whose BMI values fall in the "overweight" classification (i.e., BMI above 95th percentile). Comprehensive programs combine the expertise of physicians and dieticians and often also involve exercise physiologists and behavioral psychologists. This approach provides additional support and monitoring and can provide assessment and treatment of medical and psychological comorbidities.

Lastly, a higher level of care is recommended for the most overweight children—those whose BMI values are at or above the 99th percentile and those whom experience significant psychological and medical comorbidities that may interfere with general functioning. For these children and others for whom structured weight management and comprehensive multidisciplinary intervention were not effective, tertiary care intervention is recommended. Tertiary care approaches consist of all the features contained in previously delivered interventions plus consideration of more aggressive therapies. These more aggressive therapies may involve meal replacements, pharmacotherapy, and even bariatric surgery in selected adolescents. These interventions require close medical supervision and should be reserved for treatment resistant and medically at-risk cases.

Examining a Web-Based Approach

One aspect of stepped care which has received much less empirical and clinical attention is Internet-based interventions. We evaluated a web-based treatment approach with participants including 30, 6- to 12-year-old children (21 girls, 9 boys), and their primary caregivers. This age range was determined based on previous studies (Epstein et al., 2000). The term overweight was defined as an excess in adiposity, or body fat, in relation to lean body mass. We assessed weight status using the Center for Disease Control (2004) and American Academy of Pediatrics (2003) body mass index (BMI) definitions for at-risk for overweight and overweight in children aged 2- to 20-years-old. "Overweight" status for children was defined as a body mass index greater than the 95th percentile for age and sex; "at-risk" status was defined as a BMI at or above the 85th percentile (American Academy of Pediatrics, 2003; Centers for Disease Control, 2004). In assessing weight status, the participant's age, sex, height, pubertal status, and historical growth patterns were considered. Although BMI is recognized as an imperfect indicator of weight status, this measure was selected given the ease and reliability of data collection. Children had no medically related diet or activity restrictions and medical complications were ruled out via an unremarkable physician's visit within the last year.

Based on parent report, 90% of participating children had a BMI-for-age score within the "overweight" range; 10% of participants' BMI-for-age scores fell within the "at-risk" range. Fifty-six percent of mothers' BMI values fell within the "obese" range; 20% fell within the "overweight" range. Mothers were on average 37-years-old, with 40% from single-parent households. Of those reporting socioeconomic data (approximately 60%), families earned on average $30,000 annually and had at least some college education. Families reported their ethnicity as Caucasian (43%), Hispanic (27%), African-American (23%), Asian/Pacific Islander (6%), or Native American/Alaskan Native (6%). Participants were predominately (69%) from small, rural towns with populations of less than 50,000 persons.

A web-based intervention was evaluated via a randomized, controlled feasibility trial. This design was selected to gain information about attrition, hypothesized mechanisms of change, progress toward clinical efficacy, and participant acceptance. Given the goals and procedures of Stage 1 treatment development research (McNamara et al., 2002; Rounsaville, Carroll, and Onken, 2001), we acknowledged a priori that this design would not provide adequate statistical power to evaluate the statistical significance of our findings or draw causal inferences.

Sixty-five families indicated interest in the study. Of these, 30 families met screening criteria, consented to participation, completed baseline questionnaires, and accessed treatment materials. Children were randomly assigned, via a computer-generated sequence, to the web-based program, fitandhealthykids.com ($n = 15$), or a monitoring control group ($n = 15$). Participants randomized to the control group were offered access to the intervention at the conclusion of the study. Groups did not differ significantly at baseline in terms of demographic variables. Groups were similar on all dependent variables: BMI z score ($F = 0.21, p = $ ns); health status ($F = 0.66, p = $ ns); and knowledge of behavioral weight control skills ($F = 0.57, p = $ ns).

This protocol was approved by the University of Nevada, Reno Institutional Review Board. Participants were recruited by communication with pediatricians' offices, school, and community organizations in California and Nevada and web-based advertisements. Eligible families were identified via a computer screening process. Families provided informed consent and assent electronically, were informed that they could withdraw from the study at anytime, and were provided with the contact information of the investigators and the Institutional Review Board for questions or comments about the study.

At baseline, ethnicity, income, education, family composition, and geographical location were gathered via parent report. Parents reported their child's current health status, using the Children's Health Status Question (Landgraf et al., 1996) and provided the child's BMI by entering his or her height, weight, age, and sex into an online BMI calculator. BMI was calculated using the formula: $BMI(kg/m^2) = $ (weightinpounds $\times$ 703)/heightininches^2 (American Academy of Pediatrics, 2003; Centers for Disease Control, 2004). The Health Promotion Behavior Assessment was used as a self-report measure of dietary behavior and physical activity (adapted from Epstein et al., 2001). The Weight Control Skills Inventory assessed knowledge of cognitive, behavioral, and environmental factors theoretically associated with readiness (Rollnick, 1996), adherence skills (Baumeister et al., 1994), and relapse prevention skills (Parks and Marlatt, 2000). Measures were administered at baseline and at 6-week follow-up. Randomization occurred after collection of baseline data. Participants randomized to the control condition received web-based psychoeducation (www.AAP.org/obesity). Families randomized to the experimental condition received web-based psychoeducation plus individually tailored, family-based, behavioral weight control skills training. Participants in both groups were instructed to review program materials both independently and with their children for 1.5 h/week for 6 weeks.

Intervention

Families assigned to the web-based program interfaced with five, interactive modules addressing readiness, family-based weight control, nutrition, physical activity, and relapse prevention. Parents chose to either complete the modules in a successive fashion, with advancement contingent on meeting mastery criteria, or in any order. Families underwent a treatment readiness self-assessment and were provided with tailored feedback. Those indicating low motivation or ambivalence were directed to a motivation enhancement module (American Academy of Pediatrics, 2003; DiLillo et al., 2003; Miller and Rollnick, 2002). Families were provided with family-based, behavioral weight control treatment, including (1) behavior modification skills training (e.g., self-monitoring, stimulus control); (2) nutrition education; (3) lifestyle physical activity promotion; and (4) child management skills training (Kazdin and Weisz, 1998). Lastly, a relapse prevention module (Parks and Marlatt, 2000) provided families with skills to identify, predict, prevent, and cope with divergences from treatment. Families were taught problem solving to prepare for and manage diverse, weight control challenges (Cooper et al., 2003; Epstein et al., 2000; Harvey-Berino et al., 2004). In addition to these modules, families were provided with monitoring logs, recipes, journals, games, slideshows, and self-help resources. At post-test, parents completed an adapted version of the Treatment Evaluation Inventory (Kelley et al., 1989).

Repeated measures analyses of variance using the statistical package SPSS (Version 11.0; SPSS, Inc. Chicago, Illinois) were conducted to examine changes with experimental condition ($n = 2$) as a between-subjects variable and time ($n = 2$) as a within-subjects factor. In the presence of a significant time × group interaction, repeated measures ANOVAs were used to evaluate change over time within group. Missing values were approximately evenly distributed across groups.

Findings

Thirty-three percent accessed all treatment materials and completed post-test measures, resulting in a final sample of 10 children and indicating a retention rate similar to other studies (Cote et al., 2004). To determine the most significant factors contributing to attrition, we conducted a retention analysis and identified three primary barriers: (1) insufficient knowledge of treatment prior to enrollment; (2) provision of personal information to determine eligibility; and (3) assessment burden.

The following data must be interpreted with caution as they represent the behavior of a select and highly motivated sample. Furthermore, given this small sample size and short assessment period, it is unclear if these trends may be replicated with a larger sample over time.

BMI

BMI z scores remained stable from pre-test ($M = 2.35$, SD $= 0.33$) to post-test ($M = 2.35$, SD $= 0.33$) for children in both groups. The group × time interaction was not statistically significant ($F(1, 9) = 0.11, p = $ ns). Children remained classified as "moderately obese" throughout their participation in treatment.

Global Health Status Question

Children in both groups demonstrated stability on health status from pre-test to post-test, with no statistically significant group $\times$ time interaction ($M = 3.5$, $SD = 0.95; F(1,9) = 1.9, p =$ ns). Parents described their child's health as "good" throughout the study.

Diet

During both pre- and post-test measurements, 10% of children across groups met daily nutritional guidelines. Consumption of fruits and vegetables was notably low (10%) and consumption of sweets was high (60%). Repeated measures ANOVA did not demonstrate statistically significant differences over time ($F(1,9) = 2.23, p =$ ns) or overtime as a function of group status ($F(1,9) = 1.4, p =$ ns).

Physical Activity

Children in both groups engaged in greater amounts of physical activity at post-test than during baseline assessment ($F(1,9) = 3.32, p < 0.10$). Whereas no differences existed within or between groups in the time spent (approximately 30 min) in physical activity from pre-test ($M = 1.8, SD = 1.1$) to post-test ($M = 2.3, SD = 1.3; F(1,9) = 0.35, p =$ ns), children in both groups were active more often. Children in the experimental condition increased physical activity from 1.5 days per week at baseline ($M = 1.4, SD = 1.2$) to 3 days per week at post-test ($M = 2.8, SD = 1.6$). Children in the control group increased physical activity from 3 days per week at baseline ($M = 3.0, SD = 1.2$) to 4 days per week at post-test ($M = 4.0, SD = 0$). Repeated measures ANOVA demonstrated a group $\times$ time interaction in the expected direction ($F(1,9) = 0.14, p =$ ns). This finding was not statistically significant, but approaches clinical significance as children in the experimental group changed from physically "inactive" to a "moderately active" over time.

Skill Acquisition

Parents in the control condition demonstrated no differences in skill knowledge from baseline ($M = 60.4, SD = 10.6$) to post-test ($M = 59.6, SD = 18.5$). Parents in the experimental condition demonstrated increased skill knowledge from baseline ($M = 48.9, SD = 17.2$) to post-test ($M = 54.1, SD = 17.0$). Although not significant, the group $\times$ time interaction term was in the expected direction ($F(1,9) = 4.61$,

$p = $ ns), with parents in the experimental condition demonstrating increased knowledge of specific weight control skills from baseline ($M = 30.0, \text{SD} = 27.4$) to post-test ($M = 55.0, \text{SD} = 44.7$) and greater knowledge of cognitive behavioral skills (i.e., motivation enhancement, self-control, and relapse prevention skills) at post-test ($M = 52, \text{SD} = 14.8$) than controls ($M = 43, \text{SD} = 20.4$).

Treatment Satisfaction

Overall, parents indicated a moderately high degree of satisfaction ($M = 3.9$, $\text{SD} = 0.74; \text{high} = 5$) by endorsing statements regarding the acceptability and effectiveness of the Internet-based intervention. Overall, 70% of the total sample reported that they had a positive reaction to this treatment. However, these findings must be interpreted cautiously due to the high rate of attrition.

Discussion

The development and evaluation of the web-based intervention provided valuable information about attrition, hypothesized mechanisms of change, trends toward efficacy, and treatment acceptance. Our results replicate and extend those obtained in studies evaluating the acceptability of pediatric obesity treatment when delivered in the clinic setting (Cote et al., 2004). Extensions include the sampling of diverse participants, evaluation of hypothesized mechanisms of change, the development and evaluation of a cost-effective and disseminable approach, and the systematic evaluation of participant satisfaction using the TEI. Similar to results of extant research, this intervention experienced a high rate of attrition, produced modest improvement in health promotion behavior, modest improvement in weight management skills, and observed stability in health status over time.

These results should be considered in light of some limitations. For example, these findings represent the behavior of a select and motivated sample. This study demonstrated that the problems of attrition and adherence in pediatric obesity treatment are significant. Given the small sample size and insufficient statistical power, the generalizability of the program is unknown. This study also utilized a short, 6-week assessment period. Further research is needed to explore the long-term outcomes of such an approach. Pediatric obesity is a problem of public health proportions (Dietz, 2004). This study aimed to develop a treatment approach that could address the limitations of existing care, including high cost, limited access, and limited efficacy. Although the present treatment involved a less resource-intensive approach to treatment, it appears that low professional involvement may not be sufficient to address this epidemic. The utility of this program as an adjunctive treatment in primary care warrants further research. These limitations notwithstanding, this study adds to evidence suggesting that family-based behavioral weight loss, delivered via the web, can be a useful first-line treatment.

References

American Academy of Pediatrics. Policy Statement: prevention of pediatric overweight and obesity. Pediatrics. 2003;112(2):424–30.

Barlow S, Dietz W. Obesity evaluation and treatment: expert committee recommendations. Pediatrics. 1998;102(3):e29.

Barlow S, Dietz W. Management of child and adolescent obesity: summary and recommendations based on reports from pediatricians, pediatric nurse practitioners and registered dieticians. Pediatrics. 2002;110(1):236–8.

Campbell K, Waters E, O'Meara S, Summerbell C. Interventions for preventing obesity in children (Cochrane review). Cochrane Database Syst Rev. 2001;1:CD001871.

Centers for Disease Control and Prevention. Overweight and Obesity: defining overweight and obesity. Nutrition and Physical Activity. 2004. http://www.cdc.gov/nccdphp/dnpa/obesity/defining.htm. Accessed August 1, 2009.

Cote MP, Byczkowski T, Kotagal U, Kirk S, Zeller M, Daniels S. Service quality and attrition: an examination of a pediatric obesity program. Int J Qual Health C. 2004;16(2):165–73.

Dietz WH. Overweight in childhood and adolescence. New Engl J Med. 2004;350(9):855–7.

Dietz WH. Health consequences of obesity in youth: childhood predictors of adult disease. Pediatrics. 1998;101(3):554–70.

DiLillo V, Siegfried N, West D. Incorporating motivational interviewing into behavioral obesity treatment. Cogn Behav Pract. 2003;10(2):120–30.

Ebbeling CB, Pawlak D, Ludwig D. Childhood obesity: public-health crisis, common sense cure. Lancet. 2002;10(360):473–83.

Epstein LH, Gordy C, Raynor H, Beddome M, Kilanowski C, Paluch R. Increasing fruit and vegetable intake and decreasing fat and sugar intake in families at risk for childhood obesity. Obes Res. 2001;9(3):171–8.

Epstein LH, Klein KR, Wisniewski L. Child and parent factors that influence psychological problems in obese children. Int J Eat Disord. 1994;15:151–7.

Epstein LH, McCurley J, Wing RR, Valoski A. Five-year follow up of family based behavioral treatments for childhood obesity. J Consult Clin Psychol. 1990;58:661–4.

Epstein LH, Myers MD, Raynor HA, Saelens BE. Treatment of pediatric obesity. Pediatrics. 1998;101(3):554–70.

Epstein LH, Paluch RA, Gordy C, Saelens BE, Ernst MM. Problem solving in the treatment of childhood obesity. J Consult Clin Psychol. 2000;68(4):717–21.

Epstein LH, Valoski A, Wing RR, McCurley J. Ten-year outcomes of behavioral family-based treatment for childhood obesity. Health Psychol. 1994;13:373–83.

Epstein LH, Wing RR, Koeske R, Valoski A. Effects of parent weight on weight loss in obese children. J Consult Clin Psychol. 1986;54:400–1.

Fagot-Campagna A, Pettitt D, Engelgan M, Burrow N, Geiss L, Valdez R, et al. Type 2 diabetes among North American children and adolescents: an epidemiologic review and a public health perspective. J Pediatr. 2000;136(5):664–72.

Goldfield G, Epstein L, Kilanowski C, Paluch R, Kogut-Bossler B. Cost-effectiveness of group and mixed family-based treatment for childhood obesity. Int J Obes Relat Metabol Disord. 2001;25(12):1843–9.

Haddock CK, Shadish WR, Klesges RC, Stein RJ. Treatments for childhood and adolescent obesity. Ann Behav Med. 1994;16(3):235–44.

Harvey-Berino J, Pintauro S, Buzzell P, Gold E. Effect of internet support on the long-term maintenance of weight loss. Obes Res. 2004;12:320–9. http://www.healthypeople.gov/Document/HTML/Volume2/19Nutrition.htm

Healthy People. Chapter 19, Volume 2: nutrition and overweight. 2010. Retrieved on November 3, 2004 from, http://www.healthypeople.gov/Document/HTML/Volume2/19Nutrition.htm.

Jelalian E, Saelens B. Empirically supported treatments in pediatric psychology: pediatric obesity. J Pediatr Psychol. 1999;24(3):223–48.

Kazdin AE, Weisz JR. Identifying and developing empirically supported child and adolescent treatments. J Consult Clin Psychol. 1998;66(1):19–36.

Kelley M, Heffer R, Gresham F, Elliot S. Development of a modified treatment evaluation inventory. J Psychopathol Behav Assessment. 1989;11:235–47.

Kirk S, Scott BJ, Daniels S. Pediatric obesity epidemic: treatment options. Suppl J Am Diet Assoc. 2005;105:S44–51.

Landgraf JL, Abetz L, Ware JE. The CHQ user's manual. The Health Institute, New England Medical Center, Boston, MA; 1996.

McNamara C, et al. Setting the stage: an introduction to NIDA's stage model for behavioral treatment development research. Symposium presented at the annual meeting of the association for the advancement of behavior therapy, Reno, NV; 2002.

Miller WR. Rollnick S. Motivational interviewing: preparing people for change. 2nd ed. New York: Guilford; 2002.

Nader PR, O'Brien M, Houts R, Bradley R, Belsky J. et al. Identifying risk for obesity in early childhood. Pediatrics. 2006;118:594–601.

National Center for Health Statistics. 2002. Retrieved on October 30, 2004 from, http://www.cdc.gov/nchs/nhanes.htm.

Parks GA, Marlatt GA. Relapse prevention therapy: A cognitive-behavioral approach. Natl Psychol. 2000;9(5). http://nationalpsychologist.com/articles/art_v9n5_3.htm.

Perri MG. The maintenance of treatment effects in the long-term management of obesity. Clin Psychol Sci Pract. 1998;5:526–43.

Rollnick S. Behavior change in practice: targeting individuals. Int J Obes Relat Metabol Disord. 1996;20(1):22–6.

Rounsaville BJ, Carroll KM, Onken LS. A stage model of behavioral therapies research: getting started and moving from stage 1. Clin Psychol Sci Pract. 2001;8:133–42.

Wadden T, Sarwer D, Berkowitz R. Behavioral treatment of the overweight patient. Balliere's Clin Endocrinol Metabol. 1999;13:93–107.

Young-Hyman D, Schlundt DG, Herman L, DeLuca F, Counts D. Evaluation of the insulin resistance syndrome in 5- to 10-year old overweight/obese African-American children. Diabetes Care. 2001;24:1359–64.

Chapter 9
Chronic Disease Management

Victoria Mercer

Introduction

Chronic diseases such as heart disease, cancer, stroke, chronic lower respiratory diseases, diabetes, Alzheimer's disease, and kidney disease account for seven of the top ten causes of death and account for billions of dollars of health-care expenditures annually in the United States (Center for Disease Control, 2005; Weingarten et al., 2002). In 2007, 11% of the US population suffered from the number one killer in the United States diagnosed heart disease (National Center for Health Statistics, 2008; 2009). The cost of medical management of heart disease alone is staggering, in 2006 it accounted for 43% of all Medicare expenditures and 1–2% of total US health care (Foote, 2003; Stewart, 2005; Thorn et al., 2006). The management of chronic disease (CD) strains the psychological well-being of chronically diseased individuals and their families (Levy et al., 2007; de Ridder et al., 2008), particularly with problems such as heart disease where psychological factors such as stress, social isolation, anxiety, depression, and type A behavior have a role in disease progression, and management of the disease requires stressful caregiving and case management skills from unprepared family members (Hemingway and Marmot, 1999; Rozanski et al., 1999). In the early 1990s, managed care organizations began developing and implementing chronic disease management (CDM) programs in an effort to contain costs and improve health outcomes (Mayzell, 1999; Villagra, 2004). What emerged from these early programs was an understanding that quality improvement and cost reductions could be achieved through enhancing disease process understanding and attending to the psychological aspects of health and illness (Levy et al., 2007; Schneiderman et al., 2001). In more recent years, as both integrated primary care models for disease management and a wide array of commercial for-profit carve-out programs were developed, the Disease Management Association of America (DMAA; www.dmaa.org) was established as a non-profit trade association representing stakeholders in the disease management industry. The DMAA worked

V. Mercer (✉)
Department of Psychology, University of Nevada-Reno, Mail Stop 0298, Reno, NV 89557, USA
e-mail: vicmercer@gmail.com

W.T. O'Donohue, C. Draper (eds.), *Stepped Care and e-Health*,
DOI 10.1007/978-1-4419-6510-3_9, © Springer Science+Business Media, LLC 2011

to converge the different players within the DM industry, as well as to encourage more productive research, by establishing a comprehensive working definition of what key components must exist within a program for it to be considered a disease management program. The DMAA definition states

Disease management is a system of coordinated health-care interventions and communications for populations with conditions in which patient self-care efforts are significant. Disease management

- supports the physician or practitioner/patient relationship and plan of care;
- emphasizes prevention of exacerbations and complications through the use of evidence-based practice guidelines and patient empowerment strategies; and
- evaluates clinical, humanistic, and economic outcomes on an ongoing basis with the goal of improving overall health.

Disease management components include

- population identification processes;
- evidence-based practice guidelines;
- collaborative practice models to include physician and support service providers;
- patient self-management education (may include primary prevention, behavior modification programs, and compliance/surveillance);
- process and outcomes measurement, evaluation, and management; and
- routine reporting/feedback loop (may include communication with patient, physician, health plan, and ancillary providers and practice profiling).

Full-service disease management programs must include all six components. Programs consisting of fewer components are disease management support services (Disease Management Association of America, 2009).

However, even this definition is not a consistent standard for research because it has not empirically established that it includes the optimal mix of ingredients for a successful program (Krumholz et al., 2006). Overall, CDM programs are functional in nature, focusing on providing cost-effective optimization of health-care services, delivered by a coordinated, interdisciplinary clinical system such as stepped care (Levy et al., 2007; Mayzell, 1999).

Interventions targeting the psychosocial and biobehavioral aspects of the disease experience have increased in number as we have improved our understanding of psychological, genetic, and biological risk factors (Schneiderman et al., 2001). Research has provided substantial evidence that psychosocial factors including depression, anxiety, social isolation and low perceived emotional support, hostility, type A behavior, and stress have roles in whether someone develops a CD (Hemingway and Marmot, 1999; Rozanski et al., 1999). Given the significant impact of psychosocial and biobehavioral factors on disease progression, efforts to integrate psychological interventions into the medical management of CD have increased in the recent decades (Cummings et al., 2005).

Two pioneering CDM programs are the chronic care model (CCM; Wagner, 1998) and the chronic disease self-management program (CDSMP; Lorig et al., 1993). The CCM aims to make patient-centered evidenced-based care a widespread clinical reality by introducing an array of system changes to routine primary care

(Coleman et al., 2009). CCM has attempted to improve the quality of care by transforming daily care for CD patients from treatment that is acute and reactive, to treatment that is proactive, planned, and population based (Coleman et al., 2009). The CCM aims to meet these goals through four avenues: (1) integrating effective team care and planned interactions; (2) enhancing self-management principles by connecting patients with community resources and supporting their continued use of resources; (3) integrating patient and provider decision support; (4) installing and maximizing the capabilities of patient registries and other information technology medical supports (Coleman et al., 2009; Myette, 2008). Most evidence for the effectiveness of the CCM comes from research conducted by members of health-care organizations that participated in the Breakthrough Series (BTS) Collaborative (Wagner, 1998). The BTS has been the primary method by which practitioners have learned about the CCM and have received support to implement the necessary changes to health-care delivery system (Coleman et al., 2009).

Several reviews have shown that incorporation of the CCM into primary care can improve the quality of care and while reducing costs (Neumeyer-Gromen et al., 2004; Ofman et al., 2004; Weingarten et al., 2002). A variety of CD patients have demonstrated improved care when they receive care from practices that were CCM adherent (Asch et al., 2005). In a study of patients with congestive heart failure who received CCM-based practices compared to control practices, CCM patients were found to be more knowledgeable about their disease, more adherent to recommended treatment such as lipid lowering and angiotensin-converting enzyme inhibition therapy, had reduced emergency room visits, and a 35% reduction in days in the hospital (Asch et al., 2005). Asthma patients who received redesigned CCM care, compared to those in regular care, were more likely to monitor their peak flows and have a written action plan for their care, as well as demonstrate improved quality of life (Mangione-Smith et al., 2005). In a study cardiovascular disease events among diabetes patients receiving CCM redesigned care, for each 48 patients served risk declined by one cardiovascular disease event (Vargas et al., 2007). In randomized controlled trials conducted by non-collaborative CCM interventions (those that are research-based interventions and involve components such as the addition of new staff or new technology, which may facilitate CCM implementation while reducing internal practice redesign) also found that implementing CCM significantly improved at least some process and outcome measures compared to controls across a variety of diseases, including comorbid depression and cancer (Dwight-Johnson et al., 2005).

Rather than focus on systemic changes, the CDSMP was designed around the utility of Bandura's self-efficacy principles applied to individual management of CD (Lorig et al., 1999). The CDSMP focuses on community-based self-management education, generally delivered in a 7-week small group intervention that addresses common issues experienced across patients with varied CD diagnoses (Myette, 2008; Lorig et al., 1993). Outcome studies evaluating the efficacy and effectiveness of the CDSMP will be detailed in the following section on group care; an abundance of research has demonstrated statistically significant and long-lasting improvements in patients' cognitive symptom management, communication with physicians, self-efficacy, depression, health-related distress, and savings in health expenditures (Lorig et al., 2001; Lorig et al., 1999; Lorig et al., 2001).

When elements of successful chronic disease management (CDM) program guidelines were reviewed for core components, seven elements were revealed (Von Kroff and Tiemens, 2000). These elements included generation of a treatment plan (e.g., specific iteration of health behavior changes and goals, interventions schedule), patient education (e.g., disease-specific information, biopsychosocial model of disease), scheduled follow-up (e.g., usually done with nurse or care coordinator to determine appropriate and realistic care schedule), outcomes measuring (e.g., what to measure and when to measure it: A1C for diabetes patients, depression levels), adherence monitoring (e.g., measure patient success and barriers to implementing the necessary behavior change such as exercise or diet changes, pill counts), stepped therapy (e.g., start with least intrusive therapy appropriate for level of patient need, measure outcomes and adherence, and use this monitoring information to make future treatment decisions), and specialty consultation and referral (e.g., physician or nurse referral to dieticians, physical therapists, mental health specialists; inpatient care; Von Kroff and Tiemens, 2000). Research shows that adherence to these eight treatment elements improves patient outcomes; however, the elements are often inadequately organized and delivered (Wagner et al., 1996). Wagner et al. (1996) hypothesize that lack of adherence to these elements in routine primary care for chronic disease patients' results in suboptimal care for four reasons:

(1) Delays in the detection of complications or declines in health status because of irregular or incomplete assessments or inadequate follow-up;
(2) Failures in self-management of the illness or risk factors as a result of patient passivity or ignorance stemming from inadequate or inconsistent patient assessment, education, motivation, and feedback;
(3) Reduced quality of care due to the omission of effective interventions or the commission of ineffective ones; and
(4) Undetected or inadequately managed psychosocial distress (Wagner et al., 1996, p. 514)

In an effort to provide the largest number of patients with the least intrusive and lowest cost care, integration of the effective components of CDM programs such as CCM and CDSCM into a stepped-care system offers both CDM providers and consumers with a powerful quality improvement tool (Haaga, 2000; Newman, 2000).

CDM in a high-tech era must embrace empirically based techniques and enhance their dissemination through technologically enhanced coordinated care, supportive therapy, and sustained treatment. This chapter will review the common psychological components across stepped-care disease management treatment programs, highlight how technology such as telehealth (e.g., nurse phone calls), e-mail (e.g., health provider follow-up or education dissemination), and video chatting is being used to enhance traditional disease management programs, and will conclude with a focus on change agendas and future directions among triage, research, and dissemination issues.

Assessment/Triage

Assessment should focus on psychosocial and lifestyle factors that are associated with health promoting behaviors and better psychological adjustment to CD: (1) self-management; (2) cognitive processing; and (3) emotion regulation skills (de Ridder et al., 2008). Beyond health-related psychological functioning, assessment should ascertain whether the patient meets criteria for any DSM-IV diagnostic categories in order to streamline care coordination and the use of empirically supported treatments (Chambless et al., 1996). Many CDM programs may have parameters for which type of assessment tools a provider may use; therefore, the reader is referred to the numerous assessment resources available within your area of practice to ascertain which specific and sometimes proprietary self-report or structured interview you would use to gather the following information. Below is a list of domains of psychological health that chronic disease programs consider important and that researchers have established as being important for psychological adjustment to chronic disease (Cummings and Cummings, 2005; de Riddler et al., 2008):

- Overall psychological health: general psychological functioning, diagnosis, or symptoms from DSM-IV Axis I or II disorders (especially depression and anxiety) and treatment interfering behaviors
- Self-management includes health promoting and reducing lifestyle factors (e.g., diet, exercise, energy, sleep hygiene, substance use, and disease-specific factors), medication and drug use, knowledge on disease cause, course, prognosis, and treatment, problem-solving and goal-setting skills, social support, communication skills, presence of caregiver burden, stage of change, and adherence to treatment regimen
- Cognitive processing includes adaptive and maladaptive coping strategies, self-defeating thoughts, catastrophic interpretations, fear or anxiety or depression, accurate understanding and acceptance of diagnosis, and any DSM-IV Axis I disorder (e.g., panic)
- Emotion regulation includes emotional functioning (experience, processing, and modulation), emotional avoidance or inhibition, and emotional expression and acknowledgment
- Case management includes advanced planning directives, medical and legal power of attorney, and decisions regarding end-of-life issues

A stepped-care treatment plan for each patient should include a decision tree that includes disease-specific thresholds (e.g., hemoglobin A1C levels for diabetes patient) that should be used in conjunction with psychological variables (e.g., score on depression measure) to guide patient outcome monitoring and move the patient between levels of care. Based on the treatment plan the patient should then be triaged into the appropriate tier of stepped care. Skills and preferences, as well as practical issues of staff availability, patient flow, scheduling, payment, and availability of service options, influence how a patient is triaged into care. Triage of patients is based on consideration of the interplay between the severity and intrusiveness of four factors:

- Psychological distress:

    o High distress (threat to harm self or others, instability, emotion dysregulation, impaired quality of life, or occupational functioning) ⇒ upper steps of care (inpatient, individual, group)
    o Low distress (emotion regulation, stable, little impairment in functioning) ⇒ lower steps of care (psychoeducation, bibliotherapy, eHealth, group)

- Impact of psychosocial and lifestyle factors:

    o High impact (depression, anxiety, eating disorders, substance use disorder, Axis II disorder is causing a further deterioration of their physical functioning and negatively impacting their disease management) ⇒ upper steps of care (inpatient, individual, group)
    o Low impact (distress is not causing any functional impairment or disease progression and skills will help) ⇒ dictated by distress and stage of change (bibliotherapy, eHealth, group)

- Motivation:

    o High readiness and willingness ⇒ whatever step is dictated by distress and impact
    o Low readiness and or willingness ⇒ if low distress and low impact then lower steps (motivational interviewing within appropriate step of care such as psychoeducation, bibliotherapy, eHealth); if high distress and impact then higher steps (motivational interviewing within appropriate step of care such as group, individual)

- Skills and preferences:

    o High skills ⇒ whatever step dictated by distress, impact, and stage of change
    o Low skills (low literacy, low technology skills, and social anxiety) ⇒ common sense match to appropriate modality of stepped care (e.g., low literacy ⇒ no bibliotherapy but psychoeducation with DVD)

Providers need to reinforce that every step of care requires engagement and participation, even watchful waiting. Throughout all steps, patient adherence and outcomes should be monitored by case managers.

Stepped-Care Options

Watchful Waiting

Watchful waiting (WW) is the least-intrusive level of stepped care. It is an outpatient, open-ended, process in which a patient's condition is closely monitored, without engaging in new treatment, until symptoms appear or change. A central component to WW is the use of an explicit decision tree or other protocol to ensure a timely and appropriate shift from WW to another form of management (Katz et al., 1992). WW is very common in the management of slow growing cancers such as prostate and lymphocytic leukemia (Moynihan, 2008) and certain mental disorders such as depression in which baseline data has established has relatively equal rates of remitting, improving, or declining (Meredith et al., 2007). In these situations, WW without any additional intervention may be the most judicious choice form of stepped care. WW is a stepped-care option that will be repeatedly returned to throughout the course of evaluating, treating, and monitoring patient thresholds and outcomes. WW may be difficult for individuals with high levels of anxiety given that they are literally waiting for something bad to happen. It may be beneficial to teach patients' stress inoculation and relapse prevention skills prior to their entering into WW.

Psychoeducation

The content used in psychoeducation should be developed appropriately for the patient demographic, with examples and skills relevant to the unique experiences of varied treatment types, disease symptoms, or psychological experience of a disease and be written in jargon-free lay language. Psychoeducation focuses on stress management, behavior modification, and disease education. Information may be disseminated as print material (hand-outs, pamphlets, articles), media material (e.g., DVDs, TV programs, Internet resources), or verbally within more intensive steps of care. Psychoeducation is a valuable way to provide patients with referral sources, connect them to community support services, educate them on different stakeholders' roles, provide information on advanced care planning, long-term health options and care planning, and check lists for health behaviors and disease monitoring. If a patient is assessed and triaged into stepped care later in the course of their disease, then psychoeducation material may be used as an adjunct to more intensive care. This would allow the care provider to be maximally efficient within other steps of care, using developed empirically based psychoeducation materials to inform and educate new patients into treatment. Material may also be disseminated as a prevention tool in community agencies, schools, public health efforts, and within the context of routine medical and psychological care.

Outcome Data

In a systematic review of the research on psychoeducational interventions for adults and children with difficult asthma researchers found that, compared to usual or non-psychoeducational care, psychoeducational interventions reduced the relative risk (RR) of hospital admissions at follow-up in children (RR $=$ 0.64, CI $=$ $0.46 - 0.89$) and in adults (RR $=$ 0.57, CI $=$ $0.34 - 0.93$) (Smith et al., 2005). Mixed results were found for the effectiveness of psychoeducational on self-care behavior and there was a lack of quality research on cost savings (Smith et al., 2005). A meta-analysis of psychoeducational programs (health education and stress management) for coronary heart disease patients found that such programs resulted in a substantial reduction of distal health targets (34% reduction in cardiac mortality; 29% reduction in the recurrence of myocardial infarction (MI)); and a significant ($p < 0.025$) positive effect on proximal targets (blood pressure, cholesterol, body weight, smoking behavior, physical exercise, and eating habits; Dusseldorp et al., 1999).

Bibliotherapy

Bibliotherapy is a cost-effective, convenient, and less stigmatizing alternative to professional therapy (Rosen, 1987; den Boer et al., 2004). Bibliotherapy treatments exist for a number of different aspects of chronic disease self-management including the mental health components (e.g., depression, anxiety, coping, stress management) and disease-specific educational resources published by national agencies and medical service providers (Redding et al., 2008).

In an expert review of the top 50 self-help workbooks for anxiety and depression and it was suggested that consumers and practitioners follow the following heuristics when selecting self-help books: the best books focus on a limited range of problems, are authored by doctoral level mental health professionals, avoid too grandiose claims of effectiveness, and provide specific guidance for technique implementation and treatment monitoring (Redding et al., 2008). While bibliotherapy is widespread as a self-prescribed and self-administered self-help tool or an adjunct to professional treatment, the treatment is not for everyone. Bibliotherapy is well suited for patients who are motivated, willing to participate in their own treatment, and have appropriate literacy ability. Researchers who developed the self-management chronic disease program that was discussed in the introduction have published a self-help bibliotherapy resource titled *Living a Healthy Life with Chronic Conditions: Self-Management of Heart Disease, Fatigue, Arthritis, Worry, Diabetes, Frustration, Asthma, Pain, Emphysema, and Others* (Lorig et al., 2006) and is available for less than $20.00 on Amazon.com. To date they have not published any empirical study of the book's effectiveness, although much data exists on the effectiveness of their group programs.

Outcome Data

Bibliotherapy/information prescriptions/prescriptions booklets are used for a variety of problems, most researches are depression, anxiety, sexual dysfunction, panic disorders, and problem drinking (Chamberlain et al., 2008). In their summary,

Chamberlain and colleagues (2008) find that self-help resources and bibliotherapy are helpful for patients managing certain chronic diseases or issues impacting chronic diseases, such as insomnia (Mimeault and Morin, 1999), the health promoting behavior of reducing dietary salt (Hooper et al., 2003), using dietary advice to reduce blood cholesterol (Thompson et al., 2001), reducing obesity (Latner, 2001), and when used as a follow-up to individual therapy for patients with head and neck cancer (Semple et al., 2006).

A study on assisted bibliotherapy (8-week self-help treatment package with limited therapist contact of 20-min therapy sessions) in primary care found that such an intervention provided significant improvement at post-treatment and 3-month follow-up for moderate stress/anxiety in an adult clinical population (Reeves and Stace, 2005). Seventy-five percent of the participants reported the assisted bibliotherapy intervention to be "very helpful" and indicated they found the intervention to be satisfying in general. Importantly, at post-treatment all of the participants said they were using the self-help strategies "often" and at 3-month follow-up 80% said they were using the strategies "often."

An earlier study compared a wait-list control group to classroom-based or home-based (video and readings) wellness programs that instructed chronically ill patients on mind–body relationships, relaxation training, cognitive restructuring, problem solving, communication, behavioral treatment for insomnia, nutrition, and exercise (Rybarczyk et al., 1999). Researchers found that both treatment groups had a significant reduction in self-reported pain, sleeping problems, depression, and anxiety. The home-based course also had a significant decrease in self-reported frequency of medical symptoms, and the classroom course had a significant decrease in "chance" health locus of control beliefs. These findings suggest that the lower cost bibliotherapy and video-based wellness program can be an effective alternative to more resource-consuming services.

In a systematic review, Morgan and Jorm (2008) summarized the evidence for the treatment of depression (not specific to a chronic disease) with bibliotherapy. A large meta-analyses of 17 trials (16 RCTs) found bibliotherapy [reading structured written material such as *Feeling Good* (Burns, 1999) or *Control Your Depression* (Lewinsohn et al., 1986)] to be more effective than either wait list or delayed treatment controls ($d = 0.77, 95\%$ CI$0.61 - 0.94$). However, the author's mention an earlier meta-analysis of a smaller number of RCTs that found no significant difference between bibliotherapy and individual therapy (Morgan and Jorm, 2008). A pilot study investigated the usefulness of primary care physician's "prescriptions" for depressed patients to read Burn's (1999) *Feeling Good* (Naylor and O'Donohue, 2007). Of the five participants who completed the study, final depression self-report scores were lower than at baseline and pre-treatment for every participant.

Computer-Based Intervention/eHealth

New technologies provide additional options to tailor-specific therapeutic approaches to patient needs. Stepped-up approaches (e.g., self-help) successfully take advantage of new media such as CD-ROM, while promising step-down approaches include strategies such as text messaging via mobile telephones or group therapy via Internet chat rooms (de Ridder et al., 2008). However, health-care systems, managed care providers, and employers vary widely in the degree to which they incorporate and provide incentives for patients to use eHealth and computer-based services. Therefore, based on the parameters of a patient's health-care system or ability to find and pay for computer-based services, individuals will have different opportunities to use eHealth services. Evidence is growing for the potential for these programs to enhance the reach of efficacious treatments to underserved populations at a relatively low cost, while also addressing scalability, efficiency, and providing the ability to tailor and customize treatment options to best meet the needs of individual patients (Ahern et al., 2006).

Outcome Data

There is substantial data for the effectiveness of telehealth technology in the medical symptom side of disease management (Meyer et al., 2002; Darkins et al., 2008). Telehealth uses telephone services, sometimes in combination with computer-based monitoring, to perform patient assessments, place medication orders, schedule appointments, place reminder phone calls, assist with adherence issues, and assist with technology problems (Barnett et al., 2006). Research across dozens of various telehealth programs have demonstrated their ability to reduce emergency room visits, hospital admissions, hospital bed days, nursing home admissions, and nursing home bed days of care (Barnett et al., 2006; Britton and Hoggard, 2008; Darkins et al., 2008; Kashem et al., 2006; Kashem et al., 2008; Meyer et al., 2002). To highlight one large-scale RCT, Britton and colleagues (2006) found that 2 years after enrollment in a care-coordinated home telehealth program for veterans with diabetes mellitus, the treatment group demonstrated a statistically significant reduction in all-cause ($38.8 - 30\%, p = 0.01$) and a 25% reduction in disease-related ($35.3 - 26.9\%, p = 0.02$) hospitalizations while these rates increased or did not change for the comparison group. Additionally, when baseline glycosylated hemoglobin levels were controlled for, the treatment group had a lower likelihood of having care coordinator-initiated visit to a primary care clinic ($59.0 - 21.0\%, p < 0.001$). Furthermore, the home telehealth implementation program implemented system wide for the Veterans Health Administration reported high satisfaction ratings and demonstrated cost-effectiveness for the treatment of chronically ill veterans (Barnett et al., 2006).

There is less research on computer-based care for the psychological issues involved in disease management. In an effort to reduce redundancy with other chapters of this text, I will not review general depression and anxiety efforts, but focus on a study conducted on computerized cognitive behavioral therapy in primary care, a computer-based psychoeducation program targeted toward young adults with cancer, and studies conducting chronic disease self-management program groups over the Internet. Years ago the pervasive supply and demand discrepancy motivated CBT researchers to develop and test a computerized version of cognitive behavioral therapy called *Beating the Blues* (CCBT; Marks et al., 2003; Proudfoot, Goldberg et al., 2003; Proudfoot et al., 2004; Proudfoot, Swain et al., 2003; Wright et al., 2002, 2005). The efficacy of the program, *Beating the Blues*, was demonstrated in a large-scale randomized controlled trial (Proudfoot, Goldberg et al., 2003; Proudfoot et al., 2004) and the effectiveness demonstrated through implementation of *Beating the Blues* into routine primary care (Cavanagh et al., 2006). The effectiveness study showed that when CCBT was implemented into routine primary care patients demonstrated statistical and clinically significant improvements with the intention-to-treat analysis indicating an uncontrolled pre–post-effect size of 0.50 on their measure of clinical outcomes and for completers of the program and outcome measures (47% of the intake sample) larger gains with uncontrolled pre–post-treatment effect size of 1.00 (Cavanagh et al., 2006). Treatment gains were maintained where data was available at a 6-month follow-up. Such demonstrated effectiveness suggests that CCBT may be an effective first-line tool within the stepped-care model of psychological treatment.

In a second study an innovative computer-assisted psychoeducation program was developed to target disease management in young adults. The study conducted a randomized control trial of a video game developed to educate and involve young people in their cancer treatment (Beale et al., 2007). The study found that young adult cancer patients using the psychoeducational video game demonstrated significantly improved cancer-related knowledge against the control group who received a regular video game. Improved disease-specific knowledge has been shown to result in better health outcomes; therefore, using video game and computer technology may be a useful tool to increase health education and health outcomes among young adults.

Researchers have had impressive success with delivering the chronic disease self-management program (CDSMP) over the Internet, using trained peers as online moderators (Lorig et al., 2006). In an early study, 958 chronic disease patients (heart, lung, type 2 diabetes) were randomized to the 6-week Internet-based intervention or to a usual care control group. At 1 year participants in the intervention group had significant improvements in health statuses compared to the usual care control ($p < 0.005$) and similar results to the original small-group CDSMP participants across health distress, pain, or self-reported measure of global health and significantly greater reductions in disability ($p < 0.05$). In an adaptation of this program into the Expert Patients Programme, used in the United Kingdom, even more significant results were found over the course of a year (Lorig et al., 2008). Researchers found that at 6 months, significant improvements ($p < 0.01$) were found across the majority of health status measures, health-related behaviors, and utilization measures except self-rated health, disability, stretching, hospitalizations, and nights in hospital (Lorig, Ritter, Dost et al., 2008). At 12 months all improvements were significant ($p < 0.01$) except decrease in disability, nights in hospital, and hospitalizations. Self-efficacy and satisfaction with the health-care system were both significantly improved ($p < 0.01$). Researchers have also adapted the group to be delivered via the Internet for arthritis or fibromyalgia patients (Lorig, Ritter, Laurent, & Plant, 2008). At 1 year, the intervention group demonstrated statistically significant improvements on four of the six health status variables ($p < 0.01$).

No significant differences were found for health behaviors or utilization variables (Lorig, Ritter, Laurent, & Plant, 2008).

Group Therapy

Chronic disease management (CDM) programs are most commonly comprised of group interventions. Psychosocial and psychoeducational groups incorporate treatment across many issues including cognitive techniques to manage stress, emotion regulation, and self-management (e.g., fatigue, sleep, medication adherence, communication strategies, problem and decision making, and stress management). Some CDM groups are illness specific and others target heterogeneous groups of CD patients. Research has demonstrated that patients with different chronic diseases have very similar symptom management problems and can be effectively treated within a heterogeneous group led by a facilitator without specialized knowledge about any certain disease per se (Dyer et al., 2004). Both types of groups can be inpatient or outpatient, conducted by individuals from a range of training backgrounds, and serve to normalize patient experiences and provide social support (Bracke and Thoresen, 1996).

Cummings and colleagues (1993) conducted seminal research on new delivery methods of behavioral health services, with an emphasis on the use of group protocols, to Medicaid and Medicare program members in Hawaii with positive results. Researchers provided services to 36,000 Medicaid patients and 92,000 federal employees in Oahu (Cummings et al., 1993). Patients in the control group were eligible for 52 annual psychological and psychiatric sessions by any state licensed provider. Patients in the experimental group were eligible for services through the Biodyne Centers, by self-referral, physician referral, or through various outreach efforts. The Biodyne Centers provided services through numerous different group protocols, delivered by trained moderators. Results from this study found that for all three treatment groups accessing services within the Biodyne Centers demonstrated decreased utilization in terms of medical dollars, while the traditional system increased medical dollars (Cummings et al., 1993). Patients with psychological distress and no medical comorbidity saved over $200 annually per patient seen, while the control group exhibited an almost $200 increase. Biodyne patients exhibiting psychological stress and chronic disease comorbidity saved almost $550 annually per patient, while control patients increased costs by almost $500. Biodyne patients whose primary problem was substance use or addiction exhibited a medical savings of $700 savings, while control patients raised costs by almost $900. In an expansion of this Biodyne model, the Hawaii Project II, behavioral services were fully integrated (colocated) into primary care services in three community health centers (Laygo et al., 2003). The Hawaii Project II demonstrated similar medical utilization and cost offsets to the Hawaii Project I (Laygo et al., 2003).

The Biodyne model of individual and group behavioral interventions have been detailed in a number of different books (Cummings and Cummings, 2000; Cummings et al., 1997) and only key parts of their group protocols are mentioned here. The model included six chronic disease group programs: asthma, diabetes, emphysema and chronic obstructive pulmonary disease (COPD), hypertension, ischemia, and rheumatoid arthritis including fibromyalgia (Cummings et al., 1997). There were eight group programs for psychological conditions and four for addictive and substance-abuse patients (Cummings et al., 1997). Each group protocol has three aspects with disease-specific emphasis: *treatment* of the medical psychological components of each condition, *management* of the chronic aspects, and *prevention* of relapse or serious untoward developments (Cummings and Cummings, 2005). Each group protocol also included key characteristics: (1) educational component, (2) pain management, (3) relaxation techniques, (4) stress management, (5) support systems, (6) self-evaluation components, (7) homework, (8) treatment of depression, (9) self-efficacy components, (10) learned helplessness protocols, (11) sense of coherence, (12) exercise protocols, and (13) modular formatting of protocols to promote mixing and matching (Cummings and Cummings, 2005).

Examples of other heterogeneous chronic disease management groups are those developed on principles within the chronic care model (CCM; Wagner, 1996) and those overseen by the chronic disease self-management program (CDSMP; Lorig et al., 1993) discussed in the Introduction. Under the guidance of self-efficacy principles, the CDSMP targets six skills that I will briefly review below (Lorig and Holman, 2003). *Problem-solving skills* include strategies and practice with problem definition, generation of alternate solutions, solution implementation, and evaluation of results. *Decision making* is identified as a separate skill that focuses on how to make day-to-day decisions around changes in disease condition. *Resource utilization skills* include teaching patients techniques to locate, seek out, establish contact, and evaluate resources available to them. The *formation of patient–provider partnerships* is a skill that frequently requires a paradigm shift in many patients' conceptualization of their patient–provider roles; the provider role shifts from expert to a teacher, partner, and professional supervisor. *Action planning* is characterized by skill mastery and implementation and includes learning to develop a short-term action plan, carry it out, reevaluate it, and make any necessary changes to modify it or make it more "doable." *Self-tailoring* is described as the skill that sets self-management programs apart from traditional health promotion or education efforts. Self-tailoring stems from literature that has established the importance of assessing and addressing a patient's readiness to learn, stage of change, and health belief model (Prochaska and DiClemente, 1986; Rosenstock, 1974).

Outcome Data

The impressive results of the coordinated services offered by the Hawaii project have already been mentioned above, those studies demonstrated the ability of nontraditional group-based integrated behavioral health interventions to reduce health utilization and health cost offsets for services provided to various chronically diseased individuals with comorbid psychological distress (Cummings et al., 1993; Cummings and Cummings, 2005).

Much research has been conducted on Lorig and colleagues (1999) CDSMP. In a 6-month randomized controlled trial of 952 patients with diagnosed heart disease, lung disease, stroke, or arthritis, participating in either a CDSMP or a wait-list control, CDSMP group participants showed improvements in weekly minutes of exercise, frequency of cognitive symptom management, communication with physicians, self-reported health, health distress, fatigue, disability, and social/role activities. CDSMP participants also had fewer hospitalizations and hospital days (Lorig et al., 1999). In a continuing study of 489 CD patients, comparisons of base-line and follow-up data found that at 1 year participants in the CDSMP experienced statistically significant improvements in health behaviors (e.g., exercise, cognitive symptom management, and communication with physicians), self-efficacy, health status (e.g., fatigue, shortness of breath, pain, role function, depression, and health distress), and reduced emergency department visits ($p < 0.05$; Lorig et al., 2001). Researchers estimated program costs to be about $200 per participant (Lorig et al., 2001). In an additional study of 831 participants with heart disease, lung disease, stroke, and arthritis in CDSMP groups, Lorig and colleagues (2001) compared participants against baseline for 2 years and demonstrated statistically significant reductions in ER/outpatient visits, health-related distress, and improved self-efficacy ($p < 0.05$).

Individual Therapy

Patients may need to work with an individual therapist for one of two reasons: (1) they have high levels of psychological distress or deficient skill repertoires that prohibit them from participating and gaining benefit from alternative less intensive steps of care or (2) they lack motivation or commitment to behavior change and require early individual therapy that may then permit them to gain the benefits of less intensive self-management alternatives.

- Problem-solving therapy can be helpful if the patients need assertiveness training, communication strategies, decision-making techniques, prioritization techniques, skills regarding interaction with the medical system and have difficulty performing necessary self-monitoring skills, decision support around treatment options, adherence and treatment compliance, gaining social support, and barriers to lifestyle changes.
- Behavior therapy can be helpful if a patient needs one-on-one assistance with health-related behavior modification (e.g., stimulus control, reinforcement strategies, and self-monitoring for behaviors such as exercise, diet, smoking cessation, alcohol reduction, and adherence).
- Empirically based protocols should be followed when available such as when providing clients with strategies for pain management, stress management, relaxation, anxiety and depression, or addressing problems with motivation (Arkowitz and Miller, 2008).

- Relapse prevention skills are useful if the patient is stable, stepping down in treatment or terminating, or anticipating participation in a stressful event.
- Cognitive behavior therapy is appropriate if a patient is struggling with depression or anxiety, expressing maladaptive thoughts or beliefs, catastrophizing, or would benefit from learning about the biopsychosocial model of illness or the ABCs of behavior.
- Emotion regulation techniques are appropriate if a patient is avoiding emotional processing or experiencing.
- Mindfulness and acceptance-based techniques may be helpful if the patient is struggling with anxiety, avoiding limitations/restrictions caused by their diagnosis or having trouble accepting their CD status or impaired functioning.
- Caregiver skills and support to family and friends may be warranted to shore up social support.

Outcome Data

While the outcome data on individual therapy for the treatment of mental disorders in general is extensive, the research available on individual therapy for the treatment of mental disorders specific to chronic disease is much more sparse. Below I will review how the different treatment techniques mentioned above have been used to treat different CD in the literature. For example, research on problem-solving therapy and the management of diabetes has been equivocal (Hill-Briggs, 2003). Hill-Briggs (2003) suggests this is largely because of widely varied conceptualization and measurement of problem solving in the context of chronic disease. The essential role of problem solving is widely accepted clinically and remains an important component of chronic disease management (Paterson and Thorne, 2000; Bonnet et al., 1998).

Research on emotion regulation techniques and chronic disease management has shown that avoidance and inhibition of emotions are associated with maladaptive outcomes such as increased disease occurrence and risk of disease progression, while there is increasing evidence that routine acknowledgment and expression of emotions can promote good disease adjustment (Austenfeld and Stanton, 2004). Research found that emotional expression in chronic diseases led to improved psychological adjustment as evidenced by decreased distress, improvement in mood, and a reduction in intrusions for several months following the intervention (Kelley et al., 1997; Stanton, Danoff-Burg, Sworoski et al., 2002; Warner, Lumley, Casey et al., 2006; Wetherell, Byrne-Davis, Dieppe et al., 2005; Zakowski et al., 2004). Emotional expression also led to improved physical adjustment as evidenced by reduced health-care use, improved physical functioning, fewer reported symptoms, reduced self-perceived disease activity for several months following the intervention (De Moor, Sterner, Hall et al., 2002; Kelley et al., 1997; Rosenberg, Rosenberg, Ernstoff et al., 2002; Stanton et al., 2002; Taylor et al., 2003; Warner et al., 2006; Wetherell et al., 2005). The expression of emotions also led to improved clinical and laboratory observations (e.g., pulmonary function in asthma, joint score in rheumatoid arthritis, CD4+ lymphocyte counts in HIV) for several months following the intervention (Broderick et al., 2004; Rosenberg et al., 2002; Taylor et al., 2003; Warner et al., 2006; Wetherell et al., 2005).

Research on mindfulness and acceptance strategies has found that accepting responses to chronic pain are positively associated with more successful adaptation to that pain: less depression, less overt pain and less pain-related suffering (Schmitz et al., 1996), adaptively coping with pain (McCracken et al., 1999), less disability, pain-related anxiety, more daily up-time, and better work status (McCracken and Eccleston, 2003).

Research on the benefits of caregiver skills and support interventions and chronic disease has shown that the caregiving role to Alzheimer's patients (whether continuing or former) results in long-term physiological consequences in the form of significantly poorer response by natural killer cells to cytokines in older adults than for control groups (Esterling et al., 1994). With the known physiological and psychological consequences of caregiving, it is important to provide adequate support and skills to caregivers in order to ensure that a healthy and well-functioning social support system exists for the chronically diseased individual. Such efforts include education about the stress of caregiving, behavioral solutions to frequent caregiving challenges, communication training, and emotion regulation techniques for caregivers (Dobrof, Ebenstein, Dodd et al., 2006; Hepburn et al., 1991).

Research on cognitive behavioral therapy (CBT) and chronic disease has shown the effectiveness of CBT for patients presenting at cardiac clinics with non-cardiac chest pain who were offered to participate in a trial of cognitive behavioral therapy if they continued to have symptoms at their 6-week follow-up (Mayou et al., 1997). Of the small number ($N = 37$) that agreed to participate, patients were randomized to a treatment group who received 12 sessions of individual therapy from a counseling psychologist or an assessment-only control. At the 6-month follow-up, the cognitive behavioral therapy treatment group experienced significantly lower symptom severity ($F(1, 34) = 4.82, p < 0.05$), significantly higher social activity levels ($F(1, 34) = 5.19, p < 0.05$), and lower percentage of patients meeting criteria for DMS-IV diagnosis (Mayou et al., 1997). In a randomized controlled crossover trial researcher's compared CBT for adherence and depression (CBT-AD) and enhanced treatment as usual (ETAU: single-session intervention for adherence and a letter to the patient's provider documenting their continued depression) in 45 HIV-infected individuals (Safren et al., 2009). Participants in the intervention group received 10–12 sessions of CBT-AD, and both the groups received ETAU. At outcome assessment (3 months), the CBT-AD group demonstrated statistically significant improvements in change scores for adherence ($F(1, 42) = 21.94, p<0.0001$) and depression as measured by the Clinical Global Impression ($F(1, 42) = 9.68, p < 0.01$), the Hamilton Depression Rating Scale ($F(1, 42) = 6.32, p < 0.02$), and the Beck Depression Inventory ($F(1, 42) = 9.78, p < 0.01$). Comparison cross-over patients demonstrated similar improvements, and by the end of the follow-up period, the original CBT-AD group also demonstrated improvements in plasma HIV RNA concentrations ($p < 0.05$).

Medication

Psychopharmacologic management of psychological symptoms and neuropsychiatric symptoms consequent to disease is a central part of a patient's treatment battery. It is critical that any prescribing provider realize that the psychotropic(s) being suggested will be added to a complex medication regimen including things such as antibiotics, analgesics, antacids, steroids, anti-convulsive agents, bronchodilators, cardiovascular agents, hormone replacement, hypoglycemic agents, and potentially numerous disease-specific pharmacologic agents (Leipzig, 1990). Given the complexity of a patient's medication routine the physician's credo "do no harm" becomes particularly relevant when considering factors such as potential drug interactions, polypharmacy, excess disability, problems with malnutrition or dehydration, very young or very advanced age, and possible deficiencies of metabolizing enzymes (Kalash, 1998; Leipzig, 1990).

Steps should be taken that minimize the chance of causing harm to the patient including performing a comprehensive review of the patient's current medication, consulting with a pharmacologist to review the safety and risk associated with adding/modifying any medication, providing education on adherence, proper use, handling, symptom monitoring, and guidance on when to seek help for problems associated with new medication.

Outcome Data

In a feasibility study of antidepressant drug therapy to treat depression in elderly chronic obstructive pulmonary disease patients the findings reflect the potential ineffectiveness and therapeutic concerns of treating depression in CD patients with drug therapy alone (Yohannes et al., 2001). In the single-blind study of 137 symptomatic irreversible moderate to severe COPD patients, 57 were diagnosed with criteria meeting depression. Fourteen agreed to undergo drug therapy (fluoxetine, 20 mg/day for 6 months) and 36 refused to take the antidepressant. Of the seven completers, four responded positively to the fluoxetine therapy on their depression measure at 6 weeks ($t = 2.05, p = 0.02$) without any further improvement at 3 or 6 months. When 22 of the patients who refused antidepressant therapy were interviewed, 19 endorsed still being depressed. The study concluded that patient acceptance of fluoxetine was poor and the untreated depression in the COPD patients often became chronic. The authors concluded that offering antidepressant medication to depressed COPD patients is not an effective depression management strategy (Yohannes et al., 2001).

A larger ($N = 1801$) randomized controlled trial of antidepressant medication versus 6–8 sessions of problem-solving focused psychotherapy for depression against usual care (generally usual care consisted of antidepressant medication and if deemed necessary by primary care providers referral to specialty mental health services) found positive results for the more comprehensive care program (Lin et al., 2003). In addition to lower depressive symptoms, at 12 months the intervention group also had lower pain intensity scores (between group difference $p < 0.009$), lower interference with daily activities due to arthritis (between group difference $p < 0.004$), lower interference with daily activities due to pain (between group difference $p < 0.002$), and overall health and quality of life were also improved for intervention patients relative to the control group (Lin et al., 2003). The study highlights the benefits of treatment above and beyond usual care with antidepressant medication for depression in older adults with arthritis (Lin et al., 2003).

In a study that assessed antidepressant use before and after initiation of diabetes mellitus treatment, researchers found that antidepressant and benzodiazepine use was increased 2 months before and 3 months after initiation of diabetes treatment, usually medication (Knol et al., 2009). The strongest increase in medication use was seen in the month after treatment initiation (antidepressant incident rate ratio of 2.4: 95% CI 2.0–3.0; benzodiazepine incident rate ratio of 3.4: 95% CI 3.0–3.8), suggesting that depression may be a frequent consequent (rather than antecedent) to the burden of diabetes disease, starting diabetes medication, or being diagnosed with diabetes (Knol et al., 2009). The study highlights the importance of solicitous and early detection of psychological health following initial diagnosis of a chronic disease and the potential role of medication in the management of psychological adjustment symptoms (Knol et al., 2009).

Inpatient Treatment

Inpatient treatment for the persons with a chronic disease could take one of two forms: (1) treatment while within a hospital or care facility setting that would simply entail the earlier steps of care delivered within that setting and (2) a person requiring intensive treatment in a secure and regulated setting for acute and severe psychological distress associated with or consequent to coping with their chronic disease. Most commonly this would include severe depression or threat to harm self or others. Inpatient treatment should adhere to empirically established protocols for the management of the presenting problem, with a focus on establishing and implementing support structures and skills for the patient's return to the community. Disease self-management, stress inoculation, and relapse prevention should be a focus of treatment. Prior to releasing a patient from inpatient treatment, efforts should be made to enhance their social and professional supports, and new decision point thresholds should be established for guiding future clinical decisions.

Outcome Data

In a study of patients with chronic pain and severe disuse syndrome, positive long-term outcomes were found for an inpatient multidisciplinary cognitive behavioral program (van Wilgen et al., 2009). The authors stated that for severe chronic pain and disuse syndrome patients, inpatient treatment may be warranted if the duration or severity of physiological, psychological, and social adaptations of the pain, combined with previous treatment failures, warrants treatment beyond that available in primary care (van Wilgen et al., 2009). For the 32 patients who participated in the inpatient program, long-term significant ($p < 0.001$) improvements were documented in reported pain severity, fatigue, walking distance, muscle strength, anxiety, depression, somatization, negative self-efficacy, and catastrophizing in the intervention period (van Wilgen et al., 2009).

Consumer Preferences and Cultural Sensitivity

While some empirical studies have been conducted on patient preferences within certain disease types; choice options are usually disease specific and therefore cannot be generalized to other consumer groups (Torgerson et al., 1996; Klaber-Moffett et al., 1999; Williams et al., 1999; Janevic et al., 2003). While sparse, existing research shows that consumer preference or choice of intervention does seem to effect health-related outcomes (Bakker, Spinhoven, van Balkom, Vleugel, van Dyck, 2000; Rovers et al., 2001). In a study by Clark and colleagues (2008) it was found that when consumer choice was permitted for a group or self-directed heart disease management program patients, those individuals showed a preference for group format and this group showed enhanced psychological and physical functioning at 1 year. Interestingly, despite a preference for group format, cardiac symptoms were fewer over 18 months follow-up for patients assigned to the self-directed format, perhaps due to the self-discipline required to complete the self-directed program. These findings suggest that while permitting consumer-directed choice for intervention increases adherence and attendance; it may not be the best strategy to increase program efficacy. This finding suggests that disease management programs may increase efficacy and adherence by targeting patient motivation and stages of change first within the preferred patient step and then facilitating program efficacy by assisting patients' completion of the more demanding self-directed programs.

Studies have shown that self-management skills are recognized and appreciated by patients from varying cultures, suggesting that they are a valuable and preferential component to CDM protocols (Walker et al., 2005). Notably, minority chronic disease patients often receive brief infrequent health visits that result in their providers demonstrating an incomplete understanding and monitoring of a patient's culturally based explanatory model of their disease, adherence to self-management, barriers to adherence, and patient functioning (Katon et al., 2001). This deficiency results in an incomplete understanding of a patient's functional deficits and a lack of appreciation of a patient's need for rehabilitative, supportive, and educational services.

Disease Management Industry Outcome Data

Outcome research conducted on disease management programs is highly variable in terms of methodological quality (e.g., lack of control populations, reliance on longitudinal pre/post-study design, and poor control of selection bias and regression to the mean) and, because of an overall focus on process rather than costing metrics, the causal linkages between disease management programs and any positive return on investment have remained elusive (Geyman, 2007; Levy et al., 2007). Reviews of the literature consistently conclude that disease management programs improve the quality of care delivered to the patient; however, the same programs may not also improve the cost effectiveness of care (Geyman, 2007; Ouwens et al., 2005). Cost savings has indeed been demonstrated across numerous studies; however, these studies are criticized for not factoring in the full cost of the disease management interventions themselves (Geyman, 2007). Furthermore, there are very few studies that compare the outcomes of chronic disease management programs integrated within primary care, like the chronic care model's of Group Health Cooperative in Seattle and Kaiser Permanente in Northern California, with the commercial programs such as those carved out private for-profit companies that are contracted on a per-member-per-month fee for a package of services to employers or health-care providers or public sector providers such as Medicaid (Casalino, 2005; Geyman, 2007; Landro, 2006). This lack of comparison leaves consumers without direction in terms of a preferred model for implementation.

Empirically sound studies published by the Group Health Cooperative in Seattle; which, as mentioned above adopted Wagner's chronic care model in the mid-1990s, demonstrated a 2-year 11% overall cost reduction for 15,000 diabetic patients (except for pharmacy costs which increased by 16%) and a 25% reduction in specialty visits and hospital admissions (Geyman, 2007; McCulloch et al., 2004). During this 2-year period the program also demonstrated an improvement in quality, evidenced by sustained reductions of glycosylated hemoglobin levels (Wagner, Sandhu, Newton et al., 2001). Over a 6-year time frame, Kaiser Permanente programs in Northern California demonstrated substantial quality improvement, but without any cost savings, for their multidisciplinary program's focused on coronary artery disease, heart failure, diabetes, and asthma (Fireman et al., 2004). Results are more ambiguous when looking at the overall track record of all disease management programs, including the commercial carve outs described above that are often disconnected from primary care (Geyman, 2007). Three recent assessments cast doubt on whether disease management programs are an effective vehicle for cost containment: a 2006 analysis of numbers needed to treat, in order to decrease costs, calculated that such programs would need to decrease hospital admissions by 10–30% to cover program fees alone (Linden, 2006); in 2004 the Congressional Budget Office stated that there was insufficient evidence to conclude if such programs could generally reduce overall health spending (Holtz-Eakin, 2004); and a 2005 report on the long-term effects of such programs on cost savings in diabetes concluded that over a 30-year time frame with zero turnover (patients stay with the same plan) the net effect on diabetes-related costs would be an overall increase of about 25% (Eddy et al., 2005). A general criticism of reviews of cost savings for integrated disease management programs is that the analysis is often too short term and that the projections do not account for the full cost of the interventions (Geyman, 2007; Ouwens et al., 2005).

Quality Improvement Outcomes

Quality improvement outcomes on the individual level include things such as feeling like an active participant and partner in care, disease stability (improvement or normal trajectory), consumer/patient satisfaction, adherence to medical regimens, lifestyle improvements (health promoting behaviors), reduced medical expenses, fewer costly medical procedures, reported increase in health-related quality of life, and reduced comorbid psychological distress. Quality improvement outcomes on the industry level include things such as increased patient numbers, reduced costs of services, increase consumer satisfaction and retention rates, higher reports of provider satisfaction and retention, reduction in redundant assessments/tests, improved practitioner communication, and adherence to practice guidelines.

Quality improvement has focused on the frequently fragmented, disorganized, and duplicative junction of primary care and mental health (Norris, Nichols, Caspersen et al., 2002). CDM programs have focused on strategies to deliver services differently through integrated primary care, with carefully coordinated and monitored links to community resources, employer resources, and emphasizing the efforts of self-management of CD (Myette, 2008). These models are demonstrating improved quality of care and cost-effectiveness relative to usual care (Weingarten et al., 2002; Neumeyer-Gromen et al., 2004; Ofman et al., 2004). Cavanagh and colleagues (2006) benchmarked findings from a computerized cognitive behavior therapy (CCBT) program against equivalent "completer" data sets and researchers found that CCBT program offered benefits similar to those associated with routine delivery of face-to-face depression treatment (Barkham et al., 2005).

Quality improvement of outcome measurement should focus on objective quantifiable data including health-care utilization, cost, readmission rates, length of stay, emergency department visit rate, office visit rate, and quality of life (Mayzell, 1999). Program effectiveness should include goal-oriented performance measures on the patient side, provider side, and plan side (Mayzell, 1999). Researchers have found that across varied CDM programs and diagnoses, participation in CD programs results in a combination of lower insurance expenditures, hospital admissions and readmissions, hospital days, emergency department visits, and moderate program satisfaction (Sylvia et al., 2008; Douglas et al., 2007; Afifi et al., 2007).

Triage Agenda

Psychology continues to poorly define, articulate, and evaluate principles such as clinically significant change and treatment (Davison, 2000). This lack of clarity negatively effects provider's ability to efficiently and appropriately triage patients into stepped care. Without clearly defined guidelines and markers for what clinically significant change is, it is difficult to know when to step patients up or down between levels of care (Davison, 2000; Haaga, 2000). The discipline of psychology continues to struggle with what the most effective and powerful components of our best empirically supported treatments are. We continue to have inconsistent and duplicative diagnostic symptoms and treatment components, and this duplicity makes treatment determinations difficult and subjective (Davison, 2000; Von Korff Tiemens, 2000). We consistently blame the patient and their lack of adherence and motivation rather than look toward system deficiencies (Von Korff and Tiemens, 2000). When systems are modified to reflect best chronic disease management principles, such as those discussed in Wagner's chronic care model (1998), powerful heath-related behavior change can occur. When there is enhanced collaboration between patients and providers, patients' health improves (Von Korff and Tiemens, 2000). Psychology must address these issues in order to make triage decisions based more on scientific evidence and less on subjective bias and judgment.

Research and Development Agenda

More research needs to occur on the clinical decision factors (thresholds, benchmarks, and matching) mentioned in triage above. While the efficiency of coordinated and patient-centered care programs including the CCM, CDSMP, and ICCM has been established, we need to research their effectiveness and develop strategies to manage the systemic barriers to integration (Wagner and Groves, 2002).

The literature shows that enhanced collaboration between the patient and the provider improves patient outcomes (Von Korff et al., 1997). We must research how to best implement the innovative "patient as expert" model of chronic disease management. Care management that uses structured protocols and active follow-up has produced beneficial effects for a range of chronic disease conditions (Katon et al., 1995, 1996; Alexopoulos et al., 2008; DiMatteo et al., 2000); however, research shows that systems of care often fail to follow clinical practice guidelines for key aspects of chronic disease patients (Katon et al., 2001; Wagner et al., 1996; Von Korff et al., 1997). Research needs to explore why there are such unwarranted variations in adherence to practice guidelines and variations in health-care delivery (Wennberg, 2002).

Dissemination Agenda

Disseminating empirically supported CDM protocols to a larger community of mental and physical health providers would benefit the overall population. CDM is largely bound within health-care systems and managed care operations. It seems that the rising prevalence of CD mandates CDM prevention efforts to be incorporated into community, schools, and workplace settings in order to assist the largest possible number of people. Knowledge about stepped care and its cost-saving effectiveness should be distributed to those making policy and funding decisions. Consumers should be given more information about empirically based treatments and have an opportunity to decide what type of stepped-care interventions they want/need from their providers.

Conclusion

In a review of 39 chronic care models of treatment across diseases including diabetes, congestive heart failure, and asthma, researchers found six key elements that were associated with reduced health-care costs and lowered use of health-care services (Bodenheimer et al., 2002). These six elements include (1) making chronic disease care a goal of the health-care organization; (2) provide links to community resources; (3) support patient self-management processes including defining problems, setting priorities, establishing goals, identifying barriers, creating treatment plans, and solving problems rather than just focusing on health education; (4) use evidence-based guidelines to improve provider decision making; (5) use other health-care providers such as nurse case managers, pharmacists, or health educators to deliver care; and (6) establish a register of patient case management information (Dyer et al., 2004). If practitioners and policy makers abide by these six elements as they implement the techniques and targets identified in this chapter, CDM has the potential to benefit current and future patients managing a chronic disease.

References

Afifi AA, Morisky DE, Kominski GF, Kotlerman JB. Impact of disease management on health care utilization: evidence from the "Florida: a health state (fahs)" medicaid program. Prev Med Int J Devot Pract Theory. 2007;44(6):547–553.

Ahern DK, Kreslake JM, Phalen JM. What is eHealth? Perspectives on the evolution of e-health research. J Med Internet Res. 2006;8(1):e4.

Arkowitz H, Miller WR. Applications of motivational interviewing. In: Arkowitz H, Westra HA, Miller WR, Rollnick S, editors. Motivational interviewing in the treatment of psychological problems. New York: Guilford; 2008.

Asch SM, et al. Does the collaborative model improve care for chronic heart failure? Med Care. 2005;43(7):667–675.

Bakker A, Spinhoven P, van Balkom AJ, Vleugel I, van Dyck R. Cognitive therapy by allocation versus cognitive therapy by preference in the treatment of panic disorder. Psychoth Psychosoma. 2000;69(5):240–243.

Barkham M, Connell J, Stiles WB, Miles JNV, Margison E, Evans C, Mellor-Clark, J. Dose-effect relations and responsive regulation of treatment duration: the good enough level. J Consult Clin Psychol. 2006;74:160–167.

Barnett TE, Chumbler NR, Vogel WB, Beyth RJ, Qin J, Kobb R. The effectiveness of a care coordination home telehealth program for veterans with diabetes mellitus: a 2-year follow-up. Am J Manag Care. 2006;12:467–474.

Beale IL, Kato PM, Marin-Bowling VM, Guthrie N, Cole SW. Improvement in cancer-related knowledge following use of a psychoeducational video game for adolescents and young adults with cancer. J Adolesc Health. 2007;41(3):263–270.

Bodenheimer T, Wagner EH, Grumbach K. Improving primary care for patients with chronic illness: the chronic care model, part 2. J Am Med Assoc. 2002;288(15):1909–1914.

Bonnet C, Garnayre R, d'Ivernois JF. Learning difficulties of diabetic patients: a survey of educators. Patient Educ Couns. 1998;35:139–147.

Bracke PE, Thorensen CE. Reducing type A behavior patterns: a structured-group approach. In: Allan R, Scheidt S, editors. Heart mind. The practice of cardiac psychology. Washington, D.C.: American Psychological Association; 1996. p. 255–290.

Britton BP, Hoggard A. Telehealth unbound: from home health care to population based care. Telemed e-Health. 2008;14(1):24.

Broderick JE, Stone AA, Smyth JM, Kaell AT. The feasibility and effectiveness of an expressive writing intervention for rheumatoid arthritis via home-based videotaped instructions. Ann Behav Med. 2004;27:50–59.

Burns DD. Feeling good: the new mood therapy. New York: Harper Collins; 1999.

Casalino LP. Disease management and the organization of physician practice. J Am Med Assoc. 2005;293(4):485–488.

Cavanagh K, Shapiro DA, Van Den Berg S, Swain S, Barkham M, Proudfoot J. The effectiveness of computerized cognitive therapy in routine care. Br J Clin Psychol. 2006;45:499–514.

Chamberlain D, Heaps D, Robert I. Bibliotherapy and information prescriptions: a summary of the published evidence-base and recommendations from past and ongoing books on prescription projects. J Psychiatr Ment Health Nurs. 2008;15:24–36.

Clark NM, Janz NK, Dodge JA, Mosca L, Lin X, Long Q, et al. The effect of patient choice of intervention on health outcomes. Contemp Clin Trials. 2008;29:679–686.

Cummings NA, Cummings JL. The essence of psychotherapy: reinventing the art in the era of data. San Diego, CA: Academic Press; 2000.

Cummings NA, Cummings JL. (2005) Behavioral interventions for somatisizers. In: Cummings NA, O'Donohue WT, Naylor EV, editors. Psychological approaches to chronic disease management. Reno, NV: Context Press; 2005. p. 49–70.

Cummings NA, Cummings JL, Johnson JN. Behavioral health as primary care: a guide for clinical integration. Madison, CT: Psychosocial Press; 1997.

Cummings NA, Dorken H, Pallak MS, Henke CJ. The impact of psychological interventions on health care costs and utilization: the Hawaii medicaid project. In: Cummings NA, Pallak MS, editors. Medicaid, managed behavioral health and implications for public policy. South San Francisco, CA: Foundation for Behavioral Health; 1993. p. 3–23.

Cummings NA, O'Donohue WT, Naylor EV. Psychological approaches to chronic disease management. Reno, NV: Context Press; 2005.

Darkins A, Ryan P, Kobb R, Foster L, Edmonson E, Wakefield B, Lancaster AE. Care coordination/home telehealth: the systematic implementation of health informatics, home telehealth, and disease management to support the care of veteran patients with chronic conditions. Telemed J eHealth. 2008;14(10):1118–1126.

Davison GC. Stepped care: doing more with less? J Consult Clin Psychol. 2000;68:580–585.

de Ridder D, Geenen R, Kuijer R, van Middendorp H. Psychological adjustment to chronic disease. Lancet. 2008;372:245–255.

den Boer PCAM, Wiersma D, van den Bosch RJ. Why is self-help neglected in the treatment of emotional disorders? A meta-analysis. Psychol Med. 2004;34:959–971.

De Moore C, Sterner J, Hall M, et al. A pilot study of the effects of expressive writing on psychological and behavioral adjustment in patients enrolled in a Phase II trial of vaccine therapy for metastatic renal cell carcinoma. Health Psychol. 2002;21:615–619.

Disease Management Association of America. (2009). Def disease manag. DMAA downloaded from http://www.dmaa.org/definition.html retrieved September 12, 2009.

Dobrof J, Ebenstein H, Dodd S-J, Epstein I, Christ G, Blacker S. Caregivers and professionals partnership caregiver resource center: assessing a hospital support program for family caregivers. J Palliat Med.2006;9(1):196–205.

Douglas SL, Daly BJ, Kelley CG O'Toole E, Montenegro H. Chronically critically ill patients: health-related quality of life and resource use after a disease management intervention. Am J Crit Care. 2007;16(5):447–457.

Dusseldorp E, Van Elderen T, Maes S, Meulman J, Kraaij V. A meta-analysis of psycheducational programs for coronary heart disease patients. Health Psychol. 1999;18(5):506–519.

Dyer JR, Levy RM, Dyer RL. (2005). An integrated model for changing patient behavior in primary care. In: Cummings NA, O'Donohue WT, Nailor EV, editors. Psychological approaches to chronic disease management. Reno, NV: Context Press; 2005. p. 71–86.

Dwight-Johnson M, Ell K, Lee PJ. Can collaborative care address the needs of low-income Latinas with comorbid depression and cancer? Results from a randomized pilot study. Psychosomatics. 2005;46(3):224–232.

Eddy DM, Schlessinger L, Kahn R. Clinical outcomes and cost-effectiveness of strategies for managing people at high risk for diabetes. Anna Internal Med. 2005;143(4):251–264.

Esterling BA, Kiecolt-Glaser JK, Bodnar JC, Glaser R. Chronic stress, social support, and persistent alternations in the natural killer cell response to cytokines in older adults. Health Psychol. 1994;13(4):291–298.

Fireman B, Barlett J, Selby J. Can disease management reduce health care costs by improving quality? Health Affairs. 2004;23(6):63–75.

Foote SM. Population-based disease management under fee-for-service Medicare. Health Affiliates (Millwood), Suppl Web Exclusives. 2003;W3:342–356.

Geyman JP. Disease management: panacea, another false hope, or something in between? Anna Fam Med. 2007;5:257–260.

Haaga DAF. Introduction to the special section on stepped care models in psychotherapy. J Consult Clin Psychol. 2000;68:547–548.

Hemingway H, Marmot M. Psychosocial factors in the aetiology and prognosis of coronary heart disease: systematic review of prospective cohort studies. Br Med J. 1999; 318:1460–1467.

Hepburn K, Caron W, Mach JR. Caregivers of persons with chronic illness or impairments: strategies and interventions. In: Myers WA, editor. New techniques in the psychotherapy of older patients. Washington, DC: American Psychiatric Association; 1991. p. 39–59.

Hill-Briggs F. Problem solving in diabetes self-management: a model of chronic illness self-management behavior. Ann Behav Med. 2003;25(3):182–193.

Holtz-Eakin P. CBO Director, Testimony to Congress. October 13, 2004.

Hooper L, Bartlett C, Davey SG, et al. Advice to reduce dietary salt for prevention of cardiovascular disease. Cochrane Database Systematic Review, 1(CD003656); 2003.

Janevic MR, Janz NK, Dodge JA, Lin X, Pan W, Sinco BR, Clark NM. The role of choice in health education intervention trials: a review and case study. Soc Sci Med. 2003;56:1581–1594.

Kalash GR. Psychotropic drug metabolism in the cancer patient: clinical aspects of management of potential drug interactions. Psychoncology. 1998;7:307–320.

Kashem A, Cross RC, Santamore WP, Bove AA. Management of heart failure patients using telemedicine communication systems. Current Cardiol Report. 2006;8(3):171–179.

Kashem A, Droogan MT, Santamore WP, Wald JW, Bove AA. Managing heart failure care using an internet-based telemedicine system. J Cardiac Failure. 2008;14(2):121–126.

Katon W, Von Korff M, Lin E, et al. Collaborative management to achieve treatment guidelines impact on depression in primary care. J Am Med Assoc. 1995;273:1026–1031.

Katon W, Robinson P, Von Korff et al. A multifaceted intervention to improve treatment of depression in primary care. Arch Gen Psychiatry. 1996;53:924–932.

Katon W, Von Korff M, Lin E, Simon G. Rethinking practitioner roles in chronic illness: the specialist, primary care physician, and the practice nurse. Gen Hosp Psychiatry. 2001;23:138–144.

Katz DA, Littenberg B, Cronenwett JL. Management of small abdominal aortic aneurysms. Early surgery vs watchful waiting. J Am Med Assoc. 1992;268(16):2678–2686.

Kelley JE, Lumley MA, Leisen JC. Health effects of emotional disclosure in rheumatoid arthritis patients. J Clin Oncol. 1997;22:4184–4192.

Klaber-Moffett J, Torgerson D, Bell-Syer S, Jackson D, Llewlyn-Phillips H, Farrin A, Barber J. (1999). Randomised controlled trial of exercise for low back pain: clinical outcomes, costs, and preferences. Br Med J. 1999;319:279–283.

Knol MJ, Geerlings MI, Grobbee DE, Egberts ACG, Heerdink ER. Antidepressant use before and after initiation of diabetes mellitus treatment. Diabetologia. 2009;52:425–432.

Krumholz HM, Currie PM, Riegel B, Phillips CO, Peterson ED, Smith R, Yancy CW, Faxon DP. A taxonomy for disease management: a scientific statement from the American heart association disease management taxonomy writing group. Circulation. 2006;114:1432–1445.

Landro J. Eliminating conflicts in medical treatment. Wall Street J. February 8, 2006;D5.

Latner, J.D. Self-help in the long term treatment of obesity. Obesity Res. 2001;2:87–97.

Laygo R, O'Donohue WT, Hall S, Kaplan A, Wood R, Cummings J, et al. Preliminary report from the Hawaii integrated healthcare project II. In: Cummings NA, O'Donohue WT, Ferguson K, editors. Behavioral health as primary care: Beyond efficacy to effectiveness. Reno, NV: Context Press; 2003. p. 111–114.

Levy P, Nocerini R, Grazier K. Paying for disease management. Disease Manag. 2007;10(4): 235–244.

Lewinsohn PM, Munoz RF, Youngren MA, Zeiss AM. Control your depression. New York: Simon Schuster; 1986.

Lin EHB, Katon W, Von Korff M, Tang L, Williams JW, Kroenke K, et al. Effect of improving depression care on pain and functional outcomes among older adults with arthritis: a randomized controlled trial. J Am Med Assoc. 2003;290(18):2428–2434.

Linden AL. What will it take for disease management to demonstrate a return on investment? New perspectives on an old theme. Am J Manag Care. 2006;12(4):251–264.

Lorig KR, Holman HR. Self-management education: history, definition, outcomes, and mechanisms. Ann Behav Med. 2003;26(1):1–7.

Lorig KR, Holman HR, Sobel DS, Laurent DD, Gonzalez VM, Minor M. Living a healthy life with chronic conditions. Boulder, CO: Bull Publishing Company; 2006.

Lorig KR, Ritter PL, Dost A, Plant K, Laurent DD, McNeil I. The expert patient programme online, a 1-year study of an Internet-based self-management programme for people with long-term conditions. Chronic Illness. 2008;4:247–256.

Lorig KR, Ritter PL, Laurent DD, Plant K. Internet-based chronic disease self-management. A randomized trial. Med Care. 2006;44(11):964–971.

Lorig KR, Ritter PL, Laurent DD, Plant K. The internet-based arthritis self-management program: a one-year randomized trial for patients with arthritis or fibromyalgia. Arthrit Rheum. 2008;59(7):1009–1017.

Lorig KR, Ritter P, Stewart AL, Sobel DS, Brown BW, Bandura A, Gonzalez VM, Laurent DD, Holman HR. (2001). Chronic disease self-management program: 2-year health status and health care utilization outcomes. Med Care. 2001;39(11):1217–1223.

Lorig KR, Sobel DS, Ritter PL, Laurent D, Hobbs M. Effect of self-management program on patients with chronic disease. Effect Clin Pract. 2001;4:256–262.

Lorig KR, Sobel DS, Stewart AL, Brown BW, Bandura A, Ritter P, Gonzalez VM, Laurent DD, Holman HR. Evidence suggesting that a chronic disease self-management program can improve health status while reducing hospitalization. Med Care. 1999;37(1):5–14.

Mangione-Smith R, et al. Measuring the effectiveness of a collaborative for quality improvement in pediatric asthma care: does implementing the chronic care model improve processes and outcomes of care? Ambulatory Pediatr. 2005;5(2):75–82.

Mayou RA, Sanders BD, Bass C, Klimes I, Forfar C. A controlled trial of cognitive behavioral therapy for non-cardiac chest pain. Psychol Med. 1997;27:1021–1031.

Mayzell G. Disease management. Jacksonville Medicine. 1999;50:380–382.

McCracken LM, Eccleston C. Coping or acceptance: what to do about chronic pain? Pain. 2003;105(1–2):299–306.

McCracken LM, Spertus IL, Janeck AS, Sinclair D, Wetzel FT. Behavioral dimensions of adjustment in persons with chronic pain: pain-related anxiety and acceptance. Pain. 1999;80 (1–2):283–289.

McCulloch D, Davis C, Austin B, Wagner E. Constructing a bridge across the quality chasm: a practical way to get healthier, happier patients, providers, and health care systems. Diabetes Spect. 2004;17:92–96.

Meredith LS, Cheng WJY, Hickey SC, Dwight-Johnson M. Factors associated with primary care clinicians' choice of a watchful waiting approach to managing depression. Psychiatr Serv. 2007;58:72–78.

Mimeault V, Morin CM. Self-help treatment for insomnia: bibliotherapy with and without professional guidance. J Consult Clin Psychol. 1999;67:511–519.

Morgan AJ, Jorm AF. Self-help interventions for depressive disorders and depressive symptoms: a systematic review. Ann Gen Psychiatry. 2008;7(13).

Moynihand T. (2008). Podcast: watchful waiting and cancer therapy. MayoClinic.com downloaded from http://www.mayoclinic.com/health/watchful-waiting/MY00403 retrieved March 5, 2009.

Myette TL. Integrated management of depression: improving system quality and creating effective interfaces. J Occup Environ Med. 2008;50:482–491.

National Center for Health Statistics. Health, United States, 2008 with chartbook. Hyattsville, MD: U.S. Government Printing Office. Downloaded from http://www.cdc.gov/nchs/fastats/heart.htm retrieved May 24, 2009.

National Center for Health Statistics. Deaths: final data for 2006. National Vital Statistics reports. 2009;57(14):19–22. Downloaded from http://www.cdc.gov/nchs/fastats/heart.htm retrieved May 24, 2009.

Naylor EV, O'Donohye WT. A pilot study investigating behavioral prescriptions for depression. J Clin Psychol Med Sett. 2007;14:152–159.

Neumeyer-Gromen A, Lampert T, Stark K, Kallischnigg G. Disease management programs for depression: a systematic review and meta-analysis of randomized controlled trials. Med Care. 2004;42:1211–1221.

Newman MG. Recommendation for a cost-offset model of psychotherapy allocation using generalized anxiety disorder as an example. J Consult Clin Psychol. 2000;68:549–555.

Norris SL, Nichols PJ, Caspersen CJ, Glasgow RE, Engelgau MM, Jack L, Snyder SR, et al. Increasing diabetes self-management education in community settings: a systematic review. Am J Prev Med. 2002;22(Suppl4):39–66.

Ofman JJ, Badamagarav K, Henning JM, et al. Does disease management improve clinical and economic outcomes in patients with chronic diseases? A systematic review. Am J Med. 2004;117:182–192.

Ouwens M, Wollersheim H, Hermens R, Hulsher M, Grol R. Integrated care programmes for chronically ill patients: a review of systematic reviews. Int J Quality Health Care. 2005;17(2):141–146.

Paterson B, Thorne S. Expert decision making in relation to anticipated blood glucose levels. Res Nurs Health 2005;23:147–157.

Prochaska J, DiClemente C. Toward a comprehensive model of change. In: Miller W, Healther N, editors. Treating addictive behavior. New York: Plenum; 1986. p 3–27.

Proudfoot J, Goldberg DP, Mann A, Everitt B, Marks I, Gray JA. Computerised, interactive, multimedia cognitive behaviour therapy for anxiety and depression in general practice. Psychol Med. 2003;33:217–227.

Proudfoot J, Ryden C, Everitt B, Shapiro DA, Goldberg D, Mann A, Tylee A, Marks I, Gray JA. Clinical efficacy of computerised cognitive-behavioural therapy for anxiety and depression in primary care: randomised controlled trial. Br J Psychiatry. 2004;185:46–54.

Reeves T, Stace JM. Improving patient access and choice: assisted bibliotherapy for mild to moderate stress/anxiety in primary care. J Psychiatr Ment Health Nurs. 2005;12: 341–346.

Redding RE, Herbert JD, Forman EM, Gaudiano BA. Popular self-help books for anxiety, depression, and trauma: how scientifically grounded and useful are they? Prof Psychol Res Pr. 2008;39(5):537–545.

Rosen GM. Self-help treatment books and the commercialization of psychotherapy. Am Psychol. 1987;57:677–689.

Rosenberg HJ, Rosenberg SD, Ernstoff MS, et al. Expressive disclosure and health outcomes in prostate cancer population. Int J Psychiatr Med. 2002;32:37–53.

Rosenstock I. The health belief model and preventive health behavior. Health Educ Monographs. 1974;2:254–386.

Rovers MM, Straatman H, Ingels K, van der Wilt GJ, van den Broek P, Zielhuis GA. Generalizability of trial results based on randomized versus nonrandomized allocation of OME infants to ventilation tubes or watchful waiting. J Clin Epidemiol. 2001;54(8):789–794.

Rozanski A, Blumenthal JA, Kaplan J. Impact of psychological factors on the pathogenesis of cardiovascular disease and implications for therapy. Circulation. 1999;99:2192–2217.

Rybarczyk B, De Marco G, De La Cruz M, Lapidos S. Comparing mind-body wellness interventions for older adults with chronic illness: classroom versus home instruction. Behav Med. 1999;24(4):181–191.

Safren SA, O'Cleirigh C, Tan JY, Raminani SR, Reilly LC, Otto MW, Mayer KH. A randomized controlled trial of cognitive behavioral therapy for adherence and depression (CBT-AD) and HIV-infected individuals. Health Psychol. 2009;28(1):1–10.

Schneiderman N, Antoni MH, Saab PG, Ironson G. Health psychology: psychosocial and biobehavioral aspects of chronic disease management. Ann Rev Psychol. 2001;52:555–580.

Schmitz U, Saile H, Nilges P. Coping with chronic pain: flexible goal adjustment as an interactive buffer against pain-related distress. Pain. 1996;67(1):41–51.

Semple CJ, Dunwoody L, Sullivan K, et al. Patients with head and neck cancer prefer individualized cognitive behavior therapy. Eur J Cancer Care. 2006;15:220–227.

Smith JR, Mugford M, Holland R, Candy B, Noble MJ, Harrison BDW, Koutantji M, Upton C, Harvey I. A systematic review to examine the impact of psycho-educational interventions on health outcomes and costs in adults and children with difficult asthma. Health Technol Assessment. 2005;9(23).

Stanton AL, Danoff-Burg S, Sworowski LA, et al. Randomized, controlled trial of written emotional expression and benefit finding in breast cancer patients. J Clin Oncol. 2002;20: 4160–4168.

Stewart S. Financial aspects of heart failure programs of care. Eur J Heart Failure. 2005;7: 423–428.

Sylvia ML, Griswold M, Dunbar L, Boyd CM, Park M, Boult C. Guided care: cost and utilization outcomes in a pilot study. Disease Manag. 2008;11(1):29–36.

Taylor LA, Wallander JL, Anderson D, Beasley P, Brown RT. Improving health care utilization, improving chronic disease utilization, health status, and adjustment in adolescents and young adults with cystic fibrosis: a preliminary report. J Clin Psychol Med Sett. 2003;10:9–16.

Thom T, Haase N, Rosamond W, et al. Heart disease and stroke statistics, 2006 update: a report from the American Heart association statistics committee and stroke statistics subcommittee. Circulation. 2006;113:e85–e151.

Thompson RL, Summerbell CD, Hooper L, et al. Dietary advice given by a dietician versus other health professional or self-help resources to reduce blood cholesterol. Cochrane Database of Systematic Reviews, 1(CD001366); 2001.

Torgerson DJ, Klaber-Moffett J, Russell IT. Patient preferences in randomized trials: threat or opportunity? J Health Serv Res Policy. 1996;1:194–197.

Van Wilgen CP, Dijkstra PU, Versteegen GJ, Fleuren MJ, Stewart R, van Wijhe M. Chronic pain and severe disuse syndrome: long-term outcomes of an inpatient multidisciplinary cognitive behavioral programme. J Rehabil Med. 2009;41(3):122–128.

Vargas R.B, et al. Can a chronic care model collaborative reduce heart disease risk in patients with diabetes? J Gen Intern Med. 2007;22(2):215–222.

Villagra VG. (2004). Integrating disease management into the outpatient delivery system during and after managed care. Health affiliates (Millwood), supplemental web exclusives: W4; 2004. p. 281–283.

Von Korff M, Grunssan J, Schaefer J, Curry S, Wagner E. Collaborative management of chronic illness: essential elements. Ann Intern Med. 1997;127:1097–1102.

Von Kroff M, Tiemens B. Individualized stepped care of chronic illness. Western J Med. 2000;172:133–137.

Wagner EH. Chronic care management: what will it take to improve care for chronic illness? Effect Clin Pract. 1998;1:1–4.

Wagner E, Austin B, Von Korff M. Organizing care for patients with chronic illness. Milbank Q. 1996;74:511–544.

Wagner EH, Groves T. Care for chronic diseases. Br Med J. 2002;325:913–914.

Wagner EH, Sandhu N, Newton K.M, et al. Effect of improved glycemic conrol on health care costs and utilization. J Am Med Assoc. 2001;285(2):182–189.

Walker C, Weeks A, McAvoy B. Exploring the role of self-management programmes in caring for people from culturally and linguistically diverse backgrounds in Melbourne, Australia. Health Expect. 2005;8:315–323.

Warner LJ, Lumley MA, Casey R.J, et al. Health effects of written emotional disclosure in adolescents with asthma: a randomized, controlled trial. J Pediatr Psychol. 2006;31:557–568.

Weingarten SR, Henning JM, Badamgarav E, Knight K, Hasselblad V, Gano A, Ofman JJ. Interventions used in disease management programs for patients with chronic illness—which ones work? Meta-analysis of published reports. Br Med J. 2002;325:925.

Wennberg J. Unwarranted variations in healthcare delivery: implications for academic medical centres. Br Med J. 2002;325:961–964.

Wetherell MA, Byrne-Davis L, Dieppe P, et al. Effects of emotional disclosure in psychological and physiological outcomes in patients with rheumatoid arthritis: an exploratory home-based study. J Health Psychol. 2005;10:277–285.

Williams ACdeC, Nicholas MK, Richardson PH, Pither CE, Fernandes J. Generalizing from a controlled trial: the effects of patient preference versus randomization on the outcome of inpatient versus outpatient chronic pain management. Pain. 1999;83:57–65.

Yohannes AM, Connolly MJ, Baldwin RC. A feasibility study of antidepressant drug therapy in depressed elderly patients with chronic obstructive pulmonary disease. Int J Geriatr Psychiatry. 2001;16:451–454.

Zakowski SG, Ramati A, Morton C, Johnson P, Flanigan R. Written emotional disclosure buffers the effects of social constraints on distress among cancer patients. Health Psychol. 2004;23:555–563.

Chapter 10
Oppositional Defiant Disorder

Bruce M. Gale

Primarily a childhood diagnosis, oppositional defiant disorder (ODD), refers to a category of negativistic child[1] behaviors that impair social functioning and learning opportunities. It was first identified in 1966 and appeared initially as a formalized diagnosis in the *Diagnostic and Statistical Manual of Mental Disorders*, 3rd edition (American Psychiatric Association, 1980). ODD has been reported to affect 2–16% of children, with boys more likely to be diagnosed than girls and most children developing symptoms by age 8 (American Psychiatric Association, 2000; Steiner and Remsing, 2007).

Along with more serious disruptive behavior disorders, ODD is the most common reason children are referred for mental health services. Yet, less than 20% of children who meet criteria are referred for services (Lavigne et al., 2008; Walker et al., 2004). Heflinger and Humphreys (2008) found that, in examining the course of treatment for children in Tennessee's Medicaid System over 5 years, ODD was the third single most commonly diagnosed psychiatric disorder, present in 3% of their enrolled population. In summarizing related research, the authors reported that a previous ODD diagnosis predicted an increase in mental health services for adolescent males. Studies have found that, left untreated, some children outgrow these early problems. However, the majority continue to exhibit social difficulties and negative behavior, leading to academic failure and increased conflicts with peers and adults. This sets the stage for the development of more serious conduct disorders and antisocial behavior. The most alarming and costly final path for a subset of children and teens occurs when these behaviors are maintained and progress into adulthood. At this stage, antisocial behavior patterns have been reported to result in school dropout, vocational maladjustment, interpersonal problems, social isolation, and criminal behavior. In order to prevent such socially and financially costly negative outcomes, a significant literature base has developed focused on prevention.

B.M. Gale (✉)
BehaviorTech Solutions, Inc., 16430 Ventura Blvd., Suite 107, Encino, CA 91436, USA
e-mail: bgale@behaviortech.net

[1]Unless otherwise specified, the terms "child" or "children" is used generically to refer to both children and adolescents.

W.T. O'Donohue, C. Draper (eds.), *Stepped Care and e-Health*,
DOI 10.1007/978-1-4419-6510-3_10, © Springer Science+Business Media, LLC 2011

In this chapter, we will briefly review the current literature, then focus on current specific interventions with recommendations for empirically based assessment strategies. Directions for additional research and dissemination will be discussed, including ways to use e-health elements to improve the likelihood of successful outcomes.

Assessment/Triage

It is important to distinguish between common transient developmentally expected behaviors that may include oppositionality from more chronic presentations. Harvey et al. (2009) found that using diagnostic interviews plus a rating scale with 3-year-olds effectively discriminated between transient behavior problems and those which continued and met criteria for ODD or CD for 67% of the children they assessed. Consistent with earlier research, they reported that a sizable number of participants did not go on to develop more serious symptoms. This indicates the need to balance between identifying children at risk, but without unfairly labeling them or using treatments that may result in negative side effects. In a stepped-care model, some parents whose children exhibit sub-clinical level symptoms may benefit from minimal interventions, such as online psychoeducation. This may help them develop skills to feel less overwhelmed and better able to manage normative level problems.

The "terrible twos" refers to the sudden metamorphosis toddlers undergo as they turn from cuddly babies to feisty, troublesome tykes. Suddenly, they appear to relish saying "no," laughing at almost anything, or spilling/throwing things on purpose. At this young age, with language and self-awareness skills just emerging, it represents part of a normal process by which children learn to express themselves and assert their independence. At the same time, parents typically respond to this increased autonomy by imposing rules and limits (Shaw et al., 1994; Keenan and Wakschlag, 2002). Usually, such behavior represents a normal phase of development in these little developing citizens and does not require further attention, paving the way for additional autonomy, social skills development, friendship seeking, and respect for authority. It is essential that parents avoid overreactive or inconsistently harsh strategies that may prolong or exacerbate problems.

Sometimes, these negative behaviors solidify and prosocial development becomes arrested, creating levels of distress and impairment. At this point, the diagnosis of oppositional defiant disorder (ODD) should be considered. According to the DSM-IV-TR (American Psychiatric Association, 2000), hallmark characteristics of ODD include (1) defiance (refusing to comply with adult requests or becoming argumentative); (2) negativity (chronic feelings of resentfulness, blaming others for problems, deliberately annoying others, being vindictive); and (3) reactivity ("hair-trigger" emotional responses and tantrums over minor events). Children with ODD have trouble sharing, waiting their turn, hold grudges, can become aggressive toward peers, and complain that "things are not fair." They typically have difficulty making or maintaining friendships and other children often avoid them. Academic problems are common because their behavior typically results in reduced learning time and positive teacher interaction.

ODD is not diagnosed when chronic disorders, such as mental retardation, autistic spectrum disorders, or other pervasive developmental disabilities, are present, except when the severity of behaviors is beyond what would normally be seen in children diagnosed with these disorders. Oppositionality is commonly seen as one component of the overall clinical presentation for these developmental disorders due to challenges in language and/or cognition. Children have difficulty stopping activities, exhibit narrowed attentional focus, and may not fully comprehend what is being asked.

ODD cannot be diagnosed when more serious symptoms are present that indicate the presence of conduct disorder (CD). In such cases, more serious rule infractions, aggression, and more significant antisocial acts are typically present. Many researchers view ODD as the precursor to CD (Biederman et al., 1996; Lahey et al., 2009; Olson et al., 2000).

Sometimes anxiety-based disorders, such as phobias, panic disorder, social anxiety, and obsessive-compulsive disorders, may include elements of oppositionality. This usually occurs when a child is asked to engage in activities that trigger fear and is situation specific. The resulting increased avoidance may appear similar to behavioral refusal. The same can be true for depressive disorders, where any social contact may be perceived as unpleasant and cognitive tolerance for managing stress is reduced. Also, there is significant comorbidity with children who have preexisting diagnoses of ADHD/ADD and learning disorders (Biederman et al., 2008a; Steiner and Remsing, 2007). More than half of children with ADHD also have ODD; some authors have suggested that ADHD acts as a facilitating variable in the development of ODD symptoms (Biederman et al., 2008b).

ODD is linked most significantly to parental factors during early formative years, such as parental lack of interest, little involvement in activities, minimal supervision, harsh, inconsistent punitive reactions, and family or marital stress. Accordingly, in addition to evaluating a child's functioning, clinicians must also consider how others respond and the situations that trigger oppositional reactions before proposing intervention strategies. The comprehensiveness of initial assessment can vary considerably, depending upon the nature and severity of these presenting symptoms plus the presence and complexity of psychosocial stressors (e.g., divorce, problems at school).

Referrals for treatment typically occur in one of three ways. (1) *Primary care setting initiated*: Pediatricians, upon observing or learning of excessive levels of refusal or tantrum behaviors may initially offer self-help resources, print bibliotherapy sources, or referral to a support group. If the symptoms are more serious or there is no improvement, they typically make a referral to a specialist. (2) *School initiated*: As part of federal law, schools must have a mechanism in place to identify "at-risk" students. The current model, known as "response to intervention" (RtI) consists of three increasing levels of support, similar to stepped care. They range from school-wide interventions, to select groups of students, to individual student interventions. Unfortunately, there are no standardized guidelines for conducting

these screenings, although an emerging literature base supports more standardized screening efforts (Biederman et al., 2008a; Fanton et al., 2008). Presently,
behavior disorders, such as ODD, are specifically excluded from special education.
However, as the current chapter demonstrates, there is usually associated impairment that may increase the chances a child will qualify for needed services. Whether
or not a child qualifies for special education services, they may receive behavior
management support to help them access their educational curriculum or address
social–emotional problems, including ODD. The topic of school-related services is
extremely involved and broad. It is important for private clinicians to be aware that
positive behavior supports are available for all students, whether or not they qualify
for special education services. Interested readers are advised to review *Antisocial
Behavior in School: Evidence-Based Practices* (2nd ed.) by Walker et al. (2004),
visit http://www.pent.ca.gov or http://www.rti4success.org for timely information
about assessment, treatment, and positive supports in school settings. (3) *Mental
health services initiated*: Clinicians and agencies specializing in childhood behavior
problems routinely receive calls from desperate and frustrated parents who have run
out of tolerance, patience, and options. No current published data exist regarding
the frequency parents try other alternatives, such as psychoeducation or self-help
bibliotherapy, and the degree of success.

When mental health clinicians receive referrals, it is important to consider
each of the following areas in conducting intake assessments: (1) identification
of the specific behaviors involved across settings, situations that trigger them,
their level of occurrence, and severity/level of impairment across settings; (2) how
adults and peers respond when the child exhibits these behaviors; (3) current levels of cognitive, academic, adaptive behavior, and social–emotional functioning;
(4) developmental and educational history, specially focusing on age of onset,
language development, peer relations, and presence of comorbid or preexisting
psychiatric or medical conditions; (5) review of parenting strategies and school
interventions; and 6) review of family or marital stresses.

Building therapeutic alliances with both parents and the child early on is associated with more positive treatment outcomes (Kazdin et al., 1997; Weisz et al.,
2006). Having the child present during the initial meeting may help the clinician
gain first-hand knowledge of the parent–child interaction difficulties, but it can also
increase the chance that parents will feel defensive or inadequate, especially if they
are unable to control their child's behavior. Lower stepped assessments and recommendation methods for gathering initial information appear promising, but none
could be found that followed general evidence-based guidelines for ODD. Meeting
with the parents also provides a sample of marital interaction patterns and provides
potential information about family stresses. Howes and Markman (1989) conducted
longitudinal studies with couples at pre-marriage and postbirth of their first child.
They found they were able to predict levels of child security based upon indicators
of marital satisfaction. In the first study to specifically examine the rate of marital dissolution between parents of adolescents and young adults with and without
ADHD, Wymbs et al. (2008) found that the severity of disruptive child behavior
problems (specifically, ODD/CD) increases risk of divorce, along with other unique

factors, such as parent education levels, paternal levels of antisocial behavior, child age, and race/ethnicity. Other findings have linked externalized behavior problems to parental stress and alcohol consumption (Pelham et al., 1997).

How clinicians introduce themselves and relate to families during the treatment process can have a profound effect upon the likelihood parents will complete treatment rather than prematurely terminate (Kazdin, 2008). Development of a therapeutic alliance between parents and the clinician becomes a protective factor that increases the likelihood families will follow through with treatment recommendations and was associated with greater improvements in parenting practices. It appears unrelated to socioeconomic disadvantage, parent psychopathology and stress, or levels of child dysfunction (Kazdin et al., 2005; Kazdin and Whitley, 2006). By taking the time to understand family stresses, a therapist lays the groundwork that increases the chances of a successful outcome and decreases premature termination.

During the parent interview, a brief developmental history can be obtained and specific behaviors of concern identified along with situations that precede their occurrence. It is also essential to review the types of strategies or reactions used by parents. Since harsher parenting is associated with elevated rates of child disruptive behaviors and premature treatment drop out (Kazdin et al., 1997), clinicians need to focus on creating an environment where parents feel sufficiently comfortable describing their parenting practices without feeling judged (Stormshak et al., 2000). Clinicians must also be aware of their state's child abuse reporting mandates and are advised to disclose this obligation to families as part of a practice policies statement.

To create an enticing environment, our waiting room is chock filled with child-friendly magazines for children and teens, plus there is a video game they can play. Assuming the child stays out of the session for the first 30–45 min, the clinician can meet with parents alone during this time. It is helpful to "check in" with the child periodically, but without making any requests. Once the parent segment has concluded, the child can be invited to participate and given a choice to meet alone or with his parents. Keeping the time brief, e.g., 10 min, is tolerable for most children. During this time, the child can be asked whether they wish to continue meeting or stop. If they say they wish to stop, complying with their request and ending their portion of the session immediately can be helpful in beginning to establish a relationship that does not give them reason to escalate their behavior.

Establishing the diagnosis of ODD requires that clinicians separate normative or episodic symptoms from those which are more enduring and clinically significant. Additionally, more serious disorders, such as Asperger's syndrome, need to be considered along with comorbid diagnoses, such as ADHD/ADD, learning problems, and depressive or anxiety disorders. This can be a daunting process. Early career clinicians will likely benefit from using structured interview tools, such as the Diagnostic Interview Schedule for Children-Version 4 (DISC-IV) (Shaffer et al., 2000). Composed of 358 core questions and an additional bank of 1,300 branching questions, it covers more than 30 childhood psychiatric diagnoses. Jewell et al. (2004) advised using structured interviews such as this and suggests that typical clinician diagnoses may lack adequate validity. However, the DISC-IV can be a time-consuming process and may be off-putting for a family in distress. As an alternative, Steenhuis et al. (2009) reported on the feasibility of using an Internet-based version of the DISC-IV for parents to complete at home as a self-report tool. Specially examining the similarity of results for the ADHD module, the authors concluded the diagnostic results were highly equivalent to the more traditional paper and pencil interview version.

Other surveys and questionnaires for collecting behavioral data across settings, in combination with a semi-structured clinician interview, may be more time efficient than using the DISC-IV. Commonly used tools include the Behavior Assessment System for Children-II (BASC-2) (Reynolds and Kamphaus, 1992), Child Behavior Checklist (CBCL) (Achenbach, 1991), or the Disruptive Behavior Rating Scale (DBRS) (Erford, 1998). In particular, clinicians need to be mindful of using wide-band versus narrow-band measures. Initially, it may be helpful to use a wide-band measure, such as the BASC-II or CBCL. However, a narrow-band measure, such as the DBRS, or the Behavior Rating Inventory of Executive Function (BRIEF) (Gioia et al., 2000) can track changes in ODD. If there are questions regarding cognitive functioning or academic ability, it may be necessary to conduct or refer for a psychoeducational assessment and/or complete an adaptive behavior survey or measure of social skills. There are additional tools, such as the Parenting Stress Index (Abidin, 1995), that can track the effects upon parental functioning.

It is important to assess whether language development has proceeded smoothly and to review current levels of educational success. Sometimes parents are reluctant to permit contact with the school, but this should be encouraged. Not only do teachers and counselors typically have considerable information about child and/or parent functioning that may be helpful to clinicians but also the child's school represents a potentially powerful environment and resource for addressing ODD.

Unless financial or time considerations absolutely prohibit it, conducting an observation at school or daycare, prior to meeting the child, is highly recommended as another source for collecting direct observation data (Gale, 2006). This is typically the clinician's only opportunity to observe the child before they have formally met and in the absence of the child's parents. Again, because treatment is likely to involve school staff, this is an opportunity to learn more about the child's educational program, the teacher, and administration. It is helpful to talk with the teacher during a portion of the break time to help identify any antecedent triggers and review the kinds of interventions and their level of success. Asking to review work samples of writing and basic academics can provide information about whether there is evidence to suggest some of the behavior may be linked to academic challenges at school. Alberto and Troutman (2006) describe a number of alternate data collection methodologies in their behavior analysis textbook. It also contains links for downloading sample data forms and exercises for learning data collection methods.

Stepped-Care Options

As reported by Kazdin et al. (1997), nearly 70% of children and adolescents who require mental health treatment do not receive it. Of those who do begin, approximately one-half terminate services prematurely (Kazdin, 2008). In describing therapy services usage for children diagnosed with ODD via the Tennesee Medicaid system, Heflinger and Humphreys (2008) noted, "Inpatient hospitalization or residential treatment doubled, family therapy was used nearly four times as often by the end of the time period, and use of medication management increased by sevenfold. The proportion of children with ODD who were receiving case management increased by a factor of 11. Other types of services became less frequently used for children with ODD: individual and group therapy declined by 25% and 13%, respectively. The use of day treatment or partial hospitalization dropped even more dramatically." (p. 144).

Bower and Gilbody (2005) highlighted three fundamental assumptions behind the stepped-care model: (1) minimal interventions can provide similar gains to that of traditional psychotherapy for a proportion of patients; (2) using minimal interventions permits health-care resources to be used more efficiently; and (3) these interventions must be acceptable to both patients and clinicians. The linkage between initial assessment and treatment options is critical. Treatments must be monitored systematically and changes made ("stepping up") if the current interventions are not producing satisfactory results. With this in mind, the recommendations for a 2- or 3-year old with mild to moderate oppositional behaviors are likely to be quite different from that for a 6-year old who has entrenched behaviors, no friends, and "hates school." Similarly, the presence of comorbid factors, such as ADHD, anxiety, or school refusal, can markedly alter the type of treatment(s) recommended, as well as who should be involved in implementation.

Use of a stepped-care model can balance concerns associated with "false positives," where children who do not have the disorder are wrongly identified, and "false negatives," where children with ODD are missed. Providing minimal intervention is likely to be more effective and increases parent awareness than doing nothing. Careful examination of individual risk factors as part of the initial stepped-care assessment process can help clinicians match treatments to family needs and increase the likelihood of successful outcomes (Lavigne et al., 2008).

Consumer Preferences

It used to be that individual psychotherapy or family therapy was the only option typically available to consumers. When things escalated out of control, this would sometimes result in an unplanned, extraordinarily expensive, inpatient psychiatric hospital stay to restabilize the situation. Stepped-care models have expanded significantly the array of choices available to consumers. Considered a "self-correcting, fail upwards" model (Bower and Gilbody, 2005), the least costly, less time-intensive

Fig. 10.1 This is a
stepped-care treatment
hierarchy. Each step includes
one or more components that
may be added within that
level of service (shown by
plus signs) prior to increasing
the level of treatment

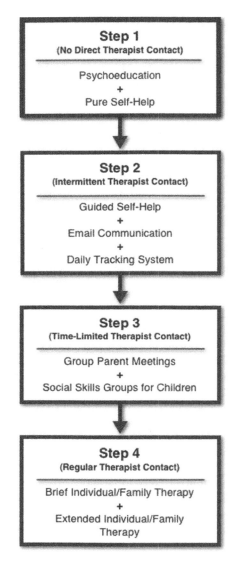

services can be considered prior to embarking on approaches that require greater levels of family commitment and cost. Figure 10.1 an adapted model based upon the one proposed by Bower and Gilbody (2005), with added "plus signs" representing adjunctive treatments for each step if significant levels of progress are not being observed. In all cases, it is recommended that outcome assessment measures be incorporated as part of the treatment process.

Currently, stepped-care alternatives for ODD have included bibliotherapy, parenting programs, combined approaches, school-based intervention, social skill programs, and medications. Considerably more research and guidelines are necessary to identify which child symptoms and family presentations fare best with specific levels of initial treatment. Kazdin (2008) has suggested that a range of treatment alternatives, including computer-based interventions, such as tele-health, be expanded in order to provide treatment to a broader range of families in need.

Outcome Data

Evidence-based treatments (EBT) require that interventions have been scientifically evaluated for efficacy. Brestan and Eyberg (1998) reviewed 82 studies of conduct disorder, categorizing promising treatments into two groups: "probably efficacious" and "well established." In general, parent training programs that focused on improving parent–child quality of interaction and teaching parents core behavior management principles, while reducing harsh or inconsistent consequences, have been found efficacious (Kazdin, 2005). Unfortunately, in longer term follow-up studies, only about 50% of children have maintained treatment gains (Schoenfield and Eyberg, 2005).

In examining the effects of family intervention programs to improve parenting skills, Lunkenheimer et al. (2008) reported that improving normative social emotional and cognitive competencies during crucial development stages, in addition to increasing parent involvement and support, were essential areas for treatment focus. They noted that success in these areas has been tied to reduction of conduct problems. Parent training programs have been well documented as providing effective interventions that can rival more traditional approaches (Lavigne et al., 2008). Webster-Stratton et al. (2008) found that poverty-related risks set the stage for children to experience challenges with emotional dysregulation, social skills, and less teacher/parent involvement. This was associated with increased conduct problems. Improvement in social competence and decreased conduct problems was noted when teachers were taught to employ social–emotionally focused curriculum training and related strategies.

The following programs have developed a significant literature base demonstrating effectiveness for treating oppositional and disruptive behaviors.

Living with children (Patterson and Gullion, 1968) has been most successful for both males and females aged 6–16. This treatment provides guidance to parents in identifying and monitoring targeted problem behaviors, using effective behavior management tools to reward for prosocial behaviors and reduce disruptive behaviors.

The incredible years (Webster-Stratton and Reid, 2007) have focused primarily on preschool populations. The program helps parents to be more positive, involved, and nurturing while reducing harsh or abusive discipline practices; helps teachers to have more positive relationships with children and their parents; plus focuses on improving social competence and self-regulation skills. Clinically significant reductions for approximately two-thirds of children with ODD have been reported.

Problem-solving skills training and parent management training: This EBT program addresses disruptive behaviors from 2 to 17 years and focuses upon teaching parents how to use essential behavior management techniques, such as stimulus control, shaping, reinforcement, extinction, and punishment. The program has strong literature-based support for its efficacy. There is a 12-session core program that includes verbatim statements for therapists to use (Kazdin, 2005).

Parent–child interaction therapy (PCIT) is a behavioral family intervention treatment focused on treating disruptive behaviors in 2- to 7-year-old populations. It incorporates elements of social learning theory, traditional play therapy, and attachment theory. PCIT is designed to enhance and improve parent–child relationships, increase children's pro-social behaviors, and increase parent behavior management skills (Brinkmeyer and Eyeberg, 2003; Querido and Eyeberg, 2005). It incorporates elements of ongoing assessment with treatment and live coaching for parents.

The *children's summer treatment program* (STP) has been described as a comprehensive intervention for children with attention-deficit/hyperactivity disorder (ADHD) and related disruptive behaviors (Pelham, 2009). STP is based on the premise that combining an intensive summer treatment program with a follow-up program during the school year is more likely to provide an effective intervention for ADHD than clinic-based treatment alone. The program combines a behavioral point system, sports and social skills training, group problem solving, and a daily report card. After the summer program, children continue during the school year. There are weekly parent behavior management sessions to generalize to the home setting.

Quality Improvement Outcomes

When a family suspects their child's behavior is out of control or has received a report of problem behaviors from school, it often creates mixed feelings. From reality shows depicting firm nannies to reports of harmful effects of medications, they typically do not know where to turn. The thought of "sending my kid to a shrink" can be enough to cause them to rethink their initial instinct to pursue assistance. As reported by Kazdin and Weisz (1998), treatment typically involves more than just meeting with a child in individual treatment sessions. In fact, parents, teachers, siblings, and peers may be involved in one or more ways as part of the treatment process. Use of stepped-care options, where less intrusive, more affordable, and less demanding approaches are tried first, may represent a more palatable option for most families.

Watchful Waiting

Current evidence for using this approach is more closely linked to the medical field in evaluating whether or not to treat ear infections and other potentially self-resolving problems. In the mental health field, the majority of studies, identified via a PsychInfo literature search (American Psychological Association), were for depression. There are presently few guidelines for clinicians who wish to use this level of service for ODD. The question of how to be "watchful" is important to consider. This approach may be best suited to those family situations where the child's behaviors are a problem, but occur within a normative range. An alternative would be to request that families complete a short questionnaire every few months to track behavior. During the initial intake, it is important to discuss what criteria will determine whether families progress to another step in treatment or discontinuing monitoring. In most cases, watchful waiting should be combined with some level of psychoeducation, discussed next.

Psychoeducation

The essential purpose of psychoeducation is to provide parents with fundamental information about effective parenting and to help them distinguish between more typical child behaviors and those that represent dysfunction. Parents can access this information via many formats: a speaker at a local hospital or parent support group may provide useful information; well-established web sites with credible, research-based information may be consulted or simply reviewing books that cover the nature of ODD symptoms and initial tips may provide a core level degree of information that helps parents recognize and begin to practice more effective strategies and how to deescalate current situations.

Families can also be encouraged to visit research-backed web sites, such as those from national organizations. Examples include the Centers for Disease Control and Prevention (http://www.cdc.gov), National Institute of Mental Health (http://www.nimh.nih.gov/topics/topic-page-children-and-adolescents.shtml), American Academy of Child & Adolescent Psychiatry (http://www.aacap.org/cs/root/facts_for_families/children_with_oppositional_defiant_disorder), the American Psychological Association (http://www.apa.org), and Parents As Teachers (http://www.parentsasteachers.org). Other than occasional anecdotal reports, these sites do not contain any research indicating their utility. While common sense indicates this information is likely to be helpful, further research is needed to determine the ultimate benefit provided by these resources.

Bibliotherapy

A plethora of bibliotherapy resources is available for helping parents manage and improve their children's oppositional behavior (Barkley and Benton, 1998; Barkley et al., 2008; Greene and Ablon, 2006; Kazdin, 2008). All of these resources were written by authors who have extensive background working with families of children with ODD. They generally follow an integrative biopsychosocial method of explaining the disorders. Lavigne et al. (2008) found that using bibliotherapy (The Incredible Years; Webster-Stratton, 1992) in a pediatric primary care setting was nearly as effective as therapist-led approaches, except in those situations where parents attended a significant number of sessions (7 or more out of a 12-session program). So, for families where the risk factors suggest that consistent attendance is unlikely, this may be a viable initial alternative. It is important to evaluate whether the family will use bibliotherapy with or without therapist guidance. If a family appears more disorganized or the situation has reached chaotic proportions, therapist guidance is likely to be necessary. Giving the family a short period of time and scheduling a check-in phone consult 1–2 weeks later will help clinicians evaluate the need for additional treatment components.

Computer-Based Assessment and Intervention/e-Health

While computer-based education for ODD appears promising, no current treatment programs that rely upon computers or the Internet have been validated. Programs have been explored as a means for teaching general social skills (Piper et al., 2006) and numerous DVDs or other multimedia are available as teaching aids for parents and teachers. This form of psychoeducation via online programs and services would appear a natural fit. In examining patient satisfaction with receiving preoperative instructions directly from a doctor or using an interactive computer program, the results indicated that patient knowledge gained from computer instruction was equivalent, as was the level of patient satisfaction (Keulers et al., 2007). This is especially important for parents who may have lowered literacy or lowered cognitive functioning. Using a computer program may likely help them review information and gain skills without feeling self-conscious. It has the advantage of being inexpensive, time efficient, and has the potential to ameliorate problems associated with parent reading difficulties. Using animation technologies, which are now quite affordable, it is possible to create more immersive experiences where children respond to scripted social situations. Programs such as "Mr. Bubb" (http://www.zoesis.com/mrbubb) use artificial intelligence to interact and teach about facial expressions and emotions.

Elgar and McGrath (2008) noted that there are few tele-health products that have been developed and evaluated for childhood disorders, other than video programs, such as the Incredible Years. Online survey programs can be a powerful vehicle for creating tutorials and data collection systems with clients. For example, simple free or low-cost survey tools (e.g., Formsite, Google Docs, Zoho, Zoomerang) can be used to create engaging interactive client tutorials where the results are stored and/or e-mailed to clinicians. There are no programming costs, as in the case of building a web site; the database is built into the survey program. The advantage of using paid services is typically the addition of features not available in free versions, plus e-mail and/or phone technical support.

Such survey tools can become a powerful, yet affordable method for creating sophisticated analysis and data reporting tools. I created a series of tools for my practice incorporating technology in assessment and treatment data collection and reporting process (Comprehensive Behavior Assessment Treatment Tools®). These tools follow the principles associated with evidence-based tools and accepted assessment protocols, but have not yet been examined in a controlled study. For example, Rapid Screener® (C-BATT RS) is an online functional behavior-based multi-rater assessment tool designed to provide a comprehensive view of behaviors across environments to help educational teams form a consensus regarding behavioral priorities (Gale, 2004). It collects detailed demographics on the unique manner in which each rater had contact with the student, the level of independence and consistency of positive school-based behaviors, and the relative frequency and severity of interfering behaviors. Based upon review of the last 260 raters (Gale, 2009), face validity measures have indicated the results were acceptable to raters 96% of the time on average and unacceptable 1% of the time. Sixty-one percent of raters completed C-BATT RS in under 30 min and 68% reported it was "easy" or "very easy" to complete; 20% indicated "no problems"; 11% reported "some problems" (typically typed password incorrectly); and 1.5% found it "difficult" or "very difficult."

Progress Communicator® (C-BATT PC) (Gale 2004) was designed as a structured online data reporting and cognitive-behavioral coaching system. Using information based upon Rapid Screener®, target behaviors are identified for inclusion. As teachers or other educational staff report on student behavior, the results are sent via email or secure links to the rest of the educational staff and family members. A separate, more friendly and immersive version guides the student through the reporting process. The system can alert others to problems at an early stage and offers to review more adaptive coping strategies with the student. Clinical experience indicates that this approach has potential for allowing students and adults to communicate to others when distress is building, setting the stage for behavior escalation. Since it can be programmed to send emails based upon specific criteria, school psychologists or outside therapists can elect to be notified under specific conditions. This has been helpful in building and maintaining a positive therapeutic alliance and in keeping the team abreast of student functioning in real time.

An example of incorporating technology with more traditional social skills training is the LUNCH Groups® program (Gale and Yamashita, 2003). It targets traditional social skills such as executive functioning, pragmatic language and social skills, academic success skills, and environmental awareness for children and teens during summer and school year sessions. Children work in large and small groups on multimedia projects and animation activities to help them practice social skills such as compliance, turn-taking, negotiation, problem solving, and consideration for others (http://www.lunchgroups.com, click on "Group Projects"). In addition to traditional parent meetings, parents fill out online data forms reporting on generalized behaviors identified by the children, which are linked to rewards in group, such as group video game time. A non-confidential blog allows parents to read about group interventions, families receive confidential audio progress notes, and they can participate in closed online parent networks. Data from the past 2 years with 49 families indicated that 92% of participants enjoyed the program and two-thirds made at least one major significant behavior change. The majority of parents (86%) reported that they were more effective at noticing their child's positive behavior, and 73% reported "things were generally better," they raised their voice less often, and used fewer negative consequences. Nearly all (88%) liked receiving audio progress notes and 77% felt the use of technology kept their child engaged. These interventions and methods have not been subjected to controlled experimental methods, but as outcome measures for a small clinical practice, parent and child feedback has been helpful in modifying and improving the program.

Group Treatment

The main purpose of group treatment has been twofold. (1) Meet with parents to increase skills, as described previously. Typically time limited, parents learn about protective factors, ways to interact with their child more successfully, and how to replace punitive methods with more positive interventions and relationship building. (2) Social skills training to help children practice behaving effectively in social situations and adjusting their behavior to avoid conflicts (Steiner and Remsing, 2007).

In discussing the quality of parent participation in behaviorally focused group therapy interventions, Nix et al. (2009) studied the notion of "meaningful participation" in a sample of 445 parents. These parents were uniformly at a lowered socioeconomic level. Approximately one-third had not completed high school, and nearly one-half were unemployed and also reported symptoms of depression that fell into a clinical range. The authors concluded that the "ability and willingness of parents to pay attention, stay on topic, participate in discussions, and enact role plays in their groups was uniquely related to improvements in parents' perceptions of children, warmth, use of nonharsh discipline, and school involvement" (p. 427).

Individual/Family Therapy

In general, the effectiveness of using individual therapy as a primary intervention approach has not been well studied. Steiner and Remsing (2007) noted that few studies exist that compared parent training interventions to individual approaches. Accordingly, recommendations regarding individual therapy are based more on "clinical wisdom and consensus rather than extensive empirical evidence" (p. 136). The main purpose of individual therapy is to help children more effectively manage their anger in order to decrease defiant behavior. In general, problem-solving therapy approaches, self-management techniques, and identifying areas of misperception are likely target areas. Individual therapy may also be indicated when comorbid conditions, such as anxiety or depression, are present. Cognitive-behavioral therapy (CBT) for anxiety or depression and interpersonal psychotherapy (IPT) for depression have been found to be most effective with adolescents (Curry and Becker, 2008).

Kendall and Braswell (1982) found that using time-limited cognitive-behavioral therapy over 12 sessions resulted in improvement, based on teacher blind behavior ratings of child self-control, as well as self-report measures. Interestingly, parent report measures did not indicate significant treatment changes. The authors concluded that 12 weeks was an insufficient amount of time and that greater emphasis would likely be necessary focusing on home-based situations. Family therapy approaches may be indicated in those situations where increased opportunities to practice positive communication and effective behavior management is indicated beyond traditional parent management training approaches. It may also be indicated if one parent has a psychiatric disorder that may require additional treatment. Barkley et al. (1992) compared behavioral therapies to structural family therapy and treatment of 12- to 18-year-olds with ODD and found no differences in the effectiveness of these treatments. The authors concluded that multimodal interventions are likely to be most effective.

Medication

In reporting on the use of medications with ODD, Phelps et al. (2002) and the American Psychological Association Working Group on Psychotropic Medications for Children and Adolescents (Meyers, 2006) reported that there are no specific medications that are used to treat the diagnosis of ODD, unless comorbid ADHD is present. This is consistent with consensus statements published by the American Academy of Child and Adolescent Psychiatry (American Academy of Child & Adolescent Psychiatry, 2009). In examining the relative efficacy of atomoxetine, Bangs et al. (2008) found the initial benefit for both symptoms associated with ADHD and ODD; however, enduring benefits were noted only for ADHD symptoms. The authors noted that they used a relatively high cutoff on the SNAP-IV (Swanson, Nolan, and Pelham Rating Scale—Revised). They hypothesized that their sample population may have had a relatively high severity of ODD symptoms and 8 weeks, the studies end point, may have been an insufficient time period to fully assess treatment effects.

More potent medications, such as risperidone, have been reported to have a positive effect on the level of disruptive behaviors. Turgay et al. (2002) examined long-term safety and efficacy of risperidone and concluded that no serious adverse events occurred, even though headaches, weight gain, and somnolence were the most commonly reported side effects. This is consistent with side effects reported by Aman et al. (2004), who also reported that subjects experienced dyspepsia, rhinitis, and vomiting when taking risperidone.

In some cases, antihypertensive drugs have been used to reduce symptoms associated with hyperarousal and aggression. Yet, the clinical use of the psychotropic medications has reportedly exceeded the research demonstrating their efficacy and safety. Additionally, significant adverse effects have included hypotension, depressive symptoms, and sedation (Phelps et al., 2002). In summarizing the research on using medications to treat ODD, Brown et al. (2008) reported that there is minimal evidence supporting psychopharmacological treatment in the management of ODD except when comorbid ADHD is present.

Inpatient Treatment

Heflinger and Humphreys (2008) reported that, despite the limited number of studies that documented the effectiveness of inpatient and residential care for children with oppositional defiant disorder, the number of children who were treated in such settings more than doubled. In reviewing factors that were linked to repeated hospitalizations, Chung et al. (2008) found that having a diagnosis of oppositional defiant disorder was one of the primary factors reported. Inpatient treatment is typically focused on symptom management and stabilization while residential treatment may be more inclusive, linking educational, social and behavioral, and family interactions. Unfortunately, no studies could be found that examined what inpatient treatment components are most likely to make meaningful differences or the overall success of this highly restrictive form of care.

Triage Agenda

The greatest challenge facing clinicians is to determine the most effective level of initial assessment and select which interventions are likely to serve as the most appropriate first-line treatments. In some cases, minimal interventions are likely to be the best match, while in other situations early intensive treatment is likely to ultimately be more clinically effective and result in the long-term lowest cost level (Bower and Gilbody, 2005). How clinicians conduct their assessments to make these determinations require initial assessment of the severity of the problem, parent motivation for treatment, plus available financial and emotional resources. Clinicians who are flexible in the range of initial contact options they offer to families (e.g., telephone, online, and face-to-face) stand the greatest chance of matching the assessment commitment to the family's needs, increasing the chances that initial contact will build a sufficient level of therapeutic alliance, and effectively minimize barriers to subsequent treatment.

In making treatment recommendations, clinicians have a range of options available to them. These include psychoeducation and/or bibliotherapy, with or without guided therapeutic assistance; parent management and social skills programs; school-based interventions; and time-limited individual or family therapy. In making recommendations for bibliotherapy, Elgar and McGrath (2008) noted that that there has been little public education regarding the effectiveness of different forms of bibliotherapy and there are no established criteria to help the public identify which books have been subjected to some level of author testing or experimental rigor. Use of medications is most likely limited to treatment of specific symptoms or comorbid ADHD.

Using online screening protocols that branch to more detailed assessments and quick contacts with appropriately skilled intake counselors or clinicians is likely to provide consumers with the most effective means for seeking and receiving help in a cost-efficient manner. In order for this to happen, the notion that all initial contacts must occur face-to-face needs to change.

Research and Development Agenda

The process of developing evidence-based treatment (EBT) programs is time consuming and is typically supported by grants and universities. Considerable progress has been made in determining the types of interventions that work. However, as noted by Kazdin (2008), the problem is not one of EBT, but for most children, receiving any treatment. To improve the quality of services, clinicians need to improve their own skills in employing measures that document the effectiveness of their own treatments. As mentioned previously, the use of online surveys makes this an affordable and manageable process, even for single practitioners. For clinicians looking to develop their own web-based assessment tools, reviewing the guidelines from the International Test Commission (http://www.intestcom.org) can be a helpful resource. Division 16 of the American Psychological Association created the Task Force on Evidence Based Interventions in School Psychology which was active from 1999 to 2008. Their coding manuals for developing EBTs in both group settings and for single subject design purposes are worth reviewing; they contain a treasure trove of information and potential questions on this subject (http://www.indiana.edu/~ebi/). In general, while many cost-effective treatments have been developed, there is a lack of integration and continuity across treatment settings. Families who are in need of help for their oppositional children require a clear path to guide them that is affordable and eliminates barriers to treatment.

Dissemination Agenda

Given that the existing EBTs are not being widely used, the question of how to best disseminate this information needs to be considered. Division 53, American Psychological Association, has conducted a limited, but useful review of EBT programs (http://sccap.tamu.edu/EST/index_files/Page775.htm). A more extensive list, complete with peer review ratings, may be found at NREPP: National Registry of Evidence-Based Programs and Practices (http://nrepp.samhsa.gov/index.asp).

Kazdin (2008) noted that EBTs presently exist, but these are not typically available in most communities and are not part of training or internship programs. "However, disseminating EBTs by itself might not reduce the burden of mental illness on the scale that is required. No doubt it will be possible to take effective interventions and integrate them with services in ways that can reach more individuals in need. Tele-health of individual psychotherapy might well be a prime example of a way in which a treatment once developed can be delivered in a new way. It will be important to proceed in another way as well in which service delivery demands are taken into consideration at the point of developing the model of treatment" (Kazdin, 2008, p. 212).

Clinicians' willingness to consider and adopt ways of systematically assessing and selecting treatment options that take into account individual family resources is likely to provide affordable services to the greatest number of families in need. Inexpensive, readily available technologies can assist in removing treatment barriers by allowing families to select treatment options that best meet their present needs, feeling confident that services may be expanded if less intensive options are unsuccessful.

References

Achenbach TM. Integrative guide for the 1991 CBCL/4-18, YSR, and TRF profiles. Burlington, VT: University of Vermont, Department of Psychiatry; 1991.

Alberto PA, Troutman AC. Applied behavior analysis for teachers. Columbus, Ohio: Pearson, Merrill Prentice-Hall; 2006.

Abidin RR. Parenting Stress Index: professional manual. 3rd ed. Odessa, FL: Psychological Assessment Resources; 1995.

Aman MG, Binder C, Turgay A. Risperidone effects in the presence/absence of psychostimulant medicine in children with ADHD, other disruptive behavior disorders, and subaverage IQ. J Child Adolesc Psychopharmacol. 2004;14(2):243–54.

American Academy of Child & Adolescent Psychiatry. (n.d.). Your Child—Oppositional Defiant Disorder. Retrieved July 7, 2009, from http://www.aacap.org/cs/root/publication_store/your_child_oppositional_defiant_disorder.

American Psychiatric Association. Diagnostic and statistical manual of mental disorders. 3rd ed (DSM-III). Washington, DC: American Psychiatric Press; 1980.

American Psychiatric Association. Diagnostic and statistical manual of mental disorders. 4th ed. Text Revision (DSM-IV-TR). Washington, DC: American Psychiatric Press; 2000.

Bangs ME, Hazell P, Danckaerts M, Hoare P, Coghill DR, Wehmeier PM, et al. Atomoxetine for the treatment of attention-deficit/hyperactivity disorder and oppositional defiant disorder. Pediatrics. 2008;121(2):e314–20.

Barkley RA, Benton CM. Your defiant child: eight steps to better behavior. New York: Guilford Press; 1998.

Barkley RA, Guevremont DC, Anastopoulos AD, Fletcher KE. A comparison of three family therapy programs for treating family conflicts in adolescents with attention-deficit hyperactivity disorder. J Consult Clin Psychol. 1992;60(3):450–62.

Barkley RA, Robin AL, Benton CM. Your defiant teen: 10 steps to resolve conflict and rebuild your relationship. New York: Guilford Press; 2008.

Biederman J, Ball SW, Monuteaux MC, Kaiser R, Faraone SV. CBCL Clinical scales discriminate ADHD youth with structured-interview derived diagnosis of oppositional defiant disorder (ODD). J Attent Disord. 2008a;12(1):76–82.

Biederman J, Faraone SV, Milberger S, Jetton JG, et al. Is childhood oppositional defiant disorder a precursor to adolescent conduct disorder? Findings from a four-year follow-up study of children with ADHD. J Am Acad Child Adolesc Psychiatry. 1996;35(9):1193–204.

Biederman J, Petty CR, Monuteaux MC, Mick E, Parcell T, Westerberg D, et al. The longitudinal course of comorbid oppositional defiant disorder in girls with attention-deficit/hyperactivity disorder: findings from a controlled 5-year prospective longitudinal follow-up study. J Dev Behav Pediatr. 2008b;29(6):501–7.

Bower P, Gilbody S. Stepped care in psychological therapies: access, effectiveness and efficiency. Narrative literature review. Br J Psychiatry. 2005;186(1):11–17.

Brestan E.V, Eyberg SM. Effective psychosocial treatments of conduct-disordered children and adolescents: 29 years, 82 studies, and 5,272 kids. J Clin Child Psychol. 1998;27(2):180–9.

Brown RT, Antonuccio DO, DuPaul GJ, Fristad MA, King CA, Leslie LK, et al. Oppositional defiant and conduct disorders. In: Childhood mental health disorders: evidence base and contextual factors for psychosocial, psychopharmacological, and combined interventions. Washington, DC: American Psychological Association; 2008. p. 33–41.

Brinkmeyer MY, Eyberg SM. Parent-child interaction therapy for oppositional children. In: Evidence-based psychotherapies for children and adolescents. New York: Guilford Press; 2003. p. 204–23.

Chung W, Edgar-Smith S, Palmer RB, Delambo D, Bartholomew E. Psychiatric rehospitalization of children and adolescents: implications for social work intervention. Child & Adolescent Social Work Journal. 2008;25(6):483–96.

Coie JD, Watt NF, West SG, Hawkins JD, Asarnow JR, Markman HJ, Ramey SL, Shure MB, Long B. The science of prevention: a conceptual framework and some directions for a national research program. Am Psychol. 1993;48:1013–22.

Cooper WO, Hickson GB, Fuchs C, Arbogast PG, Ray WA. New users of anti-psychotic medications among children enrolled in TennCare. Arch Pediatr Adolesc Med. 2004;158: 753–9.

Curry JF, Becker SJ. Empirically supported psychotherapies for adolescent depression and mood disorders. In: Handbook of evidence-based therapies for children and adolescents: bridging science and practice, Issues in clinical child psychology. Springer Science+Business Media: New York; 2008. p. 161–76.

Elgar FJ, McGrath PJ. Self-help therapies for childhood disorders. In: Handbook of self-help therapies. Routledge/Taylor Francis Group: New York; 2008. p. 129–61.

Erford BT. Technical analysis of father responses to the Disruptive Behavior Rating Scale—Parent Version (DBRS-P). Meas Eval Couns Dev. 1998;30(4):199–210.

Fanton JH, MacDonald B, Harvey EA. Preschool parent-pediatrician consultations and predictive referral patterns for problematic behaviors. J Dev Behav Pediatr. 2008;29(6):475–82.

Gale BM. Learning about the comprehensive behavior assessment & treatment tools (C-BATT). Invited Presentation, California Association for the Gifted (CAG) 42nd Annual Conference, Anaheim, California; 2004.

Gale BM. Conducting valid and defensible behavior observations, invited paper, positive environment network of trainers/california diagnostic center, 3rd annual conference, stockton, california and rancho cucamonga, California; 2006.

Gale BM. Analysis of 260 consecutive users of rapid screener. Unpublished raw data; 2009.

Gale BM, Yamashita J. L.U.N.C.H Groups: preliminary results on the efficacy of using, time-limited psychosocial and behavior treatment with integrated technological enhancements in the treatment of Asperger's Syndrome and related disorders. Poster presentation, 37th Annual Meeting of the Association for the Advancement of Behavior Therapy, Boston, MA; 2003.

Gioia GA, Isquith PK, Guy SC, Kenworthy L. Behavior rating inventory of executive function. Odessa, FL: Psychological Assessment Resources; 2000.

Greene RW, Ablon JS. Treating explosive kids: the collaborative problem-solving approach. New York: Guilford Press; 2006.

Harvey EA, Youngwirth SD, Thakar DA, Errazuriz PA. Predicting attention-deficit/hyperactivity disorder and oppositional defiant disorder from preschool diagnostic assessments. J Consult Clin Psychol. 2009;77:349–54.

Heflinger CA, Humphreys KL. Identification and treatment of children with oppositional defiant disorder: a case study of one state's public service system. Psychol Serv. 2008;5(2):139–52.

Howes P, Markman HJ. Marital quality and child functioning: A longitudinal investigation. Child Dev. 1989;60(5):1044–51.

Jewell J, Handwerk M, Almquist J, Lucas C. Comparing the validity of clinician-generated diagnosis of conduct disorder to the Diagnostic Interview Schedule for Children. J Clin Child Adolesc Psychol. 2004;33(3):536–46.

Kazdin AE. Parent management training: treatment for oppositional, aggressive, and antisocial behavior in children and adolescents. New York: Oxford University Press; 2005.

Kazdin AE. Evidence-based treatments and delivery of psychological services: shifting our emphases to increase impact. Psychol Serv. 2008;5(3):201–15.

Kazdin AE, Holland L, Crowley M. Family experience of barriers to treatment and premature termination from child therapy. J Consult Clin Psychol. 1997;65(3):453–63.

Kazdin AE, Marciano PL, Whitley MK. The therapeutic alliance in cognitive-behavioral treatment of children referred for oppositional, aggressive, and antisocial behavior. J Consult Clin Psychol. 2005;73(4):726–30.

Kazdin AE, Weisz JR. Identifying and developing empirically supported child and adolescent treatments. J Consult Clin Psychol. 1998;66(1):19–36.

Kazdin AE, Whitley MK. Pretreatment social relations, therapeutic alliance, and improvements in parenting practices in parent management training. J Consult Clin Psychol. 2006;74:346–55.

Keenan K, Wakschlag LS. Can a valid diagnosis of disruptive behavior disorder be made in preschool children? Am J Psychiatry. 2002;159(3):351–8.

Kendall PC, Braswell L. Cognitive-behavioral self-control therapy for children: a components analysis. J Consult Clin Psychol. 1982;50(5):672–89.

Keulers BJ, Welters CFM, Spauwen PHM, Houpt P. Can face-to-face patient education be replaced by computer-based patient education? A randomised trial. Patient Educ Couns. 2007;67(1–2):176–82.

Lahey BB, Van Hulle CA, Rathouz PJ, Rodgers JLD, Onofrio BM, Waldman ID. Are oppositional-defiant and hyperactive-inattentive symptoms developmental precursors to conduct problems in late childhood? Genetic and environmental links. J Abnorm Child Psychol. 2009;37(1):45–58.

Lavigne JV, LeBailly SA, Gouze KR, Cicchetti C, Pochyly J, Arend R, et al. (2008). Treating oppositional defiant disorder in primary care: a comparison of three models. J. Pediatr Psychol. 2008;33(5):449–61.

Lunkenheimer ES, Dishion TJ, Shaw DS, Connell AM, Gardner F, Wilson MN, et al. Collateral benefits of the family check-up on early childhood school readiness: indirect effects of parents' positive behavior support. Dev Psychol. 2008;44(6):1737–52.

Meyers L. Medicate or not? An APA working group reports on use of medications when treating children. Monit Psychology. 2006;37(10):24.

Nix RL, Bierman KL, McMahon RJ. How attendance and quality of participation affect treatment response to parent management training. J Consult Clin Psychol. 2009;77(3):429–38.

NREPP: National Registry of Evidence-based Programs and Practices. (n.d.). . Retrieved July 6, 2009, from http://nrepp.samhsa.gov/index.asp.

Olson SL, Bates JE, Sandy JM, Lanthier R. Early developmental precursors of externalizing behavior in middle childhood and adolescence. J Abnorm Child Psychol. 2000;28(2):119–33. doi:10.1023/A:1005166629744.

Parent-Child Interaction Therapy—Literature (2009). Parent-child interaction therapy. Retrieved June 20, 2009, from http://pcit.phhp.ufl.edu/Literature.htm.

Patterson GR, Gullion ME. Living with children: new methods for parents and teachers. Champaign, IL: Research Press; 1968.

Pelham WE, Lang AR, Atkeson B, Murphy DA, Gnagy EM, Greiner AR, et al. Effects of deviant child behavior on parental distress and alcohol consumption in laboratory interactions. J Abnorm Child Psychol. 1997;25(5):413–24.

Pelham WE. NREPP: children's summer treatment program (STP). Retrieved July 9, 2009, from http://nrepp.samhsa.gov/programfulldetails.asp?PROGRAM_ID=160.

Phelps L, Brown RT, Power TJ. Externalizing disorders. In: Pediatric psychopharmacology: combining medical and psychosocial interventions. Washington, DC: American Psychological Association; 2002. p. 101–31.

Piper AM, O'Brien E, Morris MR, Winograd T. SIDES: a cooperative tabletop computer game for social skills development. In: Proceedings of the 2006 20th anniversary conference on computer supported cooperative work (Banff, Alberta, Canada, November 04–08, 2006). CSCW '06. New York, NY: ACM; 2006. p. 1–10.

Querido JG, Eyberg SM. Parent-child interaction therapy: maintaining treatment gains of preschoolers with disruptive behavior disorders. In: Psychosocial treatments for child and adolescent disorders: Empirically based strategies for clinical practice. 2nd ed. Washington, DC: American Psychological Association; 2005. p. 575–97.

Reynolds CR, Kamphaus RW. Behavior assessment system for children (BASC). Circle Pines, MN: American Guidance Service; 1992.

Schoenfield L, Eyberg SM. Parent management training. In: Koocher GP, Norcross JC, Hill SS, editors. Psychologist's Desk Reference. 2nd ed. New York: Oxford University Press; 2005.

Shaffer D, Fisher P, Lucas CP, Dulcan MK, Schwab-Stone ME. NIMH Diagnostic Interview Schedule for Children Version IV (NIMH DISC-IV): description, differences from previous versions, and reliability of some common diagnoses. J Am Acad Child Adolesc Psychiatry. 2000;39:28–38.

Shaw DS, Keenan K, Vondra JI. Developmental precursors of externalizing behavior: ages 1 to 3. Dev Psychol. 1994;30(3):355–64.

Steenhuis M, Serra M, Minderaa RB, Hartman CA. (2009). An Internet version of the Diagnostic Interview Schedule for Children (DISC-IV): correspondence of the ADHD section with the paper-and-pencil version. Psychol Assessment. 2009;21(2):231–34.

Steiner H, Remsing L. Practice parameter for the assessment and treatment of children and adolescents with oppositional defiant disorder. J Am Acad Child Adolesc Psychiatry. 2007;46(1): 126–41.

Stormshak EA, Bierman KL, McMahon RJ, Lengua LJ. Parenting practices and child disruptive behavior problems in early elementary school. J Clin Child Psychol. 2000;29:17–29.

Training Guidelines for Parent-Child Interaction Therapy (2009). Parent-Child Interaction Therapy—Theoretical Underpinnings of PCIT. (n.d.). Retrieved June 21, 2009, from http://pcit.phhp.ufl.edu/TrainingGuidelines.htm.

Turgay A, Binder C, Snyder R, Fisman S. Long-term safety and efficacy of risperidone for the treatment of disruptive behavior disorders in children with subaverage IQs. Pediatrics. 2002;110(3):e34.

Walker HM, Ramsey E, Gresham FM. Antisocial Behavior in School: evidence-based practices. 2nd ed. Belmont, CA: Thomson Wadsworth; 2004.

Webster-Stratton CS. The incredible year. Toronto: Umbrella Press; 1992.

Webster-Stratton C, Reid MJ. Incredible years parents and teachers training series: a head start partnership to promote social competence and prevent conduct problems. In: Preventing youth substance abuse: science-based programs for children and adolescents. Washington, DC: American Psychological Association; 2007. p. 67–88.

Webster-Stratton C, Reid MJ, Stoolmiller M. Preventing conduct problems and improving school readiness: evaluation of the incredible years teacher and child training programs in high-risk schools. J Child Psychol Psychiatry. 2008;49(5):471–88.

Weisz JR, Jensen-Doss A, Hawley KM. Evidence-based youth psychotherapies versus usual clinical care: a meta-analysis of direct comparisons. Am Psychol. 2006;61(7):671–89.

Wright D. Time away: a procedure to keep task-avoiding students under instructional control. Retrieved June 22, 2009, from http://www.pent.ca.gov; http://www.pent.ca.gov/for/f8/timeaway.pdf.; 2008.

Wymbs BT, Pelham Jr, WE, Molina BSG, Gnagy EM, Wilson TK, Greenhouse JB. Rate and predictors of divorce among parents of youths with ADHD. J Consult Clin Psychol. 2008;76(5):735–44.

Chapter 11
Autism

Michele P. Steever

Autism is a complex disorder that disrupts normal functioning in the brain and causes multiple behavioral problems. Autism is one of many diagnoses under the umbrella of autism spectrum disorders (ASDs), a term which refers not to one specific problem, but rather to a variety of conditions that can affect communication, speech, social skills, emotional connection, and mental abilities. The core feature of autism is impairment in social interaction. However, this feature is also seen in other diagnoses, particularly those along the ASD spectrum. Other disorders that are considered to be on the autism spectrum are Asperger's disorder, Rett's disorder, childhood disintegrative disorder, and pervasive developmental disorder not otherwise specified (PDD NOS).

The prevalence of all pervasive developmental disorders is on the rise. Autism is the most common of these disorders and appears to be growing at an alarming rate. Thirty years ago, it was estimated that 1 in 10,000 people was autistic. In 2007, the Centers for Disease Control and Prevention (CDC) reported that when all PDDs are included, the prevalence rate may even be as high as 1 in 150 children, and rates are similar throughout the world. Often, the first professional to identify an ASD is the pediatrician. However, primary care settings do not generally allow for greater detail in assessment, and screening only is the norm. The pediatrician will then most likely refer to a psychologist, psychiatrist, or neurologist for a specific diagnosis and for differentiation of the autism spectrum disorders.

Assessment/Triage

Unfortunately, there is no perfect test to determine the presence of autism. Rather, the diagnosis is made by evaluating the presence or absence of certain behaviors. These behaviors are categorized in the DSM-IV-R and form the basis for diagnosis. The assessment process can often take time and, particularly with younger children, it can be difficult to determine whether the problem is autism or a pervasive

M.P. Steever (✉)
VA Sierra Nevada Health Care System, 1000 Locust St., Reno, NV 89502, USA
e-mail: michele.steever@va.gov

W.T. O'Donohue, C. Draper (eds.), *Stepped Care and e-Health*,
DOI 10.1007/978-1-4419-6510-3_11, © Springer Science+Business Media, LLC 2011

developmental disorder. Some providers will make a diagnosis of PDD-NOS with a rule out of autism. This can be frustrating for parents who are seeking a greater understanding of their child's problems. While a specific diagnosis is not usually necessary in order to begin treatment, as treatments are aimed at the behaviors in question rather than the diagnosis itself, a diagnosis will be needed for insurance billing and reimbursement. Even looking specifically at the diagnosis of autism, there are multiple criteria used in the diagnosis, and no two children with autism display the symptoms in exactly the same way. One child may have difficulty developing friendships and sharing enjoyment with other people. Another child may have many friends but difficulty making eye contact or using common social gestures. As different as these children appear, they may both be diagnosed with autistic disorder. This can make diagnosis, especially differentiating autistic disorder from other ASDs, quite time consuming and difficult.

Asperger's disorder, one of the ASDs, shares many features with autism and is often included in prevalence estimates of autism. The essential feature of Asperger's disorder is impairment in social interaction, a feature shared with autism. However, the marked difference is that children with Asperger's disorder want to have interaction with other people but have tremendous difficulty in doing so appropriately. Asperger's disorder does not share the problems in communication seen in autism—there are no delays in language or cognitive development. As with autism, Asperger's disorder is more common in boys than girls, with a 10:1 ratio. The diagnosis of PDD-NOS is made when there is severe impairment in social skills or communication skills, but the specific criteria for another pervasive developmental disorder are not met. The terms "atypical autism" and "high functioning autism" are descriptive labels only and refer to disorders that would fall under the diagnostic umbrella of the PDD-NOS category. Generally, when the diagnosis of PDD-NOS is given, it is for a clinical presentation of symptoms that is less severe than in other autism spectrum disorders such as autism or Asperger's.

One of the puzzling aspects of autism is that it seems to emerge suddenly, with symptoms most commonly noted at 15–20 months. Parents will often note that their children are developing normally, but then begin to regress, losing abilities, and words that they had previously learned. Other parents find that their child simply never started talking fluently or playing with other children. It may be that there were earlier signs of autism, but variation in development is normal and parents usually have no reason to believe that delays are related to autism. However, delays and autism-related problems become quite apparent around 15 months, when children are starting to take huge developmental leaps in language and play. Parents will often bring their child to the pediatrician with concerns about hearing problems, lack of babbling, or lack of social responsiveness. In these cases, it is often the pediatrician who first suspects autism after ruling out other potential problems (Johnson and Meyers, 2007; Wetherby et al., 2007).

Pediatricians routinely check whether a child is appropriately reaching developmental milestones. If a child is found to be behind in these milestones, then further assessment is often done, followed by referral to a specialist for further evaluation. The American Academy of Pediatrics recommends that all pediatricians screen for autism at 18 and 24 months of age, as well as at each well child visit. However, some research suggests that while most pediatricians (81%) routinely screen for general developmental delays, only 8% specifically screen for autism spectrum disorders due to factors such as not being familiar with screening tools and not having enough time in a visit (Dosreis et al., 2006). The AAP also recommends starting intervention and treatment as soon as the diagnosis is suspected rather than waiting for specialist diagnostic confirmation (Johnson and Meyers, 2007).

The primary measure used in primary care setting to evaluate autism is the Checklist for Autism in Toddlers (CHAT) (Baron-Cohen et al., 1992). It is a screening tool that can be used as young as 18 months. It is intended for use primarily by pediatricians and includes five questions to ask of parents that are geared at assessing social reciprocity in children. It also includes observations to be made by the pediatrician during the appointment. If two or more behaviors from either of the sections are absent, then autism is suspected. The CHAT takes less than 5 min to administer, making it ideal for the primary care setting. If autism is suspected, the pediatrician refers the child for further assessment and diagnosis. The CHAT was evaluated extensively (Baron-Cohen et al., 1996), and it was found that at 18 months of age, failure on three items from the CHAT corresponds to an 83.3% risk of autism. The measure does have a false-positive rate of 16%, but as further evaluation is required regardless, the ease of administration makes it a useful primary care screening tool. Additionally, the ability of the CHAT to screen autism in children as young as 18 months enables children to be referred for assessment and treatment at a young age, which is vital in order to obtain best outcomes from treatment. Further revision of the CHAT is currently underway with the development of the Q-CHAT or Quantitative Checklist for Autism in Toddlers (Allison et al., 2008). It is designed to better quantify the diagnosis and consists of 25 items scored on a five-point scale. Preliminary investigation has found the Q-CHAT to have good specificity and test–retest reliability, and further validity testing is in progress.

The Childhood Autism Rating Scale (CARS) is a very commonly used autism assessment measure (Schopler et al., 1980). It was developed by the Treatment and Education of Autistic and Related Communication Handicapped Children (TEACCH) program. The CARS is a behavior rating scale in which ratings are made by qualified professionals, such as a psychologist or behavior analyst, after both observing the child and talking with the parents or caregivers. Videos are available to train professionals with only minimal exposure to autism in the administration of the CARS. The child's behavior is rated on a scale from 1 to 4 in each of 15 areas, including relating to people, body use, adaptation to change, listening response, and verbal communication. The age range is 2 through adolescence, and administration takes 5–10 min, making it possible to administer the CARS in primary care settings. The CARS not only can identify children with autism but also can distinguish them from children with developmental disabilities other than autism. It has good reliability and validity and can differentiate mild to moderate from severe autism (Schopler et al., 1986).

Another measure used to evaluate the presence of autism in both children and adults is the Autism Diagnostic Interview Revised (ADI-R) (LeCouteur et al., 1989).

The ADI-R is a semi-structured standardized diagnostic interview that is based on DSM criteria for autism. A standard interview with the parents or caregivers is conducted at the home or in a clinic, and the measure is recognized as one of the best standardized instruments available to diagnose autism. A body of research has evaluated the psychometric properties of the ADI-R and found it to have good inter-rater reliability, internal consistency, and inter-class correlations (Lord et al., 1993, 1994, 1997). Unfortunately, it takes several hours to administer and score as well as extensive training to administer, both of which make it a poor choice for use in primary care settings.

A final measure that is commonly used and is appropriate for use in a primary care setting is the Gilliam Autism Rating Scale (GARS) (Gilliam, 1995). It takes approximately 10 min to administer, and score is completed by the parent, caregiver, or other person with knowledge of the child's behavior, such as a teacher. It is appropriate for individual aged 3–22 for whom autism is suspected. It covers the areas of stereotyped behaviors, communication, social interaction, and developmental disturbances. The GARS produces a total score, called the autism quotient (AQ) with a mean of 100 and a standard deviation of 15, and scores are interpreted as probable, possible, and unlikely for an autism diagnosis. Although the GARS was widely accepted and used, some authors have raised validity concerns, specifically pointing to problems with false negatives and overemphasis on restrictive and repetitive behaviors relative to communication and social impairments (Matson,2008; South et al., 2002). Partly in response to these concerns, the scale was revised and the GARS-2 was released in 2006. The GARS-2 retains the ease of use and practicality of the initial GARS, while improving significantly on psychometric properties (Gilliam, J., 2006; Montgomery et al., 2008).

Outcome Data

While a "cure" for autism that will produce a complete recovery is the hope of all parents with an autistic child, at this time such a universal cure does not exist. However, there is a good deal of evidence that a long-term, intensive treatment, known as applied behavior analysis (also referred to as intensive behavioral intervention or early behavioral intervention), can significantly impact the course of the disorder (Butter et al., 2006; Green et al., 2002; Lovaas, 1987; Maurice et al., 1996). ABA often leads to large-scale improvements in the child's language, social behavior, and general level of functioning (Anderson et al., 1987; Perry et al., 1995). In fact, long-term, intensive treatment can result in completely normal functioning for a significant minority of children diagnosed with autism.

Intensive behavioral treatment for autism was developed out of an understanding of applied behavior analysis and behavioral theory. From a behavior analytic viewpoint, autism is seen as "a syndrome of behavioral deficits and excesses that have a neurological basis, but are nonetheless amenable to change in response to specific, carefully programmed, constructive interactions within the environment" (Green, 1996, 29–30). The treatment stemming from this view is additionally informed by observations and research, indicating that while autistic children do not readily learn from typical environments as normally developing children do, they are still able to learn a great deal when the environment is altered, and skills are broken down into small, clear steps (Koegel and Koegel, 1995; Lovaas, 1987). Thus, in behavioral treatment of autism, skills are broken down into observable, small, discrete steps—as such, the primary intervention within the behavioral framework is discrete trial training.

The principles and techniques of applied behavior analysis are utilized in intensive behavioral treatment. The "intensive" in this label refers to the amount of time the child spends in treatment, which to be maximally effective, is 40 h/week. There is some evidence that while children can still improve significantly with 20 h a week, as few as 10 h is inadequate to produce meaningful changes (Anderson et al., 1987; Lovaas and Smith, 1988). Additional features of intensive behavior treatment include clear tracking or graphing of child response data and inappropriate behavior data, as well as programming for generalization, which often occurs through incidental teaching. A complete-intensive behavioral program requires careful development as well as implementation, and home programs utilizing applied behavior analysis must be implemented under the care of a trained psychologist or behavior analyst to ensure that all necessary areas are being addressed thoroughly and competently in order to maximize outcomes for the child.

ABA has now become well accepted as the best empirically evaluated treatment for autism. It has been recognized nationally as the treatment of choice for autism, and many state governments have corroborated this recommendation through autism taskforces and workgroups (National Research Council, 2001; New York State Department of Health Early Intervention Program, 1999). However, there are numerous other "treatments" that make various claims about their effectiveness in curing autism. Some of these options include dietary interventions, holding therapy, facilitated communication, applied behavior analysis, and sensory integration. These all have claims of success and testimonials, but very little controlled, scientific research evaluating their effectiveness.

On the other hand, there is a large body of research documenting the effectiveness of ABA. In one of the most well-known and thorough studies of this treatment to date, Lovaas (1987) compared a 40 h/week intensive behavioral treatment at UCLA to two control groups—one that received 10 h a week of the same treatment and a control group that received no treatment. After 2 years of treatment, 47% of the children in the intensive treatment group had completed first grade in a normal classroom and scored in the normal range on IQ tests, as compared with only one child from the other two groups. A follow-up study found that 6 years later, these gains were maintained (McEachin et al., 1993).

Since the publication of the Lovaas studies, a number of other investigators have published research detailing the improvement made by children in ABA-based intensive autism programs. Not all of these findings have been as robust; there are differing explanations for this, but the predominant explanation is that treatment was most intensive in the Lovaas research—40 h/week for 2–3 years. Additionally, more recent interventions do not use any form of aversives (not even a firm "stop that" to consequate problems behaviors). However, studies of ABA have consistently found meaningful increases in IQ scores and communicative ability, as well as in social, adaptive, and educational functioning. A review article (Smith, 1999) examined 12 peer-reviewed outcome studies on autism treatment—nine were ABA programs and three were other types of intervention. They found mean IQ gains of 7–28 points in the ABA programs (lower gains in programs of fewer hours per week of intervention over shorter time periods) compared to 3–9 points in the non-ABA programs. Green (1996) estimates intensive behavioral treatment is effective for nearly all children, with only a small portion (approximately 10%) failing to make significant improvements.

ABA is a long-term and intensive treatment. It most often continues for 3 years and to be maximally effective requires 40 h/week. There is some evidence that children can still improve significantly with 20 h a week, but that as few as 10 h is inadequate to produce meaningful changes. It was questioned whether the sole advantage of ABA is its intensive, long-term nature, but research has found this to not be the case. Autistic children who receive ABA treatment have significantly greater improvement than children who receive the same number of treatment hours of other interventions (Eikeseth et al., 2002).

ABA is most effective when begun early in the child's life, with best outcomes for children who began treatment before the age of five (Birnbrauer and Leach, 1993; Fenske et al., 1985). Emerging research in the area of pediatric neurology suggests that this is due to greater brain plasticity before age five (Altemeier and Altemeier, 2009). As such, there is urgency to begin treatment, and delays due to problems accessing treatment or with treatment availability can be quite costly.

Barriers to Treatment

There is a scarcity of autism treatment resources available to meet the ever increasing needs. Most of the treatment centers in existence are full, often due to a lack of resources such as space, funding, or an adequate number of treatment providers. This is an unfortunate state of affairs: the number of children diagnosed with autism is increasing, evidence for and acceptance of early behavioral intervention continues to grow, and yet the number of treatment providers is not sufficient to meet the need. This observation is easily confirmed by a comparison of the number of children with autism and the available treatment providers. The most comprehensive listing of ABA treatment providers and programs is maintained by a very dedicated parent online, is frequently updated, and can be obtained at the following address: http://members.tripod.com/Rsaffran/consultants.html. In it, 562 providers (both individuals and programs) were identified in the United States.

To compare this with the need, the CDC's autism and developmental disabilities monitoring (ADDM) network released data in 2007 finding that 1 in 150 8-year-old children in the United States had an autism spectrum disorder. This means that in the United States alone, over 25,000 children with autism are born each year. Early intensive treatment, to be most effective, should begin when the child is between 2 and 5 years old and usually continues for 3 years (Maurice et al., 1996). Using these estimates, if all children with autism were to receive ABA treatment for autism, each available center and provider would need to consistently serve nearly 140 children. While a few have such a capacity, most treatment centers reach maximum capacity at closer to 20 children, and an individual treatment provider would be able to serve even fewer than that, leaving thousands of children still in need of services.

To access treatment for their children, parents have been known to relocate to areas with availability in effective behavioral treatment programs. However, for many families, this is not feasible, and those living in areas without treatment programs, which are often rural areas, cannot access necessary treatments (Koegel et al., 2002; Slater & Black, 1986). The situation of people in rural areas being unable to access specialized care is not limited to autism services. Much more generally, there is a scarcity of specialized training and professionals to deliver treatments in rural areas. This phenomenon has been documented in a number of fields, including psychiatric services, specialized health care, and education (Gething, 1997).

Even if a treatment program has availability, another problem may arise, as many programs are too expensive for parents to afford. In 1998, Jacobson et al. estimated that 3 years of an early intensive behavioral intervention program for an autistic child would cost $101,445. The authors of this cost–benefit study conclude that the effectiveness of the intervention is so great that even when assuming only partial effects of treatment, cost savings for an autistic person from age 3 to 55 would be $940,118. Still, the initial cost of an intensive autism program may be too great for many families, and parents often have little assistance in meeting the costs.

By and large, insurance companies consider intensive behavioral treatment of autism educational (rather than medical or psychological) and do not cover the cost of treatment. Fortunately, there are hopeful signs that this is beginning to change. A major insurance carrier, Magellan Health Services, is now offering a program called Magellan Autism Connections, which provides comprehensive autism benefits, support services, and a specialty provider network. In each of these cases, whether due to space limitations in existing programs, cost of treatment, or geographical isolation, parents are forced to find other options.

Stepped-Care Options

Stepped care is a model of health-care delivery that may be able to overcome some of these barriers and constraints by beginning with treatments that are least intrusive and least expensive. If these less restrictive and less expensive interventions are effective, treatment is complete. If not, the patient then moves to a higher level of treatment (a higher "step") and moves up the steps of care until treatment is successful (Bower and Gilbody, 2005). Some problems are better suited to this model than others, and a stepped-care approach to treatment has been studied most extensively with mood disorders such as depression and anxiety.

In stepped-care models, determining the least intrusive level of care takes into account issues of patient cost, patient convenience, and treatment intensity which is often measured by therapist time required to administer the treatment. More intrusive treatments are only undertaken when a patient does not benefit from a lower level of care. This model allows the greatest number of people to benefit from the available resources, which are often limited. An important aspect of stepped care is evaluation of effectiveness, most often requiring ongoing assessment. This model is only useful if people actually derive benefit from treatment. If a patient fails to benefit from a lower level of care, does not have sufficient follow-up, drops out of treatment, and the problem goes untreated, then stepped care has failed. A mechanism must be in place to most patients to higher levels of care in instances when the lower steps have failed.

Stepped care when considered for the treatment of autism is a complex issue. It is a clear case in which the number of children in need of treatment greatly outweighs the number of available, trained treatment providers. For this reason, beginning with the least intrusive treatment marked by the least number of hours of treatment provided by a trained therapist makes a great deal of sense and would allow the greatest number of children to be treated. Lovaas alluded to this when writing about what is needed to provide effective treatments to all children with autism, noting "There are not enough professionals to deliver the necessary treatment. This means that we will have to give away our professional skills to lay persons, and the sooner the better" (Lovaas, 1993, p. 628).

There are important issues to consider regarding the disorders that are most appropriately treated through a stepped-care approach. It is generally accepted that stepped-care models are best for disorders in which there will not be an adverse consequence from starting on too low a step or in which having a treatment failure at a low step will not have long-term negative consequences. In the case of autism it is clear that the earlier intensive behavioral treatment is started and the more the hours per week provided, the better the outcomes. Waiting to implement intensive, one-on-one, ABA treatment while starting at lower steps of care may ultimately result in less robust outcomes. Additionally, starting at a lower level of intensity may have long-term negative consequences in the form of less effective treatment. Davison (2000) cautions against this and recommends that "it is better. . .to construct the steps according to a judgment of the minimally intensive/intrusive treatment that a given patient is likely to respond favorably to" (p. 583). Little is known about which families with autistic children will respond best to which treatments, but this is a goal worth bearing in mind as stepped care is investigated further. Regardless, there are real-world issues that parents of autistic children face issues that often result in families following a stepped-care approach naturally. As discussed earlier, many parents are not able to obtain intensive ABA for their children due to lack of trained treatment providers or cost. For this reason, they will seek out other treatments that are less expensive and easier to obtain, many of which are on the stepped-care continuum.

Watchful Waiting

"Watchful waiting" is an approach to medical or mental health problems in which a problem is suspected, but time is allowed to pass before any treatment or intervention is started. It is most appropriate for problems that spontaneously remit and, as such, is not an appropriate course of action for children strongly suspected of having autism, as spontaneous remission does not occur in autism. However, there is tremendous variability in normal child development, and missing one developmental milestone does not necessarily mean that a child has autism or another developmental disorder. In these cases, pediatricians may recommend the watchful waiting approach. However, as there is great importance in beginning intervention for autism early, no longer than 3 months should elapse between assessments, and there is little harm in over-referring children suspected of having autism for additional evaluation.

Psychoeducation

Significant changes to traditional autism treatment need to occur in order for ABA to be adapted to lower levels of stepped care, particularly those levels that are entirely patient guided. Intensive behavioral treatment for autism is not delivered in a way where the material is presented and absorbed for the person to then apply to their life. Rather, it is a dynamic, one-on-one, interactive treatment. Furthermore, the model of stepped care as used with other disorders must also be modified for application to autism. In traditional models, the patient is the person with the problem being addressed and is the person who is reading the psychoeducation or bibliotherapy materials. This presumes a certain level of self-motivation and desire for change that may be necessary for positive outcomes. In the case of autism, the identified patient is the child with autism, but the person participating in the self-help treatment is the parent.

Still, psychoeducation is a useful and, possibly necessary, component of treatment and initial step. Although public awareness of autism has increased, understanding is still incomplete. When a parent first learns that their child is autistic, they will first want to know exactly what autism is and what this means for their child's life. Psychoeducation, in the form of pamphlets, books, and web sites, allows parents to become educated consumers with a good understanding of available treatments and child outcomes under each treatment. The most important function of psychoeducation with autism is teaching parents to be educated consumers. Time is of the essence in the early treatment of autism, and parents need to understand that applied behavior analysis for autism is the most effective treatment option. Through psychoeducation, parents can make informed and educated choices for their children without wasting precious resources of time and money on treatments that do not have sufficient empirical support.

There are a number of web sites devoted to disseminating information about autism, such as the Autism Support Network (http://www.autismsupportnetwork.com/), Autism Speaks (http://www.autismspeaks.org), and the National Autism Association (http://nationalautismassociation.org). It is unknown whether and in what capacity these and other psychoeducational web sites will be useful to parents. A study of this issue is currently underway by the author, with the development and testing of a new psychoeducational web site designed for parents who recently had a child diagnosed with autism. It is hoped that the web site will be found to be useful in a number of domains, including increasing knowledge of behavioral principles, increasing parental interest in pursuing ABA treatment for their child, and improving individual well-being.

Bibliotherapy

Bibliotherapy is a more intensive step up from psychoeducation. Like psychoeducation, it generally not only provides information about the specific problem but also includes self-guided therapy exercises. It may include writing exercises or specific homework designed to address the problem. Like other stepped-care options that are entirely patient guided, motivation and comprehension are necessary factors for success. Bibliotherapy most often takes the form of written material, but can also be provided in the form of videos or DVDs.

An important use of bibliotherapy in the treatment of autism occurs when parents read a book to learn to be treatment providers for their children. Many books exist that describe the principles of intensive behavioral treatment and include sample curriculum that provides the foundation for treatment. Examples include *A Work in Progress: Behavior Management Strategies and a Curriculum for Intensive Behavioral Treatment of Autism* (Leaf and McEachin, 1999), *Teaching Developmentally Disabled Children: The Me Book* (Lovaas, 1981), and *Behavioral Intervention for Young Children with Autism: A Manual for Parents and Professionals* (Maurice et al., 1996). Bibliotherapy can also include fiction books and inspirational literature, such as *Chicken Soup for the Soul: Children with Special Needs: Stories of Love and Understanding for Those who Care for Children with Disabilities* (Canfield et al., 2007) and *Let Me Hear Your Voice: A Family's Triumph Over Autism* (Maurice, 1994).

A stepped-care treatment program incorporating bibliotherapy was evaluated in a recent parent training study (Phaneuf, 2009). Three tiers or steps of treatment were investigated: self-administered reading material, group training, and individualized video feedback sessions. The reading material was sufficient to produce change in only a small part of the sample, but did have some positive results. A similar application with parents of autistic children could have the benefit of being easily accessible and inexpensive; even if only a small portion of families derived benefit from reading materials, there is little drawback to doing such reading and it may possibly serve the function of priming for concepts presented differently in higher steps of care.

A groundbreaking type of bibliotherapy program, called Maximum Potential, has recently been released for parents of autistic children (http://www.maximumpotentialkids.com/). It is an ABA training course that was developed by behavior analysts and aims to teach parents how to implement ABA for autism with their children. It includes 17 modules on eight DVDs and covers topics such as teaching strategies, data collection, behavior management, and social skills. While the program has not yet been empirically investigated, it provides a promising and cost-effective new bibliotherapy approach to the treatment of autism. While traditional, therapist provided ABA treatment can cost over $30,000, the entire set of Maximum Potential DVDs is available for $350.

Computer-Based Interventions/e-Health

Computer-based interventions are a more intrusive intervention than psychoeducation and bibliotherapy in that they generally include some degree of interaction. Dean and Whitlock (1983) enumerated the many benefits of computer-based training, including more effective use of consumer time, training available at the learner's convenience, consistent presentation of training material, reduced consumer travel time and expenses, ability to meet practical training needs, versatility of training location, reduction or elimination of instructor involvement, and ease of programing that allows for efficient update in accordance with educational, clinical, and/or technological advancements. In particular, the Internet is a particularly useful form of computer-based technology, as web sites can be accessed immediately, have virtually limitless dissemination possibilities, and allow for the combination of written and videotape instructional materials. Educational treatments delivered through the Internet can preserve the benefits of videotape technology such as visual presentation that is ideal for modeling of skills, while allowing for individualized, self-paced instruction (Wetzel et al., 1994).

The use of computer-based interventions in the treatment of autism is a new field, and one with little empirical investigation to date. However, this is an area of great potential, offering options ranging from online courses in which parents could learn to be treatment providers for their children, to autistic children learning directly through Internet instruction, to social skills training with computerized peers. Researchers are starting to use virtual reality computer programs to teach higher functioning autistic children skills such as crossing the street safely and reciprocal conversation.

Many web sites exist that are best categorized as e-health. Most focus on providing information, but have the interactive quality of a support group through the use of forums and message boards. For example, http://www.autismfamilyonline.com/ is a web site with the stated goals of providing "practical, useable information to help families and educators improve the quality of life for those individuals with autism spectrum disorders who are in their care." It contains information about autism, video and audio clips, message boards, forums, case studies, and information about best practices. The site requires monthly membership at the rate of $19.95/month.

An interactive multimedia computerized intervention to teach children with ASDs how to better interpret and predict emotions is available at http://www. emotiontrainer.co.uk/. The Emotion Trainer program has some empirical support, with a study indicating that students who used the program improved in expression recognition and emotion understanding in non-literal stories (Silver and Oakes, 2001).

Another interesting computerized intervention is called TeachTown and is available at http://web.teachtown.com/. TeachTown is a research and technology company that has been funded by the Department of Education and has created a computer-based program to teach children with autism and other developmental disabilities. It employs both computerized lessons and naturalistic activities, and child progress is graphed automatically. TeachTown is designed for 2- to 7-year olds, and a subscription is $39.95/month. An early study of the program found that it increased the language and social behaviors of autistic children, decreased inappropriate behaviors, and increased positive affect (Whalen et al., 2006).

Group Therapy

Group therapy for autism can be viewed in one of two ways. The first is to treat groups of autistic children at once. The setting in which this occurs is at schools, whether in specific autism classrooms or in mainstreamed inclusion classrooms. While some of these classrooms and teaching strategies used within are quite effective, a review of school interventions for autism is beyond the scope of this chapter. Additionally, school treatment is not on the continuum of stepped-care treatments for autism, as children do not "move up" to a higher intensity treatment if they are not doing well in school. Finally, the most effective treatment for autism is ABA begun at a very young age, certainly before children are enrolled in school. As such, the application of stepped care to autism within group therapy is more appropriately viewed as training parents to be therapists for their children in the group setting.

The highest step of care in the treatment of autism is considered to be parents paying for a qualified ABA therapist 40 h/week. A lower step is for the parents to learn to be treatment providers themselves. Teaching parents to be treatment providers in a group setting does require the presence of a professional but at a lower level of intensity than higher steps would require. Thus, it still maintains the advantages of decreased cost and increased number of people able to receive care. It is also less personally intrusive in that a stranger is not coming into a family's house, as well as generally being less expensive. However, there are still serious financial issues to consider in parents providing treatment, such as the cost of lost income if a parent needs to quit working in order to become their child's therapist.

Many studies have examined the utility of training parents to be effective change agents, or treatment providers, for their children. Not only does this approach have the advantage of reducing costs but also improves the ability to disseminate treatment to an ever increasing number of autistic children in need of treatment. There is now much research indicating that parents can be skilled treatment providers for their children. Parents have been found to be able to learn and implement behavioral interventions effectively and were able to effect change with their children in many areas, including increasing functional language, decreasing echolalia, and decreasing behavior problems (Harris, 1986a, b). They are also effective in targeting adaptive skills, increasing desired behaviors, and decreasing noncompliance and unwanted behaviors (Moran and Whitman, 1991). Additionally, intensive behavioral treatment programs have been found to be less effective when parents are not also trained to implement the treatment (Koegel and Koegel, 1995).

A recent study of the Group Intensive Family Training (GIFT) program evaluated the effectiveness of one such group therapy treatment (Anan et al., 2008). Parents of preschool age children with autism spectrum disorders participated in the program 3 h each weekday for 12 weeks (total of 180 h). After parents completed the program, their children improved in cognitive and adaptive functioning, some even to the point of being in the "non-impaired" range on standardized tests. While this is a preliminary investigation, it does suggest that parent training implemented in a group setting can be both effective and efficient.

Individual Therapy

The traditional approach to providing intensive early behavioral treatment for autism was covered earlier in this chapter and is the highest step in ABA treatment for autism. In this model, a qualified ABA therapist or team of professionals provides intensive treatment 40 h/week, generally paid for by the family themselves. There are gradations within this step, however, in terms of both who provides the treatment and how many hours of treatment are provided each week. Within this model of individual therapy, the highest step would be paying professionals for 40 h/week of intensive behavioral intervention. A lower step would be parents providing the treatment themselves, but instead of learning to do so through bibliotherapy, e-health, or group therapy, by working individually with an outreach consultant. The consultant meets with the family and teaches them to implement the treatment in their home, generally with the assistance of a group of tutors that the family recruits.

A 4-year study of in-clinic intensive behavioral treatment provided by trained professionals versus that provided by parents individually coached by professionals found outcomes to be similar for both groups, with gains in areas of learning, standardized test scores, and success in regular education classrooms (Sallows and Graupner, 2005).

Medication

No medications are approved by the US Food and Drug Administration (FDA) for the treatment of autism. However, medications are often prescribed "off-label" to address the specific symptoms associated with autism, such as hyperactivity, self-abusive behavior, anxiety, or aggression. As many as one-quarter of all children with autism also suffer from seizures, and in those cases, medication is crucial. It has been estimated that over half of all children diagnosed with an autism spectrum disorder takes at least one psychotropic medication, primarily neuroleptics, antidepressants, and stimulants (Mandell et al., 2008).

Inpatient Treatment

Inpatient treatment, including hospitals and residential programs, is less utilized for the treatment of children with autism now than in the past. There is some evidence that residential treatment programs are no more effective in treating autistic children than is home-based care and comes at a significantly greater expense (Sherman et al., 1988). However, residential treatments and group homes are still common for adults with autism, especially lower functioning adults with autism who face many challenges in independent living. In terms of stepped care for autism, inpatient treatment for children with autism would only be considered in extreme cases. These include cases in which no other interventions have been successful, as well as those in which aggressive behavior problems are so severe that they pose a danger to other persons living in the home, such as siblings. However, there is not yet a body of research that speaks to the effectiveness of inpatient treatment for autism as the most intrusive step of care for the extreme and treatment resistant cases.

Consumer Preferences and Cultural Sensitivity

Little is known about consumer preferences for autism treatments. Consumer preference can be evaluated indirectly by looking into parent satisfaction with treatment, about which we do have some information. Generally, parents do seem to report high satisfaction with early intervention treatment for autism. There is some research into the factors that influence satisfaction; child progress, treatment outcome, and open communication with treatment providers are related to increased satisfaction, while parental stress and depression seems to reduce satisfaction with treatment (King et al., 2001, Rodger et al., 2008).

Cultural sensitivity is of particular importance in the screening and assessment of children for autism. For example, the absence of eye contact is a red flag for autism, but in many Asian cultures, direct eye contact is uncommon in young children and is culturally discouraged. Lack of reciprocal babbling often alerts pediatricians to potential problems, but some cultures do not encourage children to speak at an early age (Wallis and Pinto-Martin, 2008). Other obstacles to effective treatment with culturally diverse or immigrant families include language barriers, difficulty navigating community systems and agencies, discrimination, and lower likelihood of adequate insurance coverage (Welterlin and LaRue, 2007).

Racial disparities may exist in the diagnosis and treatment of autism, with minority and immigrant families receiving a later autism diagnosis than white families.

Mandell et al. (2002) examined a Medicaid eligible sample in Philadelphia and found that on average, white children were diagnosed with autism at 6.3 years of age versus 7.9 years of age for African-American children. Racial and cultural factors seem to play a role in whether children with autism receive psychotropic medications, with children in counties with lower percentages of white residents or greater urban density being less likely to receive these medications (Mandell et al., 2008).

Triage Agenda

In a stepped-care model, the two factors that are generally considered in the triage stage of assessment are patient preference and problem severity. In the case of autism, preference for treatment is likely to be strongly affected by the early step of psychoeducation. When parents become educated consumers and learn about the research studies supporting different treatments, it is likely that a preference for intensive behavioral treatment will develop. More research is necessary to better understand what considerations parents employ when making treatment decisions, as well as to understand parent preferences for different steps along the continuum of care.

Problem severity, however, is less of a consideration with the problem of autism than with other disorders, as the most highly supported intervention is intensive behavioral treatment, and this holds true regardless of presenting severity. Still, there are many questions that need to be answered in this domain in order to better understand how ABA for autism can be delivered through different levels of care. How many hours of weekly treatment are necessary for differing levels of problem severity? Do less severe cases respond better to lower levels of care than do more severe cases? If treatment is started at a higher level of care, must it continue for less time?

Research and Development Agenda

The aforementioned questions are all important targets for future research. The application of stepped care to autism is a new field of study, and little is yet known about the effectiveness of each step. Ultimately, a combination of steps may work best. Consider the following application: parents first read material to understand the basics of autism, behavior analysis, and ABA treatment for autism. They then view DVDs (or online videos) of ABA in action to better understand the treatment. They then work with a consultant, who assesses current excesses and deficits, and creates a curriculum for training that is provided to the parents. Parents implement treatment and submit weekly data and video to the consultant who can monitor treatment integrity. A weekly meeting can be held using webcam technology to allow the parents to discuss treatment issues with the consultant. Any problems identified with treatment integrity can be addressed through real-time feedback to parents.

This model could be applied anywhere with just the use of a computer, a webcam, and some software. Parents living in rural areas who do not have access to intensive behavioral intervention could help their children without the need to move or to sacrifice effective treatment for their child with autism. In most cases, consultants would spend about 3 h/week working with a family, greatly reducing the cost to the family over paying for 40 h/week treatment. The consultant would be able to work with many families at a time, increasing access to treatment and decreasing the number of children who do not receive needed services due to lack of availability. Whether such a program that utilizes a combination of steps would be effective is an empirical question, and hopefully research that addresses this type of program is in the future.

Dissemination Agenda

Two different issues must be addressed when dealing with the issues of dissemination of stepped-care treatments for autism. First, how do we disseminate effective treatments to families affected by autism, and, second, how do we ensure that this approach is accepted by and promoted by professionals? In both cases, we must consider delivery systems and policies in place that could support such efforts. Currently much of the distribution of autism information takes place through grassroots efforts of parents. While the importance of parents connecting with other parents cannot be overstated, educating those professionals on the front lines of autism screening, such as teachers, day-care providers, and pediatricians, about the importance of early intervention and the treatment options available may improve knowledge about and access to needed treatments. Increasing confidence in the usefulness of stepped-care treatments is also crucial for improving willingness and motivation to pursue such avenues, both by parents and professionals. Only through ongoing research examining the application of a stepped-care model to autism will we be able to build confidence in such as model and fully understand its potential in disseminating needed treatments to children with autism.

References

Altemeier WA, Altemeier LE. How can early, intensive training help a genetic disorder? Pediatr Ann. 2009;38:167–72.

Allison C, Baron-Cohen S, Wheelwright S, Charman T, Richler J, Pasco G, Brayne C. The Q-CHAT (Quantitative Checklist for Autism in Toddlers): a normally distributed quantitative measure of autistic traits at 18–24 months of age: A preliminary report. J Autism Dev Disord. 2008;38:1414–25.

Anan RM, Warner LJ, McGillivary JE, Chong IM, Hines SJ. Group intensive family training (GIFT) for preschoolers with autism spectrum disorders. Behav Intervent. 2008;23:165.

Anderson SR, Avery DL, DiPietro EK, Edwards GL, Christian WP. Intensive home-based early intervention with autistic children. Educ Treat Child. 1987;10:352–66.

Baron-Cohen S, Allen J, Gillberg C. Can autism be detected at 18 months? The needle, the haystack, and the CHAT. Br J Psychiatry. 1992;161:839–43.

Baron-Cohen S, Cox A, Baird G, Swettenham J, Drew A, Nightingale N, Morgan K, Charman, T. Psychological markers of autism at 18 months of age in a large population. Br J Psychiatry. 1996;168:158–63.

Birnbrauer JS, Leach DJ. The Murdoch early intervention program after 2 years. Behav Change. 1993;10:63–74.

Bower P, Gilbody S. Stepped care in psychological therapies: access, effectiveness, and efficiency. Br J Psychiatry. 2005;186:11–7.

Butter EM, Mulick JA, Metz B. Eight case reports of learning recovery n children with pervasive developmental disorders after early intervention. Behav Intervent. 2006;21 227–43.

Canfield J, Hansen MV, McNamara H, Simmons K. Chicken soup for the soul: children with special needs: stories of love and understanding for those who care for children with disabilities. Deerfield Beach, FL: Health Communications, Inc.; 2007.

Davison GC. Stepped care: doing more with less? J Consult Clin Psychol. 2000;68:580–5.

Dean C, Whitlock Q. A handbook of computer based training. New York: Nichols Publishing Company; 1983.

Dosreis S, Weiner CL, Johnson L, Newschaffer CJ. Autism spectrum disorder screening and management practices among general pediatric providers. J Dev Behav Pediatr. 2006;27:S88–94.

Eikeseth S, Smith T, Jarh E, Eldevik S. Intensive behavioral treatment at school for 4- to 7-year-old children with autism: a 1-year comparison controlled study. Behav Modif. 2002;26:49–68.

Fenske EC, Zalenski S, Krantz PJ, McClannahan LE. Age at intervention and treatment outcome for autistic children in a comprehensive intervention program. Anal Intervent Dev Disab. 1985;5:49–58.

Gething L. Providing services in remote and rural Australian communities. J Community Psychol. 1997;25:209–26.

Gilliam J. Gilliam Autism rating scale. Austin, TX: Pro-Ed.; 1995.

Gilliam J. GARS-2: Gilliam Autism Rating Scale—2nd ed. Austin, TX: Pro-Ed.; 2006.

Green G. Early behavioral intervention for autism: what does research tell us? In: Maurice C, Green G, Luce SC, editors. Behavioral intervention for young children with autism: a manual for parents and professionals. Austin, TX: Pro-Ed.; 1996.

Green G, Brennan LC, Fein D. Intensive behavioral treatment for a toddler at high risk for autism. Behav Modif. 2002;26:69–102.

Harris SL. Families of children with autism: issues for the behavior therapist. Behav Ther. 1986a;9:175–7.

Harris SL. Parents as teachers: a four to seven year follow up of parents of children with autism. Child Fam Behav Ther. 1986b;8:39–47.

Jacobson JW, Mulick JA, Green G. Cost-benefit estimates for early intensive behavioral intervention for young children with autism—general model and single state case. Behav Intervent. 1998;13:201–26.

Johnson CP. Meyers SM. Council on Children with Disabilities. Identification and evaluation of children with autism spectrum disorder. Pediatrics. 2007;120:1183–215.

King G, Cathers T, King S, Rosenbaum P. Major elements of parents' satisfaction and dissatisfaction with paediatric rehabilitation services. Child Health Care. 2001;30:111–34.

Koegel RL, Koegel LK. Teaching children with autism: Strategies for initiating positive interaction and improving learning opportunities. Baltimore: Paul H. Brookes Publishing Company; 1995.

Leaf R, McEachin J. A Work in Progress: Behavior Management Strategies and a Curriculum for Intensive Behavioral Treatment of Autism. DRL Books; 1999.

LeCouteur A, Rutter M, Lord C, Rios P, Robertson S, Holdgrafer M, McLennan, J. Autism diagnostic interview: a standardized investigator-based instrument. J Autism Dev Disord. 1989;19:363–87.

Lord C, Pickles A, McLennan J, Rutter M, Bregman J, Folstein S, Fombonne E, Leboyer M, Minshew N. Diagnosing autism: analyses of data from the Autism diagnostic interview. J Autism Dev Disord. 1997;27:501–17.

Lord C, Rutter M, LeCouteur A. Autism Diagnostic Interview-Revised: a revised version of a diagnostic interview for caregivers of individuals with possible pervasive developmental disorders. J Autism Dev Disord. 1994;24:659–85.

Lord C, Storoschuk S, Rutter M, Pickles A. (1993). Using the ADI-R to diagnose autism in preschool children. Inf Mental Health J. 1993;14:234–52.

O. Ivar Lovaas. Teaching developmentally disabled children: the Me Book. Pro-Ed.; 1981.

Lovaas OI. Behavioral treatment and normal educational and intellectual functioning in young autistic children. J Consult Clin Psychol. 1987;55:3–9.

Lovaas OI. The development of a treatment-research project for developmentally disabled and autistic children. J Appl Behav Anal. 1993;26:617–30.

Lovaas OI. Smith T. Intensive behavioral treatment for young autistic children. In: Lahey BB, Kazdin AE, editors. Advances in clinical child psychology. New York: Plenum Press; 1988. p. 285–324.

Mandell DS, Listerud J, Levy SE, Pinto-Martin JA. Race differences in the age at diagnosis among Medicaid-eligible children with autism. J Am Acad Child Adolesc Psychiatry. 2002;41: 1447–53.

Mandell DS, Morales KH, Marcus SC, Stahmer AC, Doshi J, Polsky DE. Psychotropic medication use among Medicaid-enrolled children with autism spectrum disorders. Pediatrics. 2008;121:E441.

Matson JL. Clinical assessment and intervention for autism spectrum disorders. Burlington, MA: Academic Press; 2008.

Maurice C. Let me hear your voice: a family's triumph over autism. New York: Random House; 1994.

Maurice C, Green G, Luce SC. Behavioral intervention for young children with autism: a manual for parents and professionals. Austin, TX: Pro-Ed.; 1996.

McEachin JJ, Smith T, Lovaas OI. Long-term outcome for children with autism who received early intensive behavioral treatment. Am J Ment Retard. 1993;4:359–72.

Montgomery JM, Newton B, Smith C. Test Reviews: Gilliam, J. (2006). GARS-2: Gilliam Autism Rating Scale—Second Edition. J Psychoeduc Assessment. 2008;26:395–401.

Moran DR, Whitman TL. Developing generalized teaching skills in mothers of autistic children. Child Fam Behav Ther. 1991;13:13–37.

National Research Council. Educating children with autism. Washington, DC: National Academy Press; 2001.

New York State Department of Health Early Intervention Program. Clinical practice guideline quick reference guide: autism/pervasive developmental disorders—assessment and intervention for young children (age 0–3 years). Health Education Services, P.O. Box 7126, Albany, NY 12224 (1999 Publication No. 4216); 1999.

Perry R, Cohen I, DeCarlo R. Case study: deterioration, autism, and recovery in two siblings. J Am Acad Child Adolesc Psychiatry. 1995;34:232–7.

Phaneuf LK. The application of a three tier model of intervention to parent training. Dissertation Abstracts International. 2009;69:2606.

Rodger S, Keen D, Braithwaite M, Cook S. Mothers' satisfaction with a home based early intervention programme for children with ASD. J Appl Res Intellect. 2008;21: 174–82.

Sallows GO, Graupner TD. Intensive behavioral treatment for children with autism: four-year outcome and predictors. Am J Ment Retard. 2005;110:417–38.

Schopler E, Reichler RJ, DeVellis RF, Daly K. Toward objective classification of childhood autism: childhood autism rating scale (CARS). J Autism Dev Disord. 1980;10:91–103.

Schopler E, Reichler R, Renner BR. The childhood autism rating scale (CARS) for diagnostic screening and classification of autism. New York: Irvington Publishers; 1986.

Sherman J, Barker P, Lorimer P, Swinson R, Factor DC. Treatment of autistic children: relative effectiveness of residential, out-patient and home-based interventions. Child Psychiatry Human Dev. 1988;19:109–25.

Silver S, Oakes P. Evaluation of a new computer intervention to teach people with autism or Asperger syndrome to recognize and predict emotions in others. Autism. 2001;5:299–316.

Slater MA, Black PB. Urban-rural differences in the delivery of community services: Wisconsin as a case in point. Ment Retard. 1986;24:153–61.

Smith T. Outcome of early intervention for children with autism. Clin Psychol Sci Pract. 1999;6:33–49.

South M, Williams BJ, McMahon WM, Owley T, Filipek PA, Shernoff E, et al. Utility of the Gilliam Autism rating scale in research and clinical populations. J Autism Dev Disord. 2002;32:593–9.

Wallis KE, Pinto-Martin J. The challenge of screening for autism spectrum disorder in a culturally diverse society. Acta Paediatr. 2008;97:539–40.

Welterlin A, LaRue RH. Serving the needs of immigrant families of children with autism. Disabil Soc. 2007;22:747–60.

Wetherby AM, Watt N, Morgan L, Shumway S. Social communication profiles of children with autism spectrum disorders late in the second year of life. J Autism Dev Disord. 2007;37: 960–75.

Wetzel CD, Radtke PH, Stern HW. Instructional effectiveness of video media. Hillsdale, NJ: Lawrence Erlbaum Associates, Publishers; 1994.

Whalen C, Liden L, Ingersoll B, Dallaire E, Liden S. Behavioral improvements associated with computer-assisted instruction for children and developmental disabilities. J Speech Lang Pathol Appl Behav Anal. 2006;1:11–26.

Chapter 12
Grief

Anthony Papa and Brett Litz

Assessment/Triage

Grief is a normal reaction to the loss of someone close. Grief reactions range from intense emotional responses involving sadness, longing, guilt, and anger with significant functional disruption lasting several months to the transitory, situational experience of sadness with little or no functional disruption that endures only for the first few weeks after the loss (e.g., Bonanno and Kaltman, 1999). Normal grief may be accompanied by acute somatic, depressive, and post-traumatic stress symptoms, or no appreciable distress or dysfunction (see Bonanno, 2004; Bonanno and Kaltman, 1999; Bonanno et al., 2002; Coifman et al., 2007; Parker and McNally, 2008). However, when they do occur, symptoms of normal grief typically remit within 6 months of the loss (Prigerson et al., 1997), though individuals may report intense sadness when reminded of their loss throughout their lifetime. It is important to emphasize that most people experience transient reactions to the loss, do not experience levels of disruption that warrant psychiatric diagnosis or intervention, are able to accommodate to loss, move on with their lives, and return to previous functioning (Bonanno et al., 2002; Bonanno, 2004). For example, Bonanno et al. (2005) looked at the grief trajectories of bereaved caretakers of individuals who died of HIV/AIDS suggests that resilient or recovered bereaved demonstrate low levels of depression within 8 weeks after the loss. Ott et al. (2007) found that it was possible to identify those people who demonstrated the most acute grief reactions as early as 4 months post-loss. These studies suggest that those that recover from the loss show significantly less grief and depression symptoms than those that do not recover relatively early after loss.

However, a relevant minority do not experience a reduction in symptoms or return to functioning and instead demonstrate a pathological response to loss characterized by persistent mourning, yearning, emotional pain, and withdrawal (see Prigerson and Jacobs, 2001; Prigerson et al., 2007). Differentiating those that return

A. Papa (✉)
Department of Psychology, University of Nevada-Reno, Mail Stop 0298, Reno, NV 89557, USA
e-mail: apapa@unr.edu

W.T. O'Donohue, C. Draper (eds.), *Stepped Care and e-Health*,
DOI 10.1007/978-1-4419-6510-3_12, © Springer Science+Business Media, LLC 2011

to functioning and those that do not is critical as a growing body of research suggests that psychotherapeutic intervention is at best inert, and at worst iatrogenic, if patients are not adequately screened for psychopathology (see Section "Outcome Data" below).

In addition to pathological grief reactions, there are a number of possible pathological outcomes associated with bereavement. The most common are Major Depressive Disorder (MDD), Post-Traumatic Stress Disorder (PTSD), and complicated or prolonged grief. Assessment and triage of MDD and PTSD are addressed in their respective chapters in this volume. Unique to bereavement, though, is the frequent comorbidity of these symptoms with the symptoms complicated or prolonged grief. The remainder of this section will review issues regarding the assessment of pathological grief reactions, review the most current conceptualization of pathological grief, called Prolonged Grief Disorder, and discuss risk factors related to pathological grieving.

Prolonged Grief Disorder

Pathological grief reactions are not recognized as a stand-alone disorder in the Diagnostic and Statistical Manual of Mental Disorders, 4th ed. (DSM-IV). However, in the last decade, research has steadily accumulated to support the construct validity of a stand-alone grief diagnosis with unique outcomes and core features. Recently, the DSM-V workgroup examining the evidence for inclusion of pathological grief reactions has proposed the diagnostic criteria for prolonged grief disorder (PGD; more commonly referred to a complicated grief in the research literature) listed in Table 12.1 (Boelen and Prigerson, 2007; Lichtenthal et al., 2004).

Table 12.1 Proposed DSM-V diagnostic criteria for prolonged grief disorder

A. Person experienced the death of an attachment figure
B. One or more of the following
   (1) Constant longing, yearning, or pining for the lost person
   (2) Intense feelings of emotional pain, sorrow, or pangs of grief related to separation distress
   (3) Intrusive thoughts about the deceased
C. If person meets criteria A and B, then five of the following must be present
   (1) Feeling stunned, shocked, or dazed by the loss
   (2) Feelings of bitterness and anger over the loss
   (3) Avoidance of reminders of the loss
   (4) Difficulty trusting others since the loss
   (5) Difficulty moving on, e.g., making new friends, pursuing new interests
   (6) Trouble accepting the loss
   (7) Confusion about role in life or a diminished sense of self
   (8) Feeling emotionally numb since the loss
   (9) Feeling that life is unfulfilling, empty, or meaningless without the deceased
D. Persons display persistent severe grief symptoms which do not remit after the first 6 months of the loss
E. Symptoms must interfere with social, occupational, or other important area of functioning

A number of factor analytic studies have found that grief symptoms form separate, coherent dimensions from depression symptoms (e.g., fatigue, loss of energy, self-blame, depressed mood, lack of enjoyment, worthlessness; Boelen and van den Bout, 2003; Boelen et al., 2003; Ogrodniczuk et al., 2003a; Prigerson et al., 1996a, 1995a) in broad-based community samples that are independently predictive of social and physical dysfunction and differential responding to psychosocial (Ogrodniczuk et al., 2003b) and antidepressant intervention (Pasternak et al., 1991; Reynolds et al., 1999; Zisook et al., 2001). Symptoms of sadness, impassivity, and psychomotor retardation are all depressive symptoms whereas symptoms of separation distress (yearning, pining, or longing for the deceased; intense feelings of emotional pain, sorrow, or pangs of grief) with specific cognitive, behavioral, or emotional indicators (avoidance of reminders, confusion about role, diminished sense of self, trouble accepting the loss, difficulty trusting others, feelings of bitterness and anger) are all specific indicators of PGD (Prigerson et al., 1996a, 1995a). Other studies found similar results in relation to the distinction between PGD symptoms and anxiety symptoms (e.g., worry, restlessness, anxiety, nervousness; Boelen and Prigerson, 2007; Boelen and van den Bout, 2003; Chen et al., 1999; Prigerson, Shear, Newsom, et al., 1996b) and PTSD (Simon et al., 2007). For example, Bonanno et al. (2007) examined whether PGD predicted functional problems above and beyond PTSD and depression in two independent samples of 73 widows and 447 people bereaved from the terrorist attacks on 9/11/2001 (family members, friends, and colleagues). They found that with depression and PTSD controlled, PGD emerged as a unique predictor of functioning, both cross-sectionally and prospectively. These findings provide convergent support for the incremental validity of prolonged grief as an independent marker of bereavement-related psychopathology. These findings also suggest that in measuring grief treatment outcomes, specific measures of grief symptoms must be used along with depression and anxiety measures. Widely used measures of grief-specific symptoms with good validity include the Texas Revised Inventory of Grief (Faschingbauer et al., 1987) or the Inventory of Complicated Grief (Prigerson et al., 1995b).

As previously alluded to, PGD is associated with considerable morbidity, adverse health behaviors (e.g., increased smoking and alcohol consumption), and functional impairments (social, familial, and occupational), and the costs of untreated PGD are enormous in terms of health-care costs, lost productivity, and quality-adjusted life years (Chen et al., 1999; Ott, 2003; Prigerson et al., 1995a, b, 1997, 1999). Multiple studies have shown enduring grief reactions to be associated with increased risk of hospitalization for mental illness (Li et al., 2005), suicidality (Latham and Prigerson, 2004; Melhem et al., 2007; Prigerson et al., 1997), impaired social functioning (Silverman et al., 2000; Simon et al., 2007), and medical comorbidity, such as cancer (Chen et al., 1999; Levav et al., 2000), cardiac events, stroke, and high blood pressure (Chen et al., 1999; Prigerson et al., 1997), and mortality (Li et al., 2003; Levav, 1982).

Prevalence rates and risk factors for PGD. Prevalence rates of PGD vary according to type of bereavement. Estimates vary from 10% following deaths from natural causes (Latham and Prigerson, 2004; Ott et al., 2007; Prigerson et al., 1999; Shear et al., 2001), to 20% of bereaved dementia caregivers evidencing PGD (Schulz et al., 2006), to 30–40% in Alzheimer's caregivers (Robinson-Whelen et al., 2001; Schulz et al., 2003), up to 41% in those bereaved by cancer (BrintzenhofeSzoc et al., 1999), to 50+% HIV+ caregivers (Bonanno et al., 2005) evidencing clinically significant levels of depression. Following ICU deaths, estimated rates of disruption are 22% displaying at least subsyndromal PGD with 34–69% meeting criteria for any mental disorder (Lautrette et al., 2007, Siegel et al., 2008). In the estimates involving caretakers, caregiver strain (involving demands on caregiver that affect finances, employment, socialization, personal time, and sometimes their own health status) appears to be a critical risk factor for varying levels of pathology reported, with high levels of psychopathology associated with high levels of pre-death caregiver strain (Schulz et al. 2001; Zhang et al., 2008). These results are attributed to the effects of caregiving disrupting individuals day-to-day lives and access to other rewarding or reinforcing aspects of their lives (e.g., Bernard and Guarnaccia, 2003; Bradley et al., 2004; Harvey and Miller, 1998; Prigerson et al., 2003).

In addition to research on caregiver strain, research on risk factors for PGD suggests that insults to secure attachment (or the ability to establish and maintain satisfying interpersonal relationships) are central to the disorder's etiology. Risk factors include childhood abuse and neglect (Silverman et al., 2001), childhood separation anxiety (Vanderwerker et al., 2006), previous loss of a significant other (Silverman et al., 2001; Zisook et al., 1985), close kinship relationship to the deceased (loss of a child puts individuals at the highest risk; Cleiren et al., 1994; van Doorn et al., 1998; Zisook and Lyons, 1989–90), interpersonal relating style characterized by over-dependency (Carr et al., 2000; Johnson et al., 2006; Johnson et al., 2007; van Doorn et al., 1998), lack of alternative social supports (Prigerson et al., 1993; Ott el al., 2007; Simon et al., 2005; Vanderwerker and Prigerson, 2004), and, in parental bereavement, the number of remaining children (Wijngaards-de Meij et al., 2005). Advance preparation for the loss (Barry et al., 2002) as well as having a good social support network (Brown et al., 2008; Vanderwerker and Prigerson, 2004) has been associated with a lower risk for PGD. Ethnicity is also likely to also play a role. In one of the few studies to compare rates of PGD between majority and minority groups (in this case US white and African-American comparison groups), found that of 346 bereaved older adults, African-American bereaved subjects were about twice as likely than European American subjects to meet criteria for PGD (odds ratio = 2.5; 95% CI, 1.1–5.4; Goldsmith et al., 2008). Taken together, these results suggest that bereaved persons with interpersonal difficulties feel unprepared for the death and/or unsupported after it is at heightened risk of PGD.

The unsupportiveness of others may be a critical area for intervention. Perceptions of social support have been related to better adjustment in grief in a number of studies (e.g., Dimond, Lund, Caserta, 1987; Prigerson et al. 1993; Vanderwerker and Prigerson, 2004), and social withdrawal is a key symptom of PGD. Research suggests that bereaved individuals experience a significant amount of unsupportive, distancing, discounting, non-genuine, and/ negative social interactions even within primary support relationships reducing access to an essential therapeutic resource (Davidowitz and Myrick; 1984; Helmrath and Steinitz,

1978; Knieper, 1999; Lehman et al., 1986; Lehman and Hemphill, 1990; Maddison and Walker, 1967; Peters-Golden, 1982; Wilsey and Shear, 2007). Ott (2003) found that those with PGD report lower levels of perceived support than those with uncomplicated grief reactions, perhaps reflecting greater incidence of negative social interactions.

There are many explanations of the personal cost for people interacting with the bereaved. For example, Lehman et al. (1986) asked 94 bereaved participants what kinds of support attempts were helpful or unhelpful and compared their responses to 100 controls as potential supporters. What is most interesting about these studies is that responses by the control participants about what kinds of support would be useful corresponded highly with the bereaved. Yet, given that the pool of potential supporters clearly indicated knowledge of what would be helpful, the bereaved reported a high amount of unhelpful support interactions. Lehman et al. (1986) speculate that the potential supporters anxiety about interacting with a person who has experienced a death, and the possibility that they may contribute to another distress, may lead them to act in an automatic or ritualized way. This is consistent with interpersonal theories of depression are largely based on the dynamic interplay between negative reactions by potential supporters and a depressed person's expressions of distress and need for support (Coyne, 1976; Joiner and Metalsky, 2001).

In the case of bereavement, unregulated expression of emotions and/or reassurance seeking may occur leading to the withdrawal of others in a similar pattern of responding, but also individuals who violate cultural assumptions of how long one should grieve are likely to be subject to negative attributions of pathology or malingering that may decreasing the likelihood that they will receive the support needed (Wortman and Silver, 1989). In addition, Terror Management Theory (TMT) and Just World theory both posit that exposure to mortality affect individuals' perception, processing, and appraisal of events; humans strive to maintain worldviews that provide a sense of security and meaning to buffer against feelings of anxiety related to reminders of mortality and the limits of control over fate and environment (see Arndt et al., 2002; Hafer and Bègue, 2005). Threats to these worldviews cause intense anxiety and, in turn, cause individuals to respond to those that evoke the threat with aggression, rejection, or withdrawal (e.g., McGregor et al., 1998).

Other Pathology and Comorbidity

As previously noted, the most common non-PGD reactions to bereavement are MDD and PTSD, though other anxiety disorders may also be present. In the majority of cases, onset of comorbid disorders usually occurs before the bereavement (e.g., Bonanno et al., 2005; Simon et al., 2007; Zisook and Schuster, 1993). Another critical issue for clinical consideration is the association of suicidal ideation with PGD. PGD has been associated with increased suicidal ideation in a number of studies and should be included in any assessment of post-loss adjustment (Boelen and Prigerson, 2007; Jacobsen et al., 2010; Johnson et al., 2008; Latham and Prigerson, 2004; Neria et al., 2007; Prigerson et al., 1995, 1999; Szanto et al., 2006).

Looking at MDD and PTSD, preliminary evidence suggests that PGD severity seems to interact with severity of PTSD and MDD symptoms indicating that concurrently addressing comorbid symptoms may be necessary to effect overall change in an individual. Simon et al. (2007) found that 32% of those that met criteria for a PGD did not display a comorbid MDD or PTSD diagnosis (51% did not have comorbid PTSD and 45% did not have comorbid MDD), but 36% met criteria for all three disorders. However, increases in PGD symptoms were typically associated with increased comorbidity. In a similar vein, among 704 bereaved friends and family members of 9/11 victims' exposure to trauma increased the risk for PGD by twofold as compared to those who experienced loss alone (Neria et al., 2007).

Incidence of PTSD is often related to the type of loss (e.g., if the loss was sudden and unexpected, if person was present at death, etc.; Boelen et al., 2008; Neria and Litz, 2004; Schut et al., 1991; Zisook et al., 1998). However, avoidance of fear-inducing stimuli associated with psychic trauma is not associated with PGD. Rather, there is a hyper-focus on the loss and reminders of the deceased, a desire for reconnection with the deceased, and the comfort felt, not aversive physiological reactivity, when exposed to symbolic cues that conjure thoughts of the deceased. Generally speaking, fear and anxiety-based responding to threat cues with hyper-vigilance play a more significant role in PTSD than in PGD (Boelen et al., 2003; Prigerson et al., 2000). This is particularly salient as PGD symptoms have often been conceptualized and treated as a PTSD variant. Interventions for PTSD focus on emotional processing and integration of the trauma event with the goal of reducing fear and hyperarousal reactions and avoidant behaviors while increasing individuals' sense of safety via increased efficacy regarding self-control. PGD symptoms are not a result of dysregulation of fear systems and avoidance of fear triggers, but rather are based on dysregulated reactions to sadness and loneliness and are associated with difficulties establishing and maintaining relationships causing significant impairment as a person withdraws from their social environment.

Pathological grieving has also been associated with increased substance use (especially alcohol and tobacco) and increased substance-related inpatient admissions (Byrne et al., 1999; Clayton, 1990; Li et al., 2005; Prigerson et al., 1997; Pfefferbaum et al., 2001; Zisook et al., 1985). Bereaved individuals may be overrepresented in substance use disorder treatment centers, may play an important role in substance use disorder development, and adjunctive treatment may be an important factors in recovery from both disorders (e.g., Blankfield, 1982–1983; Zuckoff et al., 2006).

Stepped-Care Options

Consumer Preferences

There is an enormous demand for interventions that are less resource intensive, less stigmatizing, and more widely accessible (Schopp et al., 2006). Clearly there is a vast market for information about grieving. Searching for books on Amazon.com using the keyword *grief* results in 322,432 titles. Internet chat rooms, memorial sites, and support groups as well as community-based support groups abound. As noted in Holland et al. (2008), caregivers often report that bereavement and grieving are important concerns even before their loss. However, as reviewed below, well-controlled outcome and efficacy studies are sparse. Moreover, the explicit study of consumer preferences in bereavement is rarely considered. Also, given the scarcity of professionals adequately trained to target loss-related mental health problems (Center for the Advancement of Health, 2004) and that face-to-face interventions are therapist and patient resource intensive, there are significant barriers that interfere with access to appropriate care. In this light, the growth of the Internet as source of grief information and support is not surprising as it can obviate barriers to seeking care, as well as other barriers such as shame and stigma. Moreover, many Americans already utilize the Internet for a wide range of health-related information (up to 80% of all Internet users; Fox, 2006), and the number seeking health information on the Internet continues to grow rapidly (The Harris Poll, 2004). Additionally, as a means to deliver standardized treatment, the Internet provides a promising means to deliver highly cost-effective evidence-based care to those reluctant to seek professional help (e.g., Lorig and Holman, 2003) or for whom trained professional help is unavailable. However, this rationale also applies to the need to research and develop appropriate resources on all levels of the stepped-care options reviewed below.

Outcome Data

Several meta-analyses have examined the efficacy of bereavement interventions (see Currier et al., 2007, 2008). As a whole, the grief intervention literature has many limitations that make it very difficult to draw generalizations from the existing studies. Many studies lack adequate control groups, clear differentiation between traumatic and non-traumatic losses, information about dropouts, random assignments to treatments, monitoring of treatment adherence, and standardized and blinded assessment of outcome (see Currier et al., 2008; Schut et al., 2001). As a result, the findings from study to study are often contradictory and inconclusive (see Center for the Advancement of Health, 2004; Currier et al., 2008; Jordan & Niemeyer, 2003; Schut et al., 2001). However, narrowing the range of focus to those studies with adequate experimental controls, a pattern emerges.

In adults, broadly focused interventions for anyone who has experienced loss may in fact exacerbate grief symptoms, whereas interventions designed for people with significant grief symptoms, which also includes adequate screening to ensure only those with clinically significant disruptions participate, have been associated with clinically significant reductions in psychiatric symptoms (see Currier et al., 2008; Schut et al., 2001). In children, Currier et al.'s (2007) meta-analysis did not find evidence that psychotherapeutic interventions for children were effective given the limited number of studies reviewed ($N = 13$), but secondary analysis did suggest that screening for clinically significant pathology ($N = 1$) was associated with better outcomes. In the following sections, we will describe the various stepped-care options available to clinicians focusing heavily on areas that have empirical support, highlighting areas in need of further research and development.

Quality Improvement Outcomes

As noted, the public health impact of pathological grief can be immense (e.g., Chen et al., 1999). There exists a wide range of treatment options available to people who are experiencing grief. At this time, the most pressing issue in quality improvement for pathological grief is in the area of outcome measurement. As treatments for PGD are developed and tested, it is critical that issues such as patient satisfaction, functional impairment, and health-related behaviors are also assessed so that consumers and professionals can make informed decisions about matching individuals to the least expensive, tolerable, and intrusive level of care.

Watchful Waiting

This is probably one of the most important actions that a clinician can take in the early stages of grief. The majority of those who experience bereavement display significant levels of grief-related disruption in the first 2–4 months after loss, and these symptoms do not necessarily predict later impairment (Prigerson et al., 1997, see below). There is no set way to grieve. Disruption and intense sadness is common, and inappropriate intervention may exacerbate symptoms later. As previously noted, differentiating pathological grief from normative grief can be difficult in the time period immediately after the loss, and as a result specific interventions that target the key symptoms of PGD may not be appropriate in the immediate aftermath of the death.

   While watchful waiting does not include direct intervention grief, it is important that this decision be made as a result of careful evaluation of suicidal ideation, loss precipitated mood or anxiety reactions, and substance use. Pre-existing mood or anxiety disorders may be addressed at this time to prevent the previously noted synergy between the severity of these disorders and the severity of grief. Decisions of whether to intervene for PTSD follow normal treatment guidelines as reviewed in the book. Decisions to intervene for MDD symptoms is somewhat more complicated. The DSM-IV-TR indicates that the diagnosis of major depression may not occur if the symptoms are a result of bereavement *unless* symptoms persist for more than 2 months or the individual displays severe functional impairment, intense feelings of worthlessness, suicidal ideation, psychotic symptoms, or psychomotor retardation. However, recently the validity of the bereavement rule out for major depression has been questioned as comparisons of the symptom profiles and treatment-seeking outcomes of loss-related depression and non-loss-related depression have found little difference (Karam et al., 2009; Kendler, Myers, and Zisook, 2008; Zisook and Kendler, 2007; though see Wakefield et al., 2007). Based on these recent findings and indications that MDD symptoms may be related to increased risk for pathological grief, we recommend that decisions to intervene for MDD follow non-loss-related guidelines as described in this book.

   The empirical literature suggests that two factors are critical in determining when to wait and when to intervene for PGD. First is the level of symptomology. As noted above, broad-based interventions for those that have experienced grief but have not begun to demonstrate the symptoms of prolonged grief may not be effective or may even be iatrogenic. Patients must show clear signs of prolonged functional impairment from grief symptoms before intervention.

However, the very important consideration is determining when a patient is demonstrating "prolonged" grief and when should a grief intervention be delivered is more complicated. There are no studies that have explicitly examined the optimal time for intervention. In their meta-analysis of the efficacy of grief interventions, Allumbaugh and Hoyt (1999) concluded that interventions provided early (3–4 months) had considerably greater efficacy; "In quantitative terms, each month that intervenes between the loss and the onset of treatment decreases the expected standardized mean-change score (i.e., standardized improvement in treatment group relative to control group) by .011. Delaying the onset of treatment by a year, for example, decreases the expected efficacy of treatment by .13 SD units" (p. 375, Allumbaugh and Hoyt, 1999). However, Currier et al. (2007) did not find that time lag moderated the effects of treatments in their meta-analysis. Schut et al. (2001) argued that the grief treatment literature is too inconclusive to make specific inferences due to poor experimental design, differential treatment adherence between groups, possible gender differences in response to treatment, and equivocal findings to draw any firm conclusions about timing of intervention.

Complicating this decision is the high symptom overlap between PGD and early stages of normal grief. To determine the optimal timing for intervention, it is important to find a window of opportunity when those at risk for PGD are beginning to show signs of unrelenting grief reactions differentiating them from persons demonstrating a normal grief course. However, data regarding grief trajectories are sparse. As noted above, Bonanno et al. (2005) found that resilient or recovered bereaved will demonstrate low levels of depression within 8 weeks after the loss, and Ott et al. (2007) found that it was possible to identify those people who demonstrated the most acute grief reactions as early as 4 months post-loss. Diagnostic criteria for prolonged grief (PGD) require that the symptoms of this disorder endure for at least 6 months. This criterion was chosen because it reduced the likelihood of a false-positive diagnosis and because sensitivity analyses revealed 6 months as optimal for the prediction of long-lasting dysfunction (Prigerson et al., 1997, 1999, 2007; Prigerson and Maciejewski, 2005; Zhang et al., 2006).

Psychoeducation

Empirical examination of the impact of psychoeducation on reactions to bereavement remains a critical quality improvement goal. Much of the existing literature is on college death education classes. These classes have focused on the reductions of anxiety on death or to provide education of the death and grieving process (Noppe, 2007). Other research has suggested that these classes tend to draw mainly students whom are intellectually interested in the topic matter, but some who enroll are bereaved, are close to someone with a potentially terminal illness, or are contemplating suicide (Brabant & Kalich, 2009). In terms of impact of these classes on pathological grief symptoms, outcome studies are meager.

Another area of research looking at psychoeducation is in the area of bereavement service associated with hospice and palliative care. Much of this research examines the effect of psychoeducation on caregiving. Schulz et al. (2006) found that pre-loss depression was a critical factor in determining post-loss PGD symptom, and inasmuch as psychoeducation may reduce pre-loss depression and disruption from caregiving these programs may impact post-loss PGD symptoms (see also Hebert et al., 2006; Hebert et al., 2009; Holland et al., 2009).

In terms of what psychoeducation may offer, there is a significant body of research on grief reactions, ways of coping, and grief course that would be potentially normalizing for people who are bereaved. For example, inevitably those that are bereaved make social comparisons or have received social feedback about how they may or may not be grieving compared to other people they know. Popular culture often emphasizes "stages of grief" models and the need to "work through" their grief reactions. In these cases, it is extremely helpful to emphasize that there is no "right" way to grieve, that everyone grieves differently, and that both intense emotional reactions with functional disruptions and small transient reactions and disruptions are normative early after a loss. Additionally, popular media and other sources often give very little consistent guidance regarding issues like talking with immediate family members/children about the loss, maintaining connections with deceased (described in the research literature as "continued bonds"), meaning making, what to do with possessions, planning for anniversaries, holidays, and birthdays. What information that is available often reinforces "grief work" ideas or that bereaved must go through specific stages of grief to resolve their loss.

The Internet is one source that provides a multitude of grief resources on a number of web sites (e.g., http://www.beyondindigo.com/, http://www.journeyofhearts. org/, http://www.compassionatefriends.org/, http://www.goodgriefresources.com/ linktous.htm). There is limited evidence that "technological connectedness" as measured simply by Internet and e-mail use is related to decreased grief symptoms and increased quality of life in bereaved (Vanderwerker & Prigerson, 2004). However, at this time there is no research on the efficacy of any of these sites to affect grief course, and anecdotal review of these sites indicates that the quality of the information varied widely to supporting stereotypes about "proper" grieving to more informed sites that emphasize multiple pathways for grief.

Bibliotherapy

There is a plethora of self-help books for grief on the market (e.g., Rando (1991) *How to go on living when someone you love dies*. New York: Bantam). At best, these resources may provide education about grief and steps to help move beyond loss. However, there has been no research into the efficacy of any of these resources and since there is no clear consensus in the field about how to conceptualize and treat PGD, it is unclear how helpful any of these resources may be.

Computer-Based Intervention/e-Health

PGD is characterized by distrust of and withdrawal from others, an inability to function in various roles, and stigmatization caused by a lack of recovery in a "proscribed" time period (for a review, see Wortman and Silver, 2001). Given preliminary research that indicates that the anonymity of the computer facilitates self-disclosure (Joinson, 1999, 2001, 2004) and the ability to utilize an Internet intervention at home helps reduce stigma and other barriers to traditional face-to-face care (e.g., Glueckauf et al., 2003; Kenwright et al., 2004; Lorig and Holman, 2003; Luce et al., 2003; Ritterband et al., 2003), it appears that PGD would be particularly amenable to Internet-delivered care. However, there may be some age-based and socioeconomic differences in who has access, knowledge, and skills to benefit from these interventions.

Indeed, there are preliminary indications that grief as a result of traumatic loss is amenable to Internet-based treatment. Wagner et al. (2005, 2006) report the use of a therapist-intensive, e-mail-based therapeutic writing intervention for those who experienced mostly traumatic loss and who evidenced critical levels of disruption based on response to the Impact of Events Scale (Horowitz et al., 1979). Although this group was younger than our target sample (meanage $= 37.0$, SD $= 10.2$), the intervention had large effect sizes (Cohen's d's all greater than 1.10), which were still found 1.5 years later in the treatment group (Wagner and Maercker, 2007). Moreover, 83% rated the contact as personal, 73% did not miss face-to-face contact, and 85% found that contact exclusively by e-mail was pleasant.

Group Therapy

Support Groups

Support groups are an oft-prescribed resource for recently bereaved. Support groups are used as a source of information from other people who have experienced or are experiencing grief. For example, individuals can find out how others dealt with the lost person's possessions, what they told their children or co-workers, or how they learned or are learning to cope with the same feelings that they are struggling with. These groups allow people to share experiences and get feedback from others who share the same experience. This may be especially important for people who feel like they are unique in their reactions to loss—like the difficulties they have experienced since the loss is unique to you and your situation. Many people who go to support groups are surprised by how much other people have many of the same experiences and self-doubts and can empathize with and understand the many various emotions you are feeling. Groups like these vary widely based on whether they are peer lead or lead by a professional and on spiritual orientation, type of loss addressed, etc., and it can be hard for recently bereaved to find a good "fit." There are even online support groups that range from therapist monitored (e.g., http://www.griefnet.org/support/sg2.html) to peer monitored (http://www.groww.com/). In terms of empirical evidence for the efficacy of support groups, the evidence supporting their efficacy is mixed with the programs associated with extensive outreach efforts showing the worse outcomes as are their use as early intervention (See Currier et al., 2008; Levy et al., 1993; Schut et al., 2001).

Group psychotherapy. Group therapy for bereavement can be an effective means to treat individuals that meet criteria for PGD (Currier et al., 2008). Groups range from providing problem-solving skills and emotion support for parents (e.g., Murphy et al., 1998), to short-term psychodynamic intervention (e.g., Piper et al., 1992), to cognitive-behavioral-based groups for AIDS' survivors with HIV (e.g., Sikkema et al., 2006). Meta-analysis suggests that the effectiveness of group therapies for grief is subject to the same strictures as individual therapy; broad-based intervention for anyone who has been bereaved may reduce efficacy while adequate screening for grief symptoms is related to improved outcomes (e.g., Currier et al., 2008).

Individual Therapy

As previously noted, the majority of treatment studies for grief either suffer from internal validity problems or have not adequately screened for specific grief symptoms to target in treatment. Often in these studies, when pathology is an inclusion criteria, it is measured in terms of depression symptoms or grief is conceptualized as a form of trauma to be treated by exposure techniques, as opposed to focusing on the core symptoms of functional and emotional disengagement from the person's environment (see Jacobs and Prigerson, 2000). Only recently have there been efforts to develop and test interventions specifically designed to target PGDs' unique separation distress and ruminative symptoms. Almost all of these studies use a modified exposure approach in which painful memories of the deceased are reviewed and the negative aspects are challenged with cognitive therapy techniques. In one of the most comprehensive interventions to date, Shear et al. (2005) conducted a randomized controlled clinical trail of a tertiary intervention for PGD in 95 participants with PGD about 2 years after their loss. The treatment package focused mainly on PTSD treatment-derived exposure therapy techniques (imaginal and in vivo exposure to the memory of the death and avoided people and places) and cognitive restructuring. However, Shear et al. did secondarily employ techniques from interpersonal therapy for depression (IPT; focusing on illness role and interpersonal role transitions and disputes) and reviewing positive memories of the deceased to help promote accommodation to the loss that are more specific to PGD. This impressive trial showed that the PGD therapy led to significantly faster and greater improvements in PGD symptoms and general functioning than IPT (51% in the broad treatment package were rated as treatment responders versus 28% in IPT on a single-item Likert-type scale).

Shear et al.'s result suggests that IPT may not be the most efficacious approach to treat bereavement. This is in line with the broader literature on IPT for PGD. Shear et al. (2005) found a mainly CBT exposure-based treatment augmented with some IPT techniques to be superior to IPT. In another study, Reynolds et al. (1999) compared the effects of nortriptyline and IPT alone and in combination against a placebo for bereavement-related depression and grief symptoms. Results indicated that IPT alone evidenced the lowest level of remission in bereavement-related depression (29%), scoring much lower than the placebo alone (45%), nortriptyline (56%), or nortriptyline and IPT together (69%; although participants in this condition received significantly more IPT sessions; this did not significantly differ from the nortriptyline alone condition). No treatment condition resulted in decreases in grief symptoms as measured by the Texas Revised Grief Inventory or the Inventory of Complicated Grief.

There have been a growing number of studies using CBT models in the conceptualization and treatment of PGD (e.g., Fleming and Robinson, 2001; Matthews and Marwit, 2004). For example, Boelen et al. (2007) assigned 54 participants who demonstrated high levels of prolonged grief symptoms due to both traumatic and non-traumatic losses to either; 6 sessions of exposure therapy focused on avoidance symptoms followed by 6 sessions of cognitive restructuring, 6 sessions of cognitive restructuring followed by 6 sessions of exposure therapy, or 12 sessions of supportive counseling. Results suggest that the CBT-based interventions were more effective than supportive counseling and that the exposure therapy was more effective than cognitive restructuring as a stand-alone treatment. Furthermore, exposure therapy followed by cognitive restructuring was most effective in reducing PGD symptoms at the 6-month follow-up. The authors did not report comorbidity, time since loss, nor functional impairment.

Note about "working through" grief. "Grief work" or confronting loss by going over the events before and at the time of the death, processing the loss, allowing the full experience and expression of emotions related to the loss, and as a result, ending one's investment in the attachment relationship to the lost person (see Bonanno and Kaltman, 1999) is a much discussed precursor for resolution of grief in the psychological literature. However, there is no empirical support that grief work is necessary precursor to adaptation in non-pathological grief (Bonanno and Kaltman, 1999; Wortman and Silver, 1989, 2001), especially if healthy adaptation is defined as a return to pre-bereavement functioning. In addition, it is unclear if grief work is supported in the case of PGD (Bonanno, 2004); one study suggests that emotional processing of a loss was helpful (Maciejewski et al., 2007), other data suggest it is not (Bonnnao et al., 2005). However, if the yardstick for adjustment is a return to pre-bereavement functioning, then interventions that do not focus specifically on *functioning* and rather on emotional processing will arguably be less effective.

Medication

Medication in the treatment of bereavement-related symptoms is most often prescribed for treatment for bereavement-related depression symptoms and insomnia. There have been no controlled trials examining the efficacy of medication on grief symptoms. However, a number of open-label studies looking at the effects of antidepressants on bereavement-related depression symptoms suggest that psychotropic medication may significantly reduce depression symptoms (see Hensley et al., 2009, for a review). In addition, a couple of these studies also suggest that antidepressant use may be related to reductions in PGD-specific symptoms as well (Hensley et al., 2009; Zisook et al., 2001; Zygmont et al., 1998; but see Pasternak et al., 1991). In terms of bereavement-related insomnia, use of hypnotics may not be recommended, especially for seniors, due to side effects including increased risk for fall-related injury (see Monk et al., 2008 for a review). Instead, cognitive-behavioral treatment for insomnia (CBT-I; see Ong et al., 2008, for a review) can be an effective treatment with longer lasting effects and fewer serious side effects than medication.

Inpatient Treatment

There are no specific grief-related symptomology per se that would lead to inpatient treatment. Inpatient treatment for PGD is most likely to be associated with comorbid problems such as suicidal ideation or symptoms of substance use disorder. Inpatient care should only be considered when psychological symptoms interfere with individuals' ability to care themselves or place their safety at risk. PGD is associated with interpersonal anger and bitterness, and it is not inconceivable that therapists may have to assess for homicidal ideation, though there are no empirical data to support his assertion at this time.

Cultural Sensitivity

Clearly culture plays a large role in determining how individuals grieve and what is more or less adaptive in that culture (e.g., Bonanno et al., 2005). However, while cultural differences in grief experience and expression are well documented (see Rosenblat, 2008, for review), very little research on grief has looked at the role of culture in defining pathological grief symptoms nor in developing a transcultural theory of grief course and resolution. The current conceptualization of PGD is firmly rooted in Western conceptualizations of grief and validated on Western participants' samples. As a result, practitioners have very little guidance in how to conceptualize and treat grief in persons primarily acculturated in non-Western societies.

Triage Agenda

In order to make appropriate assessment of level of care required for someone who has experienced bereavement, the following factors must be taken into consideration.

1. Time since loss: longitudinal data suggest that even resilient people experience significant disruption in first 2–3 months
2. Type of loss (sudden, caretaking, exposed to death/traumatic)

    a. If caretaking—assess strain (impact on employment, social integration, social and daily rhythms, etc.)

    b. If exposed to death, then if helplessness fear or horror.

3. Who died (child, spouse, parent, etc.)
4. Quality of the relationship (conflictual, level of dependency, etc.)
5. Bereaved person's age at time of loss

    a. If elderly—need to assess other support resources (family), level of physical and functional dependency on deceased, health status, and cognitive ability (see Stroebe and Hannson, 2007)

    b. If adolescent/child—relationships and frequency of contact with peer and family supports, conduct problems, irritability, caregiver mental status and parenting behaviors and warmth, anxiety symptoms, and fear of own death (see Luecken, 2008)

6. PGD symptoms
7. Suicidal (and homicidal) ideation
8. Substance use/abuse/dependency
9. Other comorbidity (MDD, PTSD, etc.)
10. Social resources and ability to trust others
11. Emotional reaction (Guilt, bitterness, anger)

Research and Development Agenda

Much of the necessary empirical work for a well-supported stepped-care model for pathological grief has yet to be completed. This has mainly been a result of a lack of a clear consensus on what differentiates pathological grief from normal grief reactions. As noted in the assessment section above, in the last decade an accumulating consensus has identified the symptoms outlined in Table 12.1, though it is likely that this list will be modified as work continues on this front. A positive result of this developing consensus for a working definition of pathological grief has been the completion of well-controlled, comparable clinical trials of the treatment of these symptoms (Shear et al., 2005, Boelen et al., 2007; Sikkema, et al., 2006) and the beginning of development of theories that can inform the development of new, more focused treatments (e.g., Shear and Shair, 2005; Stroebe and Schut, 1999). However, this work is only in its beginning stages. The research agenda for the establishment of a clear array of treatment options for pathological grief includes replication of randomized clinical trials for current published individual, group, and e-health therapies by researchers not associated with those that developed and piloted the treatments, and the initiation of controlled research into the effects of specific aspects of psychoeducation, bibliotherapy, and support group resources. Finally, systematic, randomized, controlled research into the efficacy of antidepressant medication on grief symptoms has yet to be completed.

Dissemination Agenda

Given the significant development needs in the area of stepped care for pathological grief, it is difficult to set a comprehensive dissemination agenda at this
time. There is a plethora of information about grief and grieving in the public
domain that does not reflect the current scientific understanding of the distinction between normal and pathological grief. While treatment development based
on current understandings of pathological grief is in its early stages, current dissemination efforts need to focus on getting this information to consumers who
might benefit from this information. In terms of health-care delivery, the Institute
of Medicine (IOM, 2001, 2002) has defined pathological grief as a critical under
addressed public health issue and has called upon medical professionals in oncol-
ogy, palliative care, trauma care, neonatal intensive care, etc. settings to provide
bereavement services to survivors. There appears to a growing recognition of
need in these institutional setting; however implementation of appropriate bereavement services has been slowed by the significant development needs described
above.

References

Allumbaugh DL, Hoyt WT. Effectiveness of grief therapy: a meta-analysis. J Counsel Psychol.
    1999;46:370–80.
Arndt J, Greenberg J, Cook A. Mortality salience and the spreading activation of worldview-
    relevant constructs: exploring the cognitive architecture of terror management. J Exp Psychol
    Gen. 2002;131:307–24.
Barry LC, Kasl SV, Prigerson HG. Psychiatric disorders among bereaved persons: the role
    of perceived circumstances of death and preparedness for death. Am J Geriatr Psychiatry.
    2002;10:447–57.
Bernard LL, Guarnaccia CA. Two models of caregiver strain and bereavement adjustment: a com-
    parison of husband and daughter caregivers of breast cancer hospice patients. Gerontologist.
    2003;43:808–16.
Blankfield A. Grief and alcohol. Am J Drug Alcohol Abuse. 1982–1983;9:435–46.
Boelen P, Prigerson HG. The influence of symptoms of prolonged grief disorder, depression, and
    anxiety on quality of life after bereavement: a prospective study. Eur Arch Psychiatry Clin
    Neurosci. 2007;257(8):444–52.
Boelen PA, de Keijser J, van den Hout MA, van den Bout J. Treatment of complicated grief:
    a comparison between cognitive-behavioral therapy and supportive counseling. J consult clin
    psychol. 2007;75(2):277.
Boelen PA, van den Bout J. Gender differences in traumatic grief symptom severity after the loss
    of a spouse. Omega: J Death Dying. 2003;46:183–98.
Boelen PA, van den Bout J, de Keijser J. Traumatic grief as a disorder distinct from bereavement-
    related depression and anxiety: a replication study with bereaved mental health care patients.
    Am J Psychiatry. 2003;160:1339–41.
Bonanno GA, Neria Y, Mancini A, Coifman KG, Litz B, Insel B. Is there more to complicated grief
    than depression and posttraumatic stress disorder? A test of incremental validity. J Abnorm
    Psychol. 2007;116(2):342–51.
Bonanno GA. (2004). Loss, trauma, and human resilience: have we underestimated the human
    capacity to thrive after extremely aversive events? Am Psychol. 2004;59:20–8.

Bonanno GA, Kaltman S. Toward an integrative perspective on bereavement. Psychol Bull. 1999;125:760–76.

Bonanno GA, Moskowitz JT, Papa A, Folkman S. Resilience to loss in bereaved spouses, bereaved parents, and bereaved gay men. J Pers Soc Psychol. 2005;88:827–43.

Bonanno GA, Papa A, Lalande K, Zhang N, Noll JG. Grief processing and deliberate grief avoidance: a prospective comparison of bereaved spouses and parents in the United States and the People's Republic of China. J Consult Clin Psychol. 2005;73:86–98.

Bonanno GA, Wortman CB, Lehman DR, Tweed RG, Haring M, Sonnega J, Carr D, Nesse RM. Resilience to loss and chronic grief: a prospective study from preloss to 18-months postloss. J Pers Soc Psychol. 2002;83:1150–64.

Brabant S, Kalich D. Who enrolls in college death education courses? A longitudinal study. Omega: J Death Dying. 2009;58:1–18

Bradley EH, Prigerson HG, Carlson M, Cherlin E, Kasl SV, Hurzeler-Johnson R. Does length of hospice enrollment affect depression among surviving caregivers? Am J Psychiatry. 2004;161:2257–62.

Brown SL, Brown RM, House JS, Smith DM. Coping with spousal loss: potential buffering effects of self-reported helping behavior. Pers Soc Psychol Bull. 2008;34:849–61.

BrintzenhofeSzoc KM, Smith ED, Zabora JR. Screening to predict complicated grief in spouses of cancer patients. Cancer Pract. 1999;7:233–9.

Byrne GJ, Raphael B, Arnold E. Alcohol consumption and psychological distress in recently widowed older men. Aust N Z J Psychiatry. 1999;33:740–7.

Carr D, House JS, Kessler RC. Marital quality and psychological adjustment to widowhood among older adults: a longitudinal analysis. J Gerontol. 2000;55:S374.

Center for the Advancement of Health. Report on bereavement and grief research. Death Stud. 2004;28:491–575.

Chen JH, Bierhals AJ, Prigerson HG, Kasl SV, Mazure CM, Jacobs S. Gender differences in the effects of bereavement-related psychological distress in health outcomes. Psychol Med. 1999;29:367–80.

Clayton PJ. Bereavement and depression. J Clin Psychiatry. 1990;51:34–38.

Cleiren M, Diekstra R, Kerkhof A, van der Wal J. Mode of death and kinship in bereavement: focusing on 'who' rather than 'how.' Crisis J Crisis Intervent Suicide Prevent. 1994;15: 22–36.

Coifman KG, Bonanno GA, Ray RD, Gross JJ. Does repressive coping promote resilience? Affective-autonomic response discrepancy during bereavement. J Pers Soc Psychol. 2007;92:745–58.

Coyne JC. Depression and the response of others. J Abnorm Psychol. 1976;85:186–93.

Currier JM, Holland JM, Neimeyer RA. The effectiveness of bereavement interventions with children: a meta-analytic review of controlled outcome research. J Clin Child Adolesc Psychol. 2007;36:253–9.

Currier JM, Neimeyer RA, Berman JS. The effectiveness of psychotherapeutic interventions for bereaved persons: a comprehensive quantitative review. Psychol Bull. 2008;134:648–61.

Davidowitz M, Myrick RD. Responding to the bereaved: an analysis of "helping" statements. Death Educ. 1984;8:1–10.

Dimond M, Lund DA, Caserta MS. The role of social support in the first two years of bereavement in an elderly sample. Gerontologist. 1987;27:599–604.

Faschingbauer TR, Zisook S, DeVaul R. The Texas Revised Inventory of Grief. In: Zisook S, editor. Biopsychosocial aspects of bereavement. Washington, DC: American Psychiatric Press; 1987. p. 109–24.

Fleming S. Robinson PJ. Grief and cognitive-behavioral therapy. In: Stroebe MS, Hansson RO, Stroebe W, Schut H, editors. Handbook of bereavement research: consequences, coping, and care. Washington, DC: American Psychological Association; 2001. p. 647–9.

Fox S. Online Health Search 2006. Retrieved 1/31/2007 from PEW Internet and American Life Project: (http://www.pewinternet.org/PPF/r/190/report_display.asp); 2006.

Glueckauf RL, Pickett TC, Ketterson TU, Loomis JS, Rozensky RH. Preparation for the delivery of telehealth services: a self-study framework for expansion of practice. Prof Psychol-Res Pr. 2003;34:159–63.

Goldsmith B, Morrison RS, Vanderwerker LC, Prigerson HG. Elevated rates of prolonged grief disorder in African Americans. Death Stud. 2008;32:352–65.

Hafer CL, Bègue L. experimental research on just-world theory: problems, developments, and future challenges. Psychol Bull. 2005;131:128–67.

Harvey JH, Miller ED. Toward a psychology of loss. Psychol Sci. 1998;9:429–34.

Hebert RS, Dang Q, Schulz R. Preparedness for the death of a loved one and mental health in bereaved caregivers of patients with dementia: findings from the REACH study. J Palliat Med. 2006;9:683–93.

Hebert RS, Schulz R, Copeland VC, Arnold RM. Pilot testing of a question prompt sheet to encourage family caregivers of cancer patients and physicians to discuss end-of-life issues. Am J Hosp Palliat Med. 2009;26:24–32

Helmrath TA, Steinitz EM. Death of an infant: parental grieving and the failure of social support. J Fam Pract. 1978;6:785–90.

Hensley PL, Slonimski CK, Uhlenhuth EH, Clayton PJ. Escitalopram: an open-label study of bereavement-related depression and grief. J Affect Disord. 2009;113:142–9.

Holland JM, Currier JM, Gallagher-Thompson D. Outcomes from the resources for enhancing alzheimer's caregiver health (REACH) program for bereaved caregivers. Psychol Aging. 2009;24:190–202.

Horowitz M, Wilner N, Alvarez W. Impact of event scale: a measure of subjective stress. Psychosom Med. 1979;41(3):209–18.

Institute of Medicine (IOM). In: Foley K, Gelband H, editors. Improving palliative care for cancer. Washington, DC: National Academy Press; 2001.

Institute of Medicine (IOM). When children die: improving palliative and end-of-life care for children and their families. Washington, DC: National Academy Press; 2002.

Jacobs SC, Prigerson HG. Psychotherapy of traumatic grief: a review of evidence for psychotherapeutic treatments. Death Stud. 2000;24:479–95.

Jacobsen JC, Zhang B, Block SD, Maciejewski PK, Prigerson HG. Distinguishing symptoms of grief and depression in a cohort of advanced cancer patients. Death Stud. 2010;34(3):257–73.

Johnson JG, Vanderwerker LC, Bornstein RF, Zhang B, Prigerson HG. Development and validation of an instrument for the assessment of dependency among bereaved persons. J Psychopathol Behav Assessment. 2006;28:263–72.

Johnson JG, Zhang B, Greer JA, Prigerson HG. Parental control, partner dependency and complicated grief among widowed adults in the community. J Nerv Ment Disease. 2007;195:26–30.

Johnson JG, Zhang B, Prigerson HG. Investigation of a developmental model of risk for depression and suicidality following spousal bereavement. Suicide Life-Threat Behav. 2008;38:1–12.

Joiner Jr., TE, Metalsky GI. Excessive reassurance seeking: delineating a risk factor involved in the development of depressive symptoms. Psychol Sci. 2001;12:371–78.

Joinson A. Social desirability, anonymity, and Internet-based questionnaires. Behav Res Meth Instrus Comput. 1999;31:433–8.

Joinson AN. Knowing me, knowing you: reciprocal self-disclosure in internet-based surveys. CyberPsychol Behav. 2001;4:587–91.

Joinson AN. Self-Esteem, interpersonal risk, and preference for E-mail to face-to-face communication. CyberPsychol Behav. 2004;7:472–8.

Jordan JR, Neimeyer RA. Does grief counseling work? Death Stud. 2003;27:765–86.

Karam EG, Tabet CC, Alam D, Shamseddeen W, Chatila Y, Mneimneh Z, Salamoun MM, Hamalian M. Bereavement related and non-bereavement related depressions: a comparative field study. J Affect Disord. 2009;112:102–10.

Kendler KS, Myers J, Zisook S. Does bereavement-related major depression differ from major depression associated with other stressful life events? Am J Psychiatry. 2008;165:1449–55.

Kenwright M, Marks IM, Gega L, Mataix-Cols D. Computer-aided self-help for phobia/panic via Internet at home: a pilot study. Br J Psychiatry. 2004;184:448–9.

Knieper A. The suicide survivors grief and recovery. Suicide Life Threat Behav. 1999;29(4): 353–64

Latham AE, Prigerson HG. Suicidality and bereavement: complicated grief as psychiatric disorder presenting greatest risk for suicidality. Suicide Life-Threat Behav. 2004;34:350–62.

Lautrette A, Darmon M, Megarbane B, Joly LM, Chevret S, Adrie C, Barnoud D, Bleichner G, Bruel C, Choukroun G, Curtis JR, Fieux F, Galliot R, Garrouste-Orgeas M, Georges H, Goldgran-Toledano D, Jourdain M, Loubert G, Reignier J, Saidi F, Souweine B, Vincent F, Barnes NK, Pochard F, Schlemmer B, Azoulay E. A communication strategy and brochure for relatives of patients dying in the ICU. New Eng J Med. 2007;356:469–78.

Lehman DR, Ellard JH, Wortman CB. Social support for the bereaved: recipients' and providers' perspectives on what is helpful. J Consult Clin Psychol. 1986;54:438–46.

Lehman DR, Hemphill KJ. Recipients' perceptions of support attempts and attributions for support attempts that fail. J Soc Pers Relat. 1990;7:563–74.

Levav I. Mortality and psychopathology following the death of an adult child: an epidemiological review. Isr J Psychiatry Relat Sc. 1982;19:23–38.

Levav I, Kohn R, Iscovich J, Abramson JH, Tsai WY, Vigdorovich D. Cancer incidence and survival following bereavement. Am J Public Health. 2000;90:1601–7.

Levy LH, Derby JF, Martinkowski KS. Effects of membership in bereavement support groups on adaptation to conjugal bereavement. Am J Community Psychol. 1993;21:361–81.

Li J, Precht DH, Mortensen PB, Olsen J. Mortality in parents after death of a child in Denmark: a nationwide follow-up study. Lancet. 2003;361:363–7

Li J, Luarensen TM, Precht DH, Olsen J, Moretensen PB. Hospitalization for mental illness among parents after the death of a child. New Eng J Med. 2005;352:1190–8.

Lichtenthal WG, Cruess DG, Prigerson HG. A case for establishing complicated grief as a distinct mental disorder in DSM-V. Clin Psychol Rev. 2004;24:637–62.

Lorig KR, Holman HR. Self-management education: history, definition, outcomes, and mechanisms. Ann Behav Med. 2003;26:1–7.

Luce KH, Winzelberg AJ, Zabinski MF, Osborne MI. Internet-delivered psychological interventions for body image dissatisfaction and disordered eating. Psychother-Theory Res Pract Train. 2003;40:148–54.

Maciejewski PK, Zhang B, Block SD, Prigerson HG. An empirical examination of the state theory of grief resolution. JAMA. 2007;297:716–23.

Maddison D, Walker WL. Factors affecting the outcome of conjugal bereavement. Br J Psychiatry. 1967;113:1057–67.

Matthews LT, Marwit SJ. Complicated grief and the trend toward cognitive-behavioral therapy. Death Stud. 2004;28:849–63.

McGregor HA, Lieberman JD, Greenberg J, Solomon S, Arndt J, Simon L, Pyszczynski T. Terror management and aggression: evidence that mortality salience motivates aggression against worldview-threatening others. J Pers Soc Psychol. 1998;74:590–605

Melhem NM, Moritz G, Walker M, Shear MK, Brent D. Phenomenology and correlates of complicated grief in children and adolescents. J Am Acad Child Adolesc Psychiatry. 2007;46:493–9.

Monk TH, Germain A, Reynolds III CF. Sleep disturbances in bereavement. Psychiatr Ann. 2008;38:671–8.

Murphy SA, Johnson C, Cain KC, Gupta AD, Dimond M, Lohan J, Baugher R. Broad-spectrum group treatment for parents bereaved by the violent deaths of their 12- to 28-yr-old children: a randomized controlled trial. Death Stud. 1998;22:209–35.

Neria Y, Litz BT. Bereavement by traumatic means: the complex synergy of trauma and grief. J Loss Trauma. 2004;9:73–87.

Neria Y, Gross R, Litz BT, Maguen S, Insel B, Seirmarco G, Rosenfeld H, Schmidt A, Jung Suh E, Cook J, Marshall RD. Prevalence and psychological correlates of complicated grief among bereaved adults 2.5–3.5 years after 9/11 attacks. J Traumat Stress. 2007;20:251–62.

Noppe IC. (2007). Historical and contemporary perspectives on death education. In: Balk D, Wogrin C, Thornton G, Meagher D, editors. Handbook of thanatology: the essential body of knowledge for the study of death, dying, and bereavement. New York, NY, US: Routledge/Taylor Francis Group; Association for Death Education and Counseling; 2007. p. 329–35.

Ogrodniczuk JS, Piper WE, Joyce AS, Weideman R, McCallum M, Azim HF, Rosie JS. Differentiating symptoms of complicated grief and depression among psychiatric outpatients. Can J Psychiatry. 2003a;48:87–93.

Ogrodniczuk JS, Joyce AS, Piper WE. Changes in perceived social support after group therapy for complicated grief. J Nerv Ment Dis. 2003b;191(8):524–30.

Ong JC, Cvengros JA, Wyatt JK. Cognitive behavioral treatment for insomnia. Psychiatr Ann. 2008;38:590–6.

Ott CH. The impact of complicated grief on mental and physical health at various points in the bereavement process. Death Stud. 2003;27:249–72.

Ott CH, Lueger RJ, Kelber ST, Prigerson HG. Spousal bereavement in older adults: common, resilient, and chronic grief with defining characteristics. J Nerv Ment Disease. 2007;195: 332–41.

Parker HA, McNally RJ. Repressive coping, emotional adjustment, and cognition in people who have lost loved ones to suicide. Suicide Life-Threat Behav. 2008;38:676–87.

Pasternak RE, Reynolds CF, Schlernitzauer M, Hoch CC, Buysse DJ, Houck PR, Perel JM. Acute open-trial nortriptyline therapy of bereavement-related depression in late life. J Clin Psychiatry. 1991;52:307–10.

Peters-Golden H. Breast cancer: varied perceptions of social support in the illness experience. Soc Sci Med. 1982;16:483–91.

Pfefferbaum B, Call JA, Lensgraf SJ, Miller PD, Flynn BW, Doughty DE, Tucker P, Dickson WL. Traumatic grief in a convenience sample of victims seeking support services after a terrorist incident. Ann Clin Psychiatry. 2001;13:19–24.

Piper WE, McCallum M, Azim HFA. Adaptation to loss through short-term group psychotherapy. New York, NY: Guilford Press; 1992.

Prigerson HG, Frank E, Reynolds CF, George CJ, et al. Protective psychosocial factors in depression among spousally bereaved elders. Am J Geriat Psychiatry. 1993;1(4):296–309.

Prigerson HG, Shear MK, Jacobs SC, Kasl SV, Maciejewski PK, Silverman GK, Narayan M, Bremner JD. Grief and its relationship to PTSD. In: Nutt D, Davidson JRT. Editors. Post Traumatic Stress Disorders: diagnosis, management and treatment. NY: Martin Dunitz; 2000; p. 163–86.

Prigerson HG, Jacobs SC. Diagnostic criteria for traumatic grief: a rationale, consensus criteria, and preliminary empirical test. Part II. Theory, methodology and ethical issues. In: Stroebe MS, Hansson RO, Stroebe W, Schut H, editors. Handbook of bereavement research: consequences, coping, and care. Washington, DC: American Psychological Association Press; 2001. p. 301–54.

Prigerson HG, Maciejewski PK. A call for sound empirical testing and evaluation of criteria for complicated grief proposed for DSM-V. Omega J Death Dying. 2005;52:9–19.

Prigerson HG, Bierhals AJ, Kasl SV, Reynolds CF III, et al. Complicated grief as a disorder distinct from bereavement-related depression and anxiety: a replication study. Am J Psychiatry. 1996a;153:1484–6.

Prigerson HG, Bierhals AJ, Kasl SV, Reynolds CF, Shear MK, Day N, Beery LC, Newsom JT, Jacobs S. Traumatic grief as a risk factor for mental and physical morbidity. Am J Psychiatry. 1997;154:616–23.

Prigerson HG, Bridge J, Maciejewski PK, et al. Influence of traumatic grief on suicidal ideation among young adults. Am J Psychiatry. 1999;156(12):1994–5.

Prigerson HG, Cherlin E, Chen JH, Kasl SV, Hurzeler R, Bradley EH. The stressful caregiving adult reactions to experiences of dying (SCARED) scale: a measure for assessing caregiver exposure to distress in terminal care. Am J Geriatr Psychiatry. 2003;11:309–19.

Prigerson HG, Frank E, Kasl SV, Reynolds CF III, Anderson B, Zubenko GS, Houck PR, George CJ, Kupfer DJ. Complicated grief and bereavement-related depression as distinct disorders: preliminary empirical validation in elderly bereaved spouses. Am J Psychiatry. 1995a; 152:22–30.

Prigerson HG, Maciejewski PK, Newsom J, Reynolds CF III, Frank E, Bierhals EJ, Miller M, Fasiczka A, Doman J, Houck PR. The inventory of complicated grief: a scale to measure maladaptive symptoms of loss. Psychiatry Res. 1995b;59:65–79.

Prigerson HG, Shear MK, Newsom J, Frank E, Reynolds CF III, Houck PR, Bierhals A, Kupfer DJ, Maciejewski PK. Anxiety among widowed elders: is it distinct from depression and grief? Anxiety. 1996b;2:1–12.

Prigerson HG, Vanderwerker LC, Maciejewski PK. Complicated grief as a mental disorder: inclusion in DSM. In: Stroebe M, Hansson R, Schut H, Stroebe W, editors. Handbook of Bereavement Research and Practice: 21st Century Perspectives. Washington, D. C.: American Psychological Association Press; 2007. p. 103–34.

Rando. How to go on living when someone you love dies. NewYork: Bantam; 1991.

Reynolds III CF, Miller MD, Pasternak RE, et al. Treatment of bereavement-related major depressive episodes in later life: a controlled study of acute and continuation treatment with nortriptyline and interpersonal psychotherapy. Am J Psychiatry. 1999;156(2):202–8.

Ritterband LM, Cox DJ, Walker LS, Kovatchev B, McKnight L, Patel K, Borowitz S, Sutphen J. An Internet intervention as adjunctive therapy for pediatric encopresis. J Consult Clin Psychol. 2003;71:910–7.

Robinson-Whelen S, Tada Y, MacCallum RC, McGuire L, Kiecolt-Glaser JK. Long-term caregiving: What happens when it ends? J Abnorm Psychol. 2001;110:573–84.

Schopp LH, Demiris G, Glueckauf RL. Rural backwaters or front-runners? Rural telehealth in the Vanguard of psychology practice. Prof Psychol Res Pr. 2006;37:165–73.

Schulz R, Boerner K, Shear K, Zhang S, Gitlin LN. Predictors of complicated grief among dementia caregivers: a prospective study of bereavement. Am J Geriatr Psychiatry. 2006;14:650–8.

Schulz R, Beach SR, Lind B, Martire LM, Zdaniuk B, Hirsch C, Jackson S, Burton L. Involvement in caregiving and adjustment to death of a spouse: findings from the caregiver health effects study. JAMA. 2001;285:3123–9.

Schulz R, Mendelsohn AB, Haley WE, Mahoney D, Allen RS, Zhang S, Thompson L, Belle SH. Resources for Enhancing Alzheimer's Caregiver Health (REACH) Investigators. End-of-life care and the effects of bereavement on family caregivers of persons with dementia. New Eng J Med. 2003;349:1936–42.

Schut HA, de Keijser J, Van den Bout J, Dijkhuis JH. Post-traumatic stress symptoms in the first years of conjugal bereavement. Anxiety Res. 1991;4:225–34.

Schut H, Stroebe MS, van den Bout J, Terheggen M. (2001). The efficacy of bereavement interventions: Determining who benefits. In: Stroebe MS, Hansson RO, Stroebe W, Schut H, editors. Handbook of bereavement research: consequences, coping, and care. Washington, DC: American Psychological Association; 2001. p. 705–37.

Shear K, Shair H. (2005). Attachment, loss, and complicated grief. Dev Psychobiol. 2005;47: 253–67.

Shear K, Frank E, Houck PR, Reynolds CF III. Treatment of complicated grief: a randomized controlled trial. J Am Med Assoc. 2005;293:2601–8.

Shear MK, Zuckoff A, Frank E. The syndrome of traumatic grief. CNS spectrums. 2001;6(4): 339–46.

Siegel MD, Hayes E, Vanderwerker LC, Loseth DB, Prigerson HG. Psychiatric illness in the next of kin of patients who die in the intensive care unit. Crit. Care Med. 2008;36(6):1722–8.

Sikkema KJ, Hansen NB, Ghebremichael M, Kochman A, Tarakeshwar N, Meade CS, Zhang H. A randomized controlled trial of a coping group intervention for adults with HIV who are AIDS bereaved: Longitudinal effects on grief. Health Psychol. 2006;25:563–70.

Silverman GK, Jacobs SC, Kasl SV, Shear MK, Maciejewski PK, Noaghiul FS, Prigerson HG. Quality of life impairments associated with diagnostic criteria for traumatic grief. Psychol Med. 2000;30:857–62.

Silverman GK, Johnson JG, Prigerson HG. Preliminary explorations of the effects of prior trauma and loss on risk for psychiatric disorders in recently widowed people. Israel J Psychiatry Relat Sci. 2001;38:202–15.

Simon NM, Shear KM, Thompson EH, Zalta AK, Perlman C, Reynolds CF, Frank E, Melhem NM, Silowash R. The prevalence and correlates of psychiatric comorbidity in individuals with complicated grief. Compr Psychiatry. 2007;48:395–9.

Simon NM, Pollack MH, Fischmann BA, Perlman CA, Muriel A, Moore CW, Nierenberg AA, Shear K. Complicated grief and its correlates in patients with bipolar disorder. J Clin Psychiatry. 2005;66:1105–10.

Stroebe M, Schut H. The dual process model of coping with bereavement: rationale and description. Death Stud. 1999;23:197–224.

Stroebe W, Stroebe MS, Abakoumkin G. Does differential social support cause sex differences in bereavement outcome? J Community Appl Soc Psychol. 1999;9:1–12.

Szanto K, Shear K, Houck PR, et al. Indirect self-destructive behavior and overt suicidality in patients with complicated grief. J Clin Psychiatry. 2006;67(2):233–9.

The Harris Poll® #98. Email, Research, News and Weather, Information about Hobbies or Special Interests Top the List of How People Use the Internet as it Continues to Grow. Retrieved 1/31/2007 from HarrisInteractive: (http://www.harrisinteractive.com/harris_poll/index.asp?PID=527); 2004.

van Doorn C, Kasl SV, Beery LC, Jacobs SB, Prigerson HG. The influence of marital quality and attachment styles on traumatic grief and depressive symptoms. J Nerv Ment Disease. 1998;186:566–73.

Vanderwerker LC, Prigerson HG. Social support and technological connectedness as protective factors in bereavement. J Loss Trauma. 2004;9:45–57.

Vanderwerker LC, Jacobs SC, Parkes CM, Prigerson HG. An exploration of associations between separation anxiety in childhood and complicated grief in later life. J Nerv Ment Disease. 2006;194:121–3.

Wakefield JC, Schmitz MF, First MB, Horwitz AV. Extending the bereavement exclusion for major depression to other losses: evidence from the national comorbidity survey. Arch Gen Psychiatry. 2007;64:433–40.

Wagner B, Knaevelsrud C, Maercker A. Internet-based treatment for complicated grief: concepts and case study. J Loss Trauma. 2005;10:409–32.

Wagner B, Knaevelsrud C, Maercker A. Internet-based cognitive-behavioral therapy for complicated grief: a randomized controlled trial. Death Stud. 2006;30:429–53.

Wagner B, Maercker A. A 1.5-year follow-up of an Internet-based intervention for complicated grief. J Traumat Stress. 2007;20:625–9.

Wijngaards-de Meij L, Stroebe M, Schut H, Stroebe W, van den Bout J, van der Heijden P, Dijkstra I. Couples at risk following the death of their child: predictors of grief versus depression. J Consult Clin Psychol. 2005;73:617–23.

Wilsey SA, Shear MK. Descriptions of social support in treatment narratives of complicated grievers. Death Stud. 2007;31:801–19

Wortman CB, Silver RC. The myths of coping with loss. J Consult Clin Psychol. 1989;57:349–57.

Wortman CB, Silver RC. The myths of coping with loss revisited. In: Stroebe Margaret S; Hansson Robert O; Stroebe Wolfgang, Schut Henk, editors. Handbook of bereavement research: consequences, coping, and care. Washington, DC, US: American Psychological Association; 2001. p. 405–29.

Zhang B, El-Jawahri A, Prigerson HG. Update on bereavement research: evidence-based guidelines for the diagnosis and treatment of complicated bereavement. J Palliat Med. 2006;9:1188–203.

Zhang B, Mitchell SL, Bambauer KZ, Jones R, Prigerson HG. Depressive symptom trajectories and associated risks among bereaved Alzheimer disease caregivers. Am J Geriatr Psychiatry. 2008;16:145–55.

Zisook S, Chentsova-Dutton Y, Shuchter SR. PTSD following bereavement. Ann Clin Psychiatry. 1998;10:157–63.

Zisook S, Kendler KS. Is bereavement-related depression different than non-bereavement-related depression? Psychol Med. 2007;37:779–94.

Zisook S, Lyons L. Bereavement and unresolved grief in psychiatric outpatients. Omega J Death Dying. 1989–1990;20:307–22.

Zisook S, Shuchter SR. Major depression associated with widowhood. Am J Geriatr Psychiatry. 1993;1:316–26.

Zisook S, Schuchter SR, Pedrelli P, Sable J, Deaciuc SC. Bupropion sustained release for bereavement: Results of an open trial. J Clin Psychiatry. 2001;62:227–30.

Zisook S, Shuchter S, Schuckit MA. Factors in the persistence of unresolved grief among psychiatric outpatients. Psychosoma J Consult Liaison Psychiatry. 1985;26:497–503.

Zuckoff A, Shear K, Frank E, Daley DC, Seligman K, Silowash R. Treating complicated grief and substance use disorders: a pilot study. J Subs Abuse Treat. 2006;30:205–11.

Zygmont M, Prigerson HG, Houck PR, Miller MD, Shear MK, Jacobs S, Reynolds III CF. A post hoc comparison of paroxetine and nortriptyline for symptoms of traumatic grief. J Clin Psychiatry. 1998;59:241–5.

Chapter 13
Sexual Disorders

M. Todd Sewell

Sexual disorders include both sexual dysfunctions and paraphilias. Sexual dysfunctions are sexual disorders characterized by problems that occur during the phases of the sexual response cycle. Paraphilias "are characterized by recurrent, intense sexual urges, fantasies, or behaviors that involve unusual objects, activities, or situations..." (DSM-IV-TR; American Psychiatric Association [APA], 2000, p. 535).

Sexual Dysfunctions

There are four stages in the human sexual response cycle: desire, sexual arousal, orgasm, and resolution (Master and Johnson, 1970). The sexual dysfunctions listed in the DSM-IV-TR (2000) are characterized by their association to these stages of the sexual response cycle. In this way, the stages of the sexual response cycle provide an important diagnostic marker for sexual dysfunctions.

Sexual Desire Disorders

Disorders associated with inhibited or absent desires for sexual activity and thoughts or fantasies of sex include hypoactive sexual desire disorder and sexual aversion disorder (Kaplan, 1977; APA, 2000). Sexual aversion disorder is characterized by active avoidance of sexual stimuli. This includes intense anxiety, fear, and/or disgust sexual stimuli (APA, 2000). Individuals who experience sexual aversion have a sense of revulsion or disgust in addition to anxiety and fear of sexual stimuli (Gold and Gold, 1993). Estimates of the prevalence of sexual aversion disorder for men and women are similar with 8% for men (Laumann et al., 1999) and 4–10% for women (Frank et al., 1978; Spector and Carey, 1990).

M.T. Sewell (✉)
Department of Psychology, University of Nevada-Reno, Mail Stop 0298, Reno, NV 89557, USA
e-mail: toddsewell@aol.com

W.T. O'Donohue, C. Draper (eds.), *Stepped Care and e-Health*,   247
DOI 10.1007/978-1-4419-6510-3_13, © Springer Science+Business Media, LLC 2011

Sexual Arousal Disorders

Sexual arousal disorders are characterized by disruptions in the sensations of sexual pleasure and the biological changes associated with sexual activity. These biological changes include the achievement of erections for men and vaginal swelling and lubrication in women (APA, 2000). Male erectile disorder may be one of the most common sexual disorders; however; findings related to the prevalence of this disorder are unclear due in part to methodological concerns (Bach et al., 2001). Laumann et al. (1999) report the prevalence of female sexual arousal disorder from 18 to 59 years as 20%; however, this disorder occurs more frequently as males age, so this is most likely a conservative number.

Sexual Orgasm Disorders

The orgasm stage of the sexual response cycle is characterized by impending ejaculation and eventual ejaculation for men and the contraction of the vaginal muscles in women (APA, 2000). Disorders associated with this stage include female orgasmic disorder, male orgasmic disorder, and premature ejaculation. Both male and female orgasmic disorders are marked by a persistent and recurrent delay or absence of an orgasm (APA, 2000). This is a broad and general definition given the variation of subjective views of expectations of the time between latency and ejaculation (Bach et al., 2001). The prevalence of premature ejaculation has been reported as high as 20–30% (St. Lawrence and Madakasira, 1992).

Sexual Pain Disorders

Dyspareunia is a sexual pain disorder associated with intense pain before, during, or after sexual intercourse. The pain can be caused by either medical or psychogenic factors. Although dyspareunia is more commonly experienced by women, the disorder may also occur within men. Vaginismus is the persistent contracting of the outer third of the vagina upon penetration. This is an involuntary reaction that occurs when attempts to penetrate the vagina are made in sexual contact, fingers, or even tampons (APA, 2000). Both dyspareunia and vaginismus can result in pain during sexual arousal and intercourse. Generally a diagnosis of dyspareunia is not given in addition to vaginismus (APA, 2004) if the pain results from the contraction of the vagina.

The Paraphilias

Paraphilia is marked by "intense sexually arousing fantasies, sexual urges, or behaviors generally involving (1) nonhuman objects, (2) the suffering or humiliation of oneself or one's partner, (3) children or other non-consenting persons that occur over a period of at least 6 months (APA, 2004, p. 566)." Another essential feature for the diagnoses of certain paraphilias is severe distress or impairment in the functioning of the individual. However, significant distress or impairment is not necessary for paraphilias like pedophilia, voyeurism, frotteurism, and exhibitionism. In the absence of impairment or distress individuals can be diagnosed if they have acted upon their urges (APA, 2000). Paraphilias are almost exclusively found in men and often times co-occur with other sexual disorders (Abel et al., 1988; Abel and Osborn, 1992; APA, 2000). Common paraphilias include exhibitionism, fetishism, frotteurism, pedophilia, sexual masochism, sexual sadism, transvestic fetishism, and voyeurism. Research focused on the etiology of paraphilias has proposed a number of different theories attempting to explain the origins of paraphilias. Freund and Kolarsky (as cited in Junginger, 1997) proposed that the normal courtship process for individuals who have paraphilias was disrupted.

Fetishism is a paraphilia in which an individual experiences strong sexual attraction to inanimate objects. Specific body parts may also be a subject of fetishism (Junginger, 1997). Exhibitionism is a paraphilia in which an individual experiences intense sexual urges to expose their genitals to strangers (APA, 2000). Abel and Osborn (1992) also found that sex offenders commonly reported past behaviors of exhibitionism.

Frotteurism is a paraphilia marked by intense sexual urges, fantasies, or the behavior of rubbing one's genitals against another individual in a public setting. For this reason frotteurism is usually identified with rape and sexual assault (Freund et al., 1997). Pedophilia is marked by intense sexual urges, fantasies, or behaviors involving children (APA, 2000). Here, urges and fantasies are listed as sufficient criteria, meaning even individuals who have not acted upon these urges may meet criteria for pedophilia even if they have not acted upon these desires. Prevalence rates for pedophilia are extremely difficult to ascertain. Many individuals who suffer from pedophilia report through the legal system, only after legal problems resulting from their disorder.

Sexual masochism is the experience of strong sexual urges, fantasies, or behaviors of being humiliated, bound, beaten, or made to suffer (APA, 2000). Acts of sexual masochism can include being bound and gagged during masturbation or with sex with a partner. Although rates of sexual masochistic behavior have been reported within the population, 5–10% of individuals studied have not clearly differentiated between individuals who enjoy masochistic sexual practices and those who suffer severe distress and disruption of functioning as a result of these behaviors and urges (Baumeister and Butler, 1997). Sexual sadism is a paraphilia in which an individual gains sexual pleasure and excitement as a result of psychological or physical suffering of others. It is possible for sexual sadists to derive pleasure at the suffering of consenting partners or non-consenting individuals (APA, 2004). Transvestic fetishism is a paraphilia in which an individual has strong sexual urges, fantasies, or behaviors involving cross-dressing. Again, this disorder is identified as a male paraphilia so that individuals who experience transvestic fetishism derive pleasure from women's clothing. A study of 2,450 participants found that 2.8% of males and 0.4% of women had experienced this disorder (Långström and Zucker, 2005). Voyeurism is marked by strong sexual urges, fantasies, or behaviors of viewing individuals who are engaged in sexual intercourse, undressing, or naked. The victims of voyeurism are non-consenting (APA, 2000). Fear of arrest and stigma prevent individuals who experience voyeurism from disclosing their behavior so prevalence rates are unknown.

Gender identity disorder is listed in the DSM-IV-TR as a sexual disorder that displays two distinct channels of symptoms that must be met prior to diagnoses (APA, 2000). Specifically, the DSM-IV-TR diagnoses of GID in children must be accompanied by "strong and persistent cross-gender identification" and a "Persistent discomfort with his or her sex" (APA, 2000, p. 581).

Assessment of Sexual Disorders

Given the broad definitions and criteria for many of the sexual dysfunctions clinical interviews may be seen as important assessment tools for the diagnoses and assessment of sexual dysfunctions. In addition, stigma and the sensitive nature of sexual dysfunctions inhibit many clients from disclosing sexual issues even with partners (Maltz, 2001), increasing the importance of a thorough clinical interview that considers, sexual history, childhood, past abuse, medical history, mental health history, and relationship factors. Bach et al. (2001) provide a thorough example of a clinical interview designed to assess sexual dysfunction. They stress the importance of collecting a complete history of client functioning in order to assess sexual dysfunction.

A quality assessment should include a discussion of normative sexual functioning in order to ensure that clients understand their situation in context of normal behavior. Bach et al. offer the following format for carrying out a clinical interview for sexual dysfunctions (2001). First, collect information regarding the client's childhood social and sexual history. In addition, the therapist will also need to collect information regarding the client's relationship history and history of any unusual experience that may have led to present sexual disruptions. For example, first encounters of arousal in reference to inanimate objects in the case of fetishism or experiences of pain while inserting tampons in cases of vaginismus. Collecting this information is important to pinpoint onset and severity of the disorder.

Etiological factors are an important consideration when developing treatment options for sexual disorders. Discovering the factors involved in the development and presentation of these disorders is an important part of the assessment process. In addition, assessment of these disorders needs to include assessment of other possible Axis 1 disorders that may account for similar presentation. For example, it is common for individuals who suffer from depression to experience a loss of interest in sexual activity; therefore, assessments of sexual dysfunction should include the assessment of mood disorders or other psychological disorders (Bach et al., 2001; APA, 2000). For example, depression-related disorders may result in disinterest in sexual activity similar to hypoactive sexual desire disorder. Assessment of these factors may drastically affect treatment planning.

In addition to an individual clinical interview an interview with the sexual partner can be useful (Bach et al., 2001; Wincze and Carey, 2001). This interview affords the clinician with an opportunity to support information received from the client and supplement information with details that the client may have avoided or not shared in previous assessments. It also allows the clinician an opportunity to gain some understanding of the stressors that may exist within the relationship from the perspective of the partner.

Self-report questionnaires may also provide a more private and efficient method of gathering way for individuals who suffer from sexual dysfunctions and disorder to report problems or troubling behavior (Spector et al., 1996). These measures offer a simple approach to obtaining data than some of the more intrusive assessment procedures that will be discussed shortly. There are a limited amount of self-report measures examining sexual disorders that have been empirically examined among clinical populations. However, there are some measures that have shown utility and reliability.

To date there are very few assessment instruments designed to measure sexual desire. The Sexual Desire Inventory (SDI) (Spector et al., 1996) examines an individual's desire for sex within a partnership and the individual's desire to engage in sexual behavior by oneself. This measure contains 14 items so it can be completed in a fairly short amount of time. Scores from individuals within a companionship can be used to examine discrepancies or differences in sexual desire; however, on average men have reported higher sexual desire scores than women on the SDI. The Brief Index of Sexual Functioning for Women (BIF-W) is a 22-item measure that examines sexual desire for women (Taylor et al., 1994). The BSF-W is designed to measure desire, arousal, orgasm, and sexual satisfaction.

The International Index of Erectile Function (IIEF; Rosen et al., 1997) is a 15-item self-report measure designed to assess for erectile functioning. The measure is able to discriminate men who suffer from erectile dysfunction from those who do not. The measure is available in several languages and with 15 items it does not take long to complete. The IIEF is also a useful instrument to measure treatment progress; however, it has not been studied among homosexual populations.

In addition to the SDI and BISF-W, instruments have been used to indirectly assess perceptions of sex and relationship factors that consider desire within a relationship. For example, the Derogatis Sexual Functioning Inventory (DSFI) was designed to provide a measure of overall sexual functioning (Derogatis and Melisar, 1979). The DSFI provides 10 subscales measured by 245 items. Because the measure has 245 items, many clinicians use the scale only when there is some question or element of a client's presentation that is unclear (Wincze and Carey, 2001). Derogatis has developed the Derogatis Interview for Sexual Functioning (DISF); this measure is intended to be a brief measure of sexual functioning (Derogatis, 1997). There are several versions of this measure for homosexual and gender-specific populations. Each measure is comprised of 25 items.

The Dyadic Adjustment Scale (DAS; Spanier, 1976) is a 32-item self-report measure that is designed to assess general functioning within couples. It does not specifically examine sexual functioning; however, this assessment can be used to examine the satisfaction within a relationship that may lead to or contribute to sexual dysfunction. The scale can be completed in 15 min and has been widely used in many research areas (Wincze and Carey, 2001).

There are other assessments of sexual dysfunction that are more intrusive. Penile plethysmographs (phallometry) are intended to measure blood flow into the penis and can be useful in measuring arousal (Seto et al., 2006; Krueger and Kaplan, 1997). This assessment provides a behavioral measure of arousal. Because individuals are often reluctant to endorse the object of arousal given the consequences of possible legal and/or social stigma, this assessment method provides important information about targets of arousal. Nocturnal penile tumescence assessment and the use of the RigiScan are used to assess the biological capabilities for males to achieve an erection. It has been proposed that if a male has the ability to obtain an erection at night then the erectile disorder must then be due to psychological factors, assuming the same male is unable to achieve or sustain an erection for sex. The Nocturnal Penile Tumescence test consists of a film that is wrapped around the shaft of a man's penis before bed. If the film is broken in the morning an erection has occurred during sleep and the man is psychically capable of achieving an erection. Nocturnal erections usually occur during REM sleep cycles, approximately 3–5 times per night. If the band is unbroken in the morning erectile problems may be caused by physical problems. This test can be done using a roll of moistened stamps, making this assessment private and inexpensive. The RigiScan is a more intrusive and involves multiple bands fitted around the penis that tighten every 15 or 30 s. A monitor is also fitted and worn throughout the night and may disrupt sleep. In addition, RigiScan assessments and other medical assessments can be expensive (Wincze and Carey, 2001).

In addition to these assessments, medical assessment should be used to examine factors like hormones, physical abnormalities, and organic disease that may account for some of the behaviors or characteristics of behaviors manifested in clients (Bach et al., 2001; Wincze and Carey, 2001; Barbaree and Seto, 1997; Graber, 1997). Medical examinations are an important aspect of treatment of sexual disorders, especially sexual dysfunction and medical causes should be ruled out before proceeding with psychological treatment.

Assessment of Paraphilias

Assessment of paraphilias can be done by collecting information from an individual about their sexual fantasies, urges, or behavior (APA, 2000). In addition, there are psychometric tests that assess for paraphilias. Finally, there are technological instruments that can be used to supplement information gained by conducting interviews and psychological assessment. Within the context of a stepped care model, these assessments may not be feasible as a first-line defense due to their invasive nature and financial cost. The use of a RigiScan or medical exam might only be needed if there is a reason to believe a patient is withholding information or there is some question about the client's presentation that needs further exploration.

As is the case with sexual dysfunctions, it is important to complete a thorough psychological interview to assess for paraphilias. Clinical interviews for paraphilias should follow the same format as discussed in regards to sexual dysfunction. The section on the information needed to complete a clinical interview has previously been reviewed. Collecting a thorough sexual, trauma, childhood, and medical history is an important aspect of the clinical interview. In addition, clinicians should consider assessing for comorbid psychological disorders as well as personality disorders. In some cases those who experience paraphilias may have significant distress that may cause depression or anxiety (APA, 2000). In the case of paraphilias it may also be important to assess for criminal history, sexual offenses, and sexual fantasies (Barbaree and Seto, 1997).

Self-report measures of sexual arousal are available and many of these measures have good validity. The Masochism Scale (Freund et al., 1982) is an 11-item scale designed to assess for sexual masochism ($\alpha = 0.83$). The Clarke Sexual History Questionnaire-Revised (CSHQ-R) is a widely use measure to assess a variety of paraphilias and sexual dysfunctions (Paitich et al., 1970; Langevin et al., 1977). The revised version consists of 508 items and has good validity and reliability. The CSHQ-R has been examined within a variety of populations and has demonstrated repeated utility.

Penile plethysmographs are also used as assessment instruments in a variety of the paraphilias. They are used to assess targets for arousal in frotteurism, exhibitionism, pedophilia, and sexual sadism and can be used to measure treatment progress and risk of re-offending (Laws, 2003). The process of phallometry includes the presentation of pictures, video, or audio stimuli that may be considered arousing to the patient. Phallometry may be used to identify paraphilias or to assess for treatment gains. However, there are researchers who feel the use of penile plethysmography needs to be done carefully, and the results of this assessment need to be considered among other assessment findings (O'Donohue and Letourneau, 1992). For example, penile plethysmography should not be used as the sole determinant for predicting recidivism. Predicting rates of recidivism is difficult, and although penile plethysmography has been shown to be a predictor of recidivism, it does not identify all reoffenders and assumes failure means a perpetrator will necessarily reoffend (Clift et al., 2009).

Stepped Care Treatment Approach

Although extensive options for empirically validated treatments of sexual disorders are limited, there are some treatment variations and types from which consumers may choose.

Watchful Waiting

Watchful waiting can be a first step for treatment options in many sexual dysfunctions. Sexual dysfunctions can arise due to situational variables like stress and performance anxiety that may remit over time. However, if these issues persist many of the dysfunctions may be treated effectively and quickly or require medical attention. For example, male erectile disorder has seen significant advances in medical treatment that is effective and efficient. However, erectile dysfunction has also been linked to vascular disease, highlighting the need for medical evaluation after a sufficient period of watchful waiting (Ponholzer et al., 2006). Paraphilias, on the other hand, represent a more difficult problem for watchful waiting strategies. Because many of these disorders are illegal, the immediacy for treatment presents a unique problem and watchful waiting would not be recommended.

Psycho-education and Bibliotherapy

Psycho-education has been employed in very few studies for the treatment of sexual dysfunction. Wincze and Barlow proposed that faulty beliefs about sex contributed to poor perceptions of sexual performance and the sexual process (1997). Some of these myths include ideas like

(1) A man should always be ready for sex.
(2) All women can have multiple orgasms.
(3) A woman's sex life ends with menopause.

This theory posited that addressing and correcting these faulty beliefs may improve sexual functioning (Bach et al., 1997). Psycho-education has been studied as an effective means of treating individuals with some types of sexual dysfunction. Women who were treated for either cervical or endometrial cancer by hysterectomy, which is associated with the experience of sexual arousal disorder, participated in a study for the treatment of sexual dysfunction with significant results (Christopherson et al., 2006). Participants were given three sessions combining cognitive behavioral therapy, mindfulness training, and education. The initial session was 20–30 min and the following two sessions were only 10–15 min. After completing these sessions, participants reported significant positive changes in arousal, desire, and orgasm. In addition, participants reported higher relationship satisfaction. These findings suggest that psycho-education can be an important part of the treatment of female sexual arousal disorder. Limitations of this study are the limited number of participants, no control group comparisons, and the confounding of treatments. It is unclear whether psycho-education was an active component of the treatment, aside from cognitive behavioral therapy or mindfulness training.

Similarly, a review of literature offering findings related to the treatment of sexual disorders and bibliotherapy yielded very little. Zeiss (1978) found that using bibliotherapy was a successful alternative to therapist-directed treatment for premature ejaculation. Van Lankveld (1998) found that the impact of bibliotherapy for sexual dysfunctions was positive. Van Lankveld used a manual he constructed based on psycho-education and sensate focus treatment (Masters and Johnson, 1970). In addition, the manual supplied participants with exercises of genital exploration and guided masturbation techniques in order to address dysfunctions of desire, arousal, and orgasm. Overall, van Lankveld supported the use of bibliotherapy based on these findings. Participants who completed the treatment felt that their problem had changed prior to treatment. However, when results included individuals who did not complete treatment ratings were not as positive. The use of psycho-education and bibliotherapy to treat these disorders offers a compelling and attractive alternative to individual treatment with a therapist, which is traditionally expensive and time consuming (Regev & Schmidt, 2004). Another issue of concern is that the manuals used by Ziess (1978) and Van Lankveld (1998) are not readily available to the general population.

In a meta-analysis of bibliotherapy for sexual dysfunction, van Lankveld found strong support for bibliotherapy for the treatment of erectile disorder, orgasmic disorders, and premature ejaculations. The analysis found an overall effect size of 0.68 (moderate effect). However, many of the studies used both bibliotherapy and other interventions within treatment. Again the results of bibliotherapy for the treatment of sexual dysfunctions seem to include other treatments. Bach et al. (2004) examine the impact of sildenafil (Viagra), combined with a manualized treatment and therapist contact. Results supported the use of bibliotherapy as a treatment for erectile dysfunction. In addition, participants reported that sildenafil was physically effective. Prior to treatment many participants stated that they did not enjoy sex, after completing the treatment protocol, which included behavioral exercises to increase sexual pleasure, participants reported higher levels for enjoying sexual activity.

Computer-Based Interventions (e-Health)

There are many Web sites that offer information regarding sexual dysfunctions and treatment options. However, currently there are no Web sites delivering empirically supported treatments for sexual disorders online. Although currently these treatments are unavailable for the treatment of sexual dysfunction, computer-based interventions have shown promise in the treatment of other psychological disorders like depression, anxiety, and social phobia (Titov, 2007). In addition, the Internet offers a treatment delivery option that may address concerns that are prominent in the treatment of sexual disorders like social stigma and shame that are common among those with sexual disorders. The Internet may be even more appealing as many individuals who suffer from paraphilias may already be accessing the Internet in order to satisfy sexual urges or fantasies (Howitt and Sheldon, 2007).

Individual and Inpatient Treatments

Cognitive behavior treatments have been supported as effective for the treatment of sexual dysfunctions (Bach et al., 2001; Bach et al., 2004; Regev and Schmidt, 2009; Waldinger, 2008). Sensate focus approaches have been used to treat premature ejaculation and sexual arousal disorders. The goals of sensate focus are to increase sexual arousal and draw attention to pleasurable sensation while diminishing the stressful demands of sex (Waldinger, 2008; Regev and Schmidt, 2009; Bach et al., 2001; Master and Johnson, 1970). In addition, the squeeze technique may be used repeatedly and can be employed for the treatment of premature ejaculation (Masters and Johnson, 1970). This technique is done by squeezing the penis behind the glans when the male feels that ejaculation is eminent, preventing ejaculation. Repeatedly use of this technique teaches males to decrease the heightened need to ejaculate.

In the case of vaginismus, the etiology of the disorder is an important consideration for treatment planning. For example, in the case of prior sexual trauma, a possible cause of vaginismus (Wincze and Carey, 2001) in vivo desensitization treatments may be supplemented with the patient private use of graduated dilators. Female sexual arousal disorder can be easily treated with over-the-counter lubrication if vaginismus is not present.

It is unlikely that an individual with a sexual dysfunction would be placed in an inpatient treatment facility unless placement is warranted by another comorbid disorder. Individuals who suffer from paraphilias like frotteurism, exhibitionism, pedophilia, and sexual sadism are often placed in prison, so treatment for these disorders is limited to the available resources within the prison system they are remanded to. Likewise many individuals who experience paraphilia are mandated to treatments by the legal system.

There are a limited number of empirically supported treatments for paraphilias, and many of them are not widely accepted among researchers or clinicians who treat these disorders (Maletzky, 1997). Cognitive therapy has been used to target the sexual urges and thoughts associated with targets of sexual arousal; however, this approach is not widely accepted (Baumeister and Butler, 1997). Behavioral treatments of paraphilia have shown mixed reviews and to date there remains an absence of consistently effective treatments (Kreuger et al., 1997). Aversion therapy, or the pairing of arousal and aversive stimuli like an electric shock, has been used with some success; however, ethical concerns and mixed results have detracted from its widespread use. Empathy training has been used with some evidence to treat sex offenders. It is designed to increase the offender's ability to empathize with their victims and then avoid victimizing others (Maletzky, 1997). Relapse prevention has focused on the use of phallometry to identify offenders who are likely to reoffend or have reoffended. Medical treatments that reduce the libido are more common among certain paraphilias.

Hormonal treatments are used in order to reduce testosterone levels in sex offenders. Rosler and Witstum (1998) showed that hormonal treatments significantly reduce sexual fantasies, desire, and abnormal sexual behavior in men with pedophilia and other paraphilias. However, questions of the use of hormonal therapy have raised ethical concerns. In addition, there are relatively few side effects of these treatments (erectile failure, hot flashes, and possible osteoporosis) and in many cases discontinuing the treatment is not accompanied by significant side effects. Flouxetine and other psychotropic medications have been used in an effort to reduce the sexual drives of individuals with paraphilias (Maletzky, 1997). In addition, antiandrogens have recently been suggested as a viable means of reducing the intensity and frequency of sexual arousal. This treatment may also serve to alter arousal in more appropriate ways for sexual offenders (Bradford, 1998).

Medical and Surgical Interventions

With the advent of Viagra (sildenafil) men who suffer from male erectile disorder have seen dramatic improvements in sexual functioning (Bach et al., 2004). Researchers have proposed using integrative approaches combining cognitive behavioral approaches and medical treatments in order to treat erectile dysfunction. While this may seem strange given the overwhelming impact of medical treatments like Viagra, it is worth mentioning that medical interventions may not treat the causes of this disorder. Stress, perceptions of relationships, and other disorders like depression may cause or impact sexual functioning. In addition, as mention previously, medical issues like vascular disease can cause erectile dysfunction (Ponholzer et al., 2006).These problems can be addressed through psychological interventions. In addition, medical interventions may place the focus of sexual processes on orgasm and climax and draw attention away from other aspects of the sexual process (Tiefer, 2002).

Other medical treatments are available for hypoactive sexual desire disorder, sexual arousal disorders, and erectile dysfunction. Endocrine therapy, hormonal treatments, and other medical treatments address many sexual disorders (Wincze and Carey, 2001; Kingsberg et al., 2008; Kresin, 1993). Medical interventions also include surgical processes that are invasive and may have adverse consequences. Although many of these procedures are successful some medical procedures report high failure rates (Wincze and Carey, 2001). Surgical procedures include treatments for vaginismus, dyspareunia, and male erectile dysfunction.

Cultural Considerations

The prevalence of sexual disorders across cultures has been of interest to researchers (Kameya, 2001). Although this research has noted many interesting differences across culture, there has been little research for alternative empirically supported treatments for sexual disorders across cultures. Religious concerns may be an important factor to consider for many patients who may present with sexual disorders. Distress that results from their disorder may in part be the result of religious beliefs that conflict with their urges. Research has shown that unique social and religious factors can influence sexual disorders. O'Sullivan (1979) found that 23 Irish women presenting with vaginismus were strongly influenced by religious and cultural beliefs of acceptable sexual behavior and feeling of guilt for sexual acts deemed unacceptable within religious and cultural views. In addition, many of the

treatments for sexual desire, arousal, and pain disorders include exercises of masturbation that may be in conflict with religious beliefs (Barlow et al., 2001). Kameya
(2001) also noted that the discussion of sexual behavior and urges is considered
a "taboo" subject for many Japanese women. It may be very difficult to proceed
with many of the behavioral techniques for treating sexual dysfunction with clients
who view sexual urges and self-stimulation in this way. Other cultural or religious
ideas of sex may influence the development and/or maintenance of sexual disorders.
Understanding the concerns of clients may impact treatment planning. For example, if religious concerns inhibit treatment plans that include masturbation exercises
in order to prevent premature ejaculation, more time should be spent explaining
the clinical relevance and importance of this treatment and addressing religious
concerns.

Triage

Initial treatment recommendations for patients with sexual disorders should include
an assessment of the severity of the problem and the least intrusive treatment that is
likely to be sufficient to alleviate the problem. In many cases, psycho-education may
be sufficient to address concerns related to the sexual response cycle. In addition,
bibliotherapy and over-the-counter sexual aids like lubrication may be sufficient to
address disorders like premature ejaculation and arousal. In any case, a thorough
assessment should be of primary importance for triage.

In the case of paraphilias triage may be more difficult and include an assessment
of legal implications and considerations. As mentioned previously many individuals who present for help with paraphilias may be ordered to do so by the legal
system. As mandated reporter implications of confidentiality are always important
for clinicians treating paraphilias, especially pedophilia.

Research Agenda

The sparse amount of research on the prevalence of sexual disorders highlights several aspects of these problems that can be addressed in future research. Stigma
associated with both sexual dysfunctions and paraphilias is a significant problem
for researchers. Because the stigma for sexual disorders is a prominent issue for
researchers, exploration of the Internet as a viable option for studying and treating
individuals within a safe and private domain has significant merit. Addressing myths
and educating consumers about the sexual response cycle may be a sufficient means
of treating many sexual dysfunctions. Continued research for psycho-educations
efforts aimed at educating individuals about treatment options and dispelling
myths is warranted. Bibliotherapy for sexual disorders also warrants continued
research. The limited amount of research devoted to this topic has been positive.
Bibliotherapy, computer-based treatments, and psycho-education offer inexpensive
and effective means of treating many disorders. Another important factor associated

with these treatment options is the privacy and avoidance of stigma that are strongly associated with sexual disorders. In addition, research on the prevention of sexual disorders is also very limited. Predictive factors for the development of identifying individuals who are likely to develop sexual disorders remain largely unknown. In addition, the development of cognitive behavior treatments for paraphilias is desperately needed.

Dissemination

Stigma and shame present a formidable problem for researchers and clinicians who treat sexual disorders. Any effort to disseminate treatments that are likely to help individual who suffer from these issues must address significant shame and social stigma concerns for individuals who need treatment. Previous research has shown the effectiveness for several sexual disorders. Research devoted to the treatment of sexual dysfunction in particular has established many effective behavioral techniques (Masters and Johnson, 1970; O'Donohue and Greer, 1993; Bach et al., 2004). Despite the fact that these treatments have been available for some time, many individuals who suffer from sexual disorders are unaware of available treatment options due in part to the shame associated with problems associated with sexual performance or sexual desires. Computer-based interventions may provide a viable means of disseminating psycho-education and information related to many of these disorders and inform consumers about potential treatment options. At higher policy level, research specific to these populations needs to be addressed on a large scale. Government funding for paraphilias is not a priority, yet disorders like pedophilia and sexual sadism remain significant problems without sufficient treatment options (Maletzky, 1997).

References

Abel GG, Becker JV, Cunningham-Rathner J, Mittelman M. Multiple paraphilic diagnoses among sex offenders. Bull Am Acad Psychiatry Law. 1988;16:153–68.

Abel GG, Osborn C. The paraphilias. The extent and nature of sexually deviant and criminal behavior. Psychiatr Clin North Am. 1992;15:675–87.

American Psychiatric Association. Diagnostic and statistical manual of mental disorders. Revised 4th ed. Washington, DC: American Psychiatric Association; 2000.

Bach AK, Barlow DH, Wincze JP. The enhancing effects of manualized treatment for erectile dysfunction among men using sildenafil: a preliminary investigation. Behav Ther. 2004;35: 55–73.

Bach AK, Wincze JP, Barlow DH. Sexual dysfunction. In: Barlow DH, editor. Clinical handbook of psychological disorders: a step-by-step treatment manual. 3rd ed. New York, Guilford Press; 2001. p. 562–608.

Barbaree HE, Seto MC. Pedophilia: assessment and treatment. In: Laws DR, O'Donohue WT, editors. Sexual deviance: theory, assessment, and treatment. New York, Guilford Press; 1997. p. 92–108.

Baumeister RF, Butler JL, Sexual masochism: deviance without pathology. In: Laws DR, O'Donohue WT, editors. Sexual deviance: theory, assessment, and treatment New York, Guilford Press; 1997. p. 92–108.

Bradford MWJ, Treatment of men with paraphilia. New Engl J Med. 1998;338:464–5.

Christopherson JM, Moore K, Foley FW, Warren KG. A comparison of written materials vs. materials and counselling for women with sexual dysfunction and multiple sclerosis. J Clin Nurs. 2006;15:742–50.

Clift RJW, Rajilic G, Gretton HM. Discriminative and predictive validity of the penile plethysmograph in adolescent sex offenders. Sex Abuse J Res Treat. 2009;21:335–62.

Derogatis LR. The Derogatis interview for sexual functioning (DISF/DISF-SR): an introductory report. J Sex Marital Ther. 1997;23:291–304.

Freund K, Seto MC, Kuban M. Frotteurism and the theory of courtship disorder. In: Laws DR, O'Donohue WT, editors. Sexual deviance: theory, assessment, and treatment New York, Guilford Press; 1997. p. 92–108.

Frank E, Anderson C, Rubinstein D. Frequency of sexual dysfunction in "normal" couples. New Eng J Med. 1978;299:111–15.

Gold SR, Gold RG. Sexual aversions: a hidden disorder. In: O'Donohue W, Jmaes H, editors. Handbook of sexual dysfunctions: assessment and treatment. Needham Heights, MA: Allyn & Bacon; 1993. p. 83–102.

Graber B. Medical aspects of sexual arousal disorders. In: O'Donohue WT, Greer JH, editors. Handbook of sexual dysfunctions: assessment and treatment. Needham Heights, Allyn & Bacon; 1997. p. 83–102.

Howitt D, Sheldon K. The role of cognitive distortions in pedophilic offending: internet and contact offenders compared. Psychol Crime Law. 2007;13:469–86.

Junginger J, Fetishism: assessment and treatment. In: Laws DR, O'Donohue WT, editors. Sexual deviance: theory, assessment, and treatment New York: Guilford Press; 1997. p. 92–108.

Kreuger RB, Kaplan MS. Frotteurism: assessment and treatment. In: Laws DR, O'Donohue WT, editors. Sexual deviance: theory, assessment, and treatment. New York: Guilford Press; 1997. p. 92–108.

Kameya Y. How Japanese culture affects the sexual functions of normal females. J Sex Marital Ther. 2001;27:151–2.

Kaplan HS. Hypoactive sexual desire. J Sex Marital Ther. 1977;3:3–9.

Kingsberg SA, Simon JA, Goldstein I. The current outlook for testosterone in the management of hypoactive sexual desire disorder in postmenopausal women. J Sex Med. 2008;5:182–93.

Kresin D. Medical aspects of inhibited sexual desire disorder. In: O'Donohue WT, Greer JH, editors. Handbook of sexual dysfunctions: assessment and treatment. Needham Heights, Allyn & Bacon; 1993. p. 83–102.

Langevin R, Paitich D, Steiner B. The clinical profile of male transsexuals living as females vs. those living as males. Arch Sex Behav. 1977;6:143–54.

Långström N, Zucker KJ. Transvestic Fetishism in the general population: prevalence and correlates. J Sex Marital Ther. 2005;31:87–95.

Laumann EO, Paik A, Rosen RC. (1999). Sexual dysfunction in the United States: prevalence and predictors. J Am Med Assoc. 1999;281:537–44.

Laws DR. Penile plethysmography: will we ever get it right? In: Ward T, Laws DR, Hudson SM, editors, Sexual deviance: issues and controversies. Thousand Oaks, CA: Sage Publications; 2003. p. 82–102.

Maletzky BM. Exhibitionism: assessment and treatment. In: Laws DR, O'Donohue WT, editors. Sexual deviance: theory, assessment, and treatment. New York: Guilford Press; 1997. p. 92–108.

Maltz W. The sexual healing journey. New York: Harper-Collins; 2001.

Master WH, Johnson VE. Human sexual inadequacy. Boston: Little, Brown; 1970.

O'Donohue WT, Geer JH (eds.). Handbook of the assessment and treatment of the sexual dysfunctions. Boston: Allyn & Bacon; 1993.

O'Sullivan K. Observations on vaginismus in Irish women. Arch Gen Psychiatry. 1979;36:824–6.

Paitch D, Langevin R, Freeman R, Mann K, Handy L. The Clarke SHQ: a clinical sex history questionnaire for males. Arch Sex Behav. 1970;6:421–36.

Ponholzer A, Temml C, Rauchenwald M, Madersbacher S. Vascular risk factors and erectile dysfunction in a cohort of healthy men. Int J Impot Res. 2006;18:489–93.

Regev L, Schmidt J. Sensate Focus. In: O'Donohue WT, Fisher JE, editors. General principles and empirically supported techniques of cognitive behavior therapy. Hoboken: Wiley; 2004. p. 584–90.

Rosen RC, Riley A, Wagner G, Osterloh IH, Kirkpatrick J, Mishra A. The international index of erectile function (IIEF): a multidimensional scale for assessment of erectile dysfunction. Urology. 1997;49:822–30.

Rosler A, Witzum E. Treatment of men with paraphilia with a long-acting analogue of gonadotropin-releasing hormone. New Engl J Med. 1998;338:416–22.

Seto MC, Cantor JM, Blanchard R. Child pornography offenses are a valid diagnostic indicator of Pedophilia. J Abnorm Psychol. 2006;115:610–5.

Spanier GB. Measuring dyadic adjustment: new scales for assessing the quality of marriage and similar dyads. J Marriage Fam. 1976;38:15–28.

Spector IP, Carey MP. Incidence and prevalence of the sexual dysfunctions: a critical review of the empirical literature. Arch Sex Behav. 1990;19:389–408.

Spector IP, Carey MP, Steinberg L. The sexual desire inventory: development, factor structure, and evidence of reliability. J Sex Marital Ther. 1996;22:175–90.

St. Lawrence JS, Madakasira S. Evaluation and treatment of premature ejaculation: a critical review. Int J Psychiatry Med. 1992;22:77–97.

Taylor JF, Rosen RC, Leiblum SR. Self-report assessment of female sexual function: psychometric evaluation of the brief index of sexual functioning for women. Arch Sex Behav. 1994;23: 627–43.

Tiefer L. Beyond the medical model of women's sexual problems: a campaign to resist the promotion of 'female sexual dysfunction. Sex Relation Ther. 2002;17:127–35.

Titov N. Status of computerized cognitive behavioural therapy for adults. Aust N Z J Psychiatry. 2007;41:95–114.

van Lankveld JJDM. Bibliotherapy in the treatment of sexual dysfunctions: a meta-analysis. J Consult Clin Psychol. 1998;66:702–8.

Waldinger MD. Premature ejaculation: different pathophysiologies and etiologies determine its treatment. J Sex Marital Ther. 2008;34:1–13.

Wincze JP, Carey MP. Sexual dysfunction: a guide for assessment and treatment. 2nd ed. New York: Guilford Press; 2001.

Zeiss RA. Self-directed treatment for premature ejaculation. J Consul Clin Psychol. 1978;46: 1234–41.

Chapter 14
Stepped Care and E-Health in Behavioral Managed Care

Ronald R. O'Donnell

Introduction

Managed care entities such as Managed Behavioral Health Care Organizations, health plans, and vendors increasingly focus on information technology, e-health, and stepped care in population-based approaches to behavioral health management. Population-based interventions, also known as disease management, involve a systematic approach to defining a population with a chronic illness. In managed care, the population is typically identified based on a combination of claims data showing utilization, diagnoses, medications, and cost of care. Once the population is identified the managed care case manager will outreach individuals and attempt to enroll them in programs designed to improve their ability to effectively manage their chronic condition. The interventions typically include telephonic contacts between the case manager and individual focused on education, monitoring treatment outcome, self-help activities and resources, and treatment adherence. These interventions are based on stepped care in which the severity of illness is matched to the least intensive intervention and outcome is closely monitored. If treatment response is sub-optimal more intensive interventions are added until the desired outcome is achieved. The premise of these efforts is that population behavioral health management will result in improved quality and clinical outcomes of care and decreased costs of medical care. Managed care entities are increasingly turning to e-health tools in an effort to enhance the effectiveness of these programs. Examples include sophisticated computer algorithms to define populations, the use of online self-assessment to track outcome, use of e-mail, instant messaging, and chat by the case manager to communicate with the individual, and web-based, interactive self-help tools to help the individual learn to manage his condition. Managed care organizations frequently partner with employers, hospitals, and physician groups on population-based health management for chronic behavioral health conditions. The purpose of this chapter is to review the critical components of managed

R.R. O'Donnell (✉)
Behavioral Health Program, School of Letters and Sciences, Arizona State University, P.O. Box 37100, Mail Code 3252, Phoenix, AZ, USA
e-mail: ronald.odonnell@asu.edu

W.T. O'Donohue, C. Draper (eds.), *Stepped Care and e-Health*,
DOI 10.1007/978-1-4419-6510-3_14, © Springer Science+Business Media, LLC 2011

care population-based disease management programs and to provide illustrative examples from the research literature

The economic burden of chronic disease in the United States is a growing problem with more than 125 million individuals having at least one chronic condition in 2000 with a projected 157 million by 2020, with 50% of these individuals having more than one condition (Wu and Green, 2000). Increases in chronic conditions are attributed to medical advances that enable those with chronic conditions to live longer, increased screening and diagnosis of chronic conditions, and the aging of Americans (Partnership for Solutions, 2008). Treatment of chronic conditions accounts for 78% of healthcare spending, 76% of all hospital admissions, 88% of all prescriptions filled, and 72% of physician visits (Partnership for Solutions, 2008). Research has shown that increases in healthcare costs are more related to increases in utilization of health services rather than an increase in unit costs of care (Loeppke et al., 2007).

The costs of chronic care fall upon private, employer-based insurance, government programs, and individual insurance premiums paid out of pocket. Over one-half of all individuals with chronic conditions have private insurance and roughly one-third are covered by Medicare or Medicaid. A 2007 survey (Claxton, 2007) found that employers spent an average of $3,785 and $8,824 for single and family plans, respectively, above employee contribution. Health insurance premiums increased 78% between 2001 and 2007. There is also increased recognition that in addition to direct medical costs, the financial impact of chronic illness on employers includes decreased work productivity and disability. The cost associated with decreased productivity and absenteeism due to illness is three times more costly than the medical costs of care (Burton et al., 1999; Collins et al., 2005; Loeppke et al., 2007, 2003; Loeppke Hymel, 2006; Stewart et al., 2003). Employees with chronic health conditions have higher medical costs and these conditions result in increased absenteeism and presenteeism (Boles et al., 2004; Burton et al., 1999, 2006; Collins et al., 2005; Loeppke et al., 2007; Stewart et al., 2003).

A major problem is that many patients with chronic illness do not receive evidence-based care for their conditions. Myette (2008) summarized a number of factors that lead to a quality of care gap between usual care and evidence-based management of chronic conditions for depression. These include

- patient reluctance to seek treatment due to stigma and other barriers
- failure to detect and diagnose depression in patients who do seek treatment
- insufficient dosage and duration of psychopharmacological interventions
- failure to recommend evidence-based psychotherapy
- limited access to behavioral health specialty clinicians
- lack of regular monitoring and relapse prevention
- failure to integrate medical and behavioral care
- underutilization of allied health professionals to assist physicians
- failure to provide psychoeducation to patients and their families on depression and promote self-management
- failure to use community resources and support

In an effort to address the quality of care gap and improve the clinical and cost of care burden of chronic illness, managed care has adopted disease management programs designed to identify chronic illness populations, outreach and enroll individuals, and provide stepped care interventions and demonstrate both clinical improvement and cost savings. The typical disease management program uses claims data such as diagnosis, service utilization, and pharmacy to segment populations into low-risk, high-risk, and chronic cases based on illness severity and cost of care. A small percentage of complex chronic patients utilize the majority of healthcare services. For example, the top 10% comprise 65% of health resources (Kathol and Clarke, 2005). The opportunity to reduce the high costs of chronic care with disease management programs has led to tremendous growth in the industry. The estimated annual revenues for the disease management industry have grown from about $78 million in 1997 to $1.2 billion in 2005 and projected to top $1.8 billion in 2008 (DM Purchasing Consortium, cited by Matheson et al., 2006).

The Chronic Care Model

Managed care has adopted the Chronic Care Model (CCM) developed by Wagner (1998), Wagner et al. (2001). The Chronic Care Model is based on (1) collaboration between a coordinated team of providers and an activated patient, promoting self-management skills so the patient can better manage his own health; (2) delivery system re-design to facilitate information sharing about patient status and treatment plan; (3) decision support tools based on evidence-based practice guidelines; (4) clinical information systems to track patient care; and (5) organization of the healthcare system and environment to improve care coordination and a focus on the community context and necessary alliances and partnerships.

An example of the chronic care model in behavioral healthcare is the collaborative care model of depression (Katon and Unutzer, 2006). This approach is designed to improve detection, diagnosis, patient education, provision of evidence-based care via collaboration between the patient, his or her primary care physician, and ancillary healthcare providers. One key component of the model is a dedicated case manager, typically a nurse or social worker, who works to engage the patient as an active partner in treatment. The case manager closely tracks treatment outcome and helps the patient learn the skills to self-manage depression. Often lifestyle changes such as behavioral activation, exercise, diet, and medication adherence are incorporated into treatment, especially for depressed patients with comorbid chronic medical conditions or risk factors.

The stepped care model is based on the acknowledgement that (1) different patients require different levels of care; (2) the most appropriate level of care is based on closely monitoring outcomes; and (3) moving from lower to more intensive levels of care based on patient response can increase the effectiveness of care while lowering overall costs (Von Korff and Tiemens, 2000). In stepped care treatment of behavioral conditions such as depression the case manager will use measures such as the Patient Health Questionnaire (PHQ-9) (Kroenke et al., 2000) to evaluate baseline severity and repeat administrations over the course of the program to monitor progress. Patients with low illness severity may initially receive educational materials, guided self-help exercise, and referral to self-help groups. More intensive treatments may range from brief interventions in the primary care site, such as wellness programs, to referral to a specialty behavioral health provider for psychotherapy or psychopharmacological intervention. A hallmark of the collaborative care model is that the care manager is typically co-located in the primary care office to assist with coordination of care and transformation of the healthcare system consistent with the Chronic Care Model (Wagner, 2002). However, other approaches to collaborative care have used remote case managers who rely on telephonic outreach and management (Wang et al., 2007).

Managed care disease management programs espouse the principles of the chronic care model but typically do not involve the significant changes in healthcare delivery system changes and transformation of physician offices to address chronic illness (Wagner, 2002). Managed care disease management programs are typically administered remotely with clinicians conducting telephonic outreach and intervention, as opposed to collaborative care interventions that are conducted within physician offices. Apart from this important difference, the stepped care clinical interventions model is nearly identical for both telephonic and collaborative care disease management. The structure of telephonic case management programs include case identification, typically using health plan claims or pharmacy date, followed by outreach. Outreach is initiated with a letter to the member describing the program and inviting them to enroll and participate.

An important distinction in enrollment is whether the program is designed as opt-in or opt-out. In the opt-in model the individual has to take action to initiate participation, such as mailing back a form or agreeing verbally in a phone call. In the opt-out model the patient is assumed to be enrolled and participating in the program unless he takes action to disenroll, via letter or phone. After the letter is sent the company initiates phone calls to the member. In many cases a non-clinician enrollment specialist with specialized training in engagement strategies will make this call. The disease manager is typically a nurse and in the initial phone call completes an assessment with brief measures such as the PHQ-9 (Kroenke et al., 2001). On the basis of the assessment the care manager will offer a stepped care intervention that is matched to the patient needs. For example, a case with severe depression and no behavioral health specialty provider for psychotherapy or psychopharmacology will routinely be referred to one or both. Follow-up calls are made by the care manager typically at 1–2 weeks, 4–6 weeks, 8–12 weeks, and 24 weeks based on repeated assessments and response to treatment.

The telephonic disease management intervention content at the initial call and follow-up includes assessment of symptoms, medication side effects, comorbid medical and behavioral conditions, suicide risk, barriers to treatment and adherence, and patient education. The assessment is heavily scripted and recorded in an information system database at baseline and follow-up. Follow-up contacts are also programmed in the information system and outreach phone calls are managed with automatic dialers for scheduled appointments. Documentation in the program may include feedback to the primary care physician or specialty behavioral care clinician, typically in the form of a patient letter or summary report.

Patient Identification and Assessment

Predictive Modeling

A commonly used approach to identifying disease management cases is predictive modeling. Predictive modeling in managed care is a technology-based statistical tool designed to systematically canvass healthcare claims data to search for combinations of clinical and service utilization variables, such as diagnosis, physician visits, and emergency room and hospitalization and using these data to predict future healthcare utilization and costs (Hodgman, 2008). A risk score is computed that is designed to indicate the likelihood that a defined population will utilize more healthcare services than a comparable group. The characteristics of the population that comprise the model are used to target specific diagnoses or related variables that are presumed to be actionable with targeted interventions. That is, specific evidence-based and stepped care interventions are expected to lead to improvements in health status and reduce the probability that the predicted cost increase will actually occur. The validity of a predictive model lies in its ability to demonstrate mitigation of costs based on targeted interventions. Predictive modeling is widely used in managed care with every major health plan or vendor promoting proprietary predictive modeling technology.

Health Risk Appraisal (HRA)

An increasingly common approach to case identification is the health risk appraisal (HRA). An HRA in managed care is a structured questionnaire completed by individuals to estimate the risk of mortality and morbidity for their particular health status profile. In addition to identifying common medical conditions, such as diabetes and hypertension, lifestyle habits that contribute to health status such as activity, diet, and stress are included. Behavioral issues such as depression and substance abuse are also included. The results of the individual's HRA are quantified and fed back to the individual either by a clinician or increasingly received by the individual in real time (Hudson and Pope, 2006).

Expert System Tailored Interventions

Once the individual is identified and enrolled in the program and the baseline assessment is completed, managed care entities increasingly use expert system tailored interventions (Velicer and Diclemente, 1993). Specific behavioral interventions are generated based on complex algorithms based on decision rules designed to match the most appropriate treatment to the patient illness severity, motivation for treatment, and readiness for change. These web-based expert systems are based on theories of behavior change that serve as a template for developing algorithms that help determine software decision rules. One of the most commonly used models in web-based behavior change programs is the Transtheoretical Model (TTM). The TTM is an integrative model of behavioral change designed to explain and predict how and when individuals change their behaviors. The TTM uses stages of change to integrate principles of behavior change across theories of behavior change intervention (Prochaska et al., 2008). The stages of change are (1) precontemplation, (2) contemplation, (3) preparation, (4) action, (5) maintenance, and (6) termination. In addition to the stage of change the TTM model incorporates theoretical constructs critical to individualized feedback: processes of change, decisional balance, self-efficacy, and temptation. The processes of change are the covert and overt actions that individuals use to progress through the stages, such as consciousness raising, contingency management, or helping relationships. Decisional balance is the individual's weighing the pros and cons of changing behavior. Self-efficacy is the situation specific confidence a person has that they have the ability to cope without relapsing to an undesirable habit (Bandura, 1982). Temptation is the intensity of a person's urges to engage in a undesirable health habit when faced with a challenging situation and is found to reflect three situations: negative affect or emotional distress, positive social situations, and craving (Prochaska et al., 2008).

Research on how individuals progress through the stages of change has been used in the development of tailored communication for disease management (Velicer and Diclemente, 1993). Stage tailoring is the application of a specific process of change based on the person's stage of change. Providing an action process such as stimulus control would not be effective for a person in precontemplation. The stage effect involves the ability to predict one's performance depending on the stage they are in at baseline. The goal becomes applying behavior change interventions that are designed to move the person to the next stage of change, rather than move from an early phase, such as precontemplation, to action. Tailored interventions in expert systems require the ongoing assessment of the person's current stage. In web-based programs the assessment is completed online and an expert report is generated to help guide people to the next stage of change. Stage-based self-help manuals are provided to individuals to guide their behavior change efforts between interventions. The reports are generated on a regular basis and are constructed form a large set of paragraphs based on decision rules derived from prior longitudinal studies of how individuals change.

Quality Improvement and Outcomes

The quality improvement designs of managed care disease management programs are robust in terms of process measures, outcome measures, clinician training and productivity, and evidence of clinical improvement and cost savings. The process measures include comprehensive descriptions of patient identification, outreach, enrollment, participation, drop-outs, and completion rates. Clinical measures include symptom assessment in clinical domains using standardized questionnaires such as the PHQ-9 for depression. In addition self-report measures of workplace productivity, absenteeism, and presenteeism are commonplace. The disease management interventions are based on regular follow-up contacts to both reassess clinical measures, address barriers to progress and motivation, and document participation. Clinicians are trained in strategies and techniques of engagement using telephone and increasingly web-based tools designed to enhance motivation. In addition the stepped care interventions are both heavily scripted and based on algorithms within information management systems that prompt care managers to complete every planned assessment and corresponding intervention. Clinician productivity is recorded in the system and includes data on measures such as caseload, call duration, number of calls completed, and completion of scheduled assessments. Many companies use live supervision of active care manager–patient phone calls or review a random selection of recordings of phone calls in order to supervise care managers on interview and engagement techniques such as motivational interviewing. The evaluation of disease management program cost savings is based on financial and actuarial models to measure return on investment (ROI). These models typically identify a medical cost trend for a time period prior to the intervention, ideally of at least 2 years duration in order to control for regression to the mean and other variables. Changes in the time period during and post-intervention are then gathered and analyzed for changes in utilization and cost of services comparing at least 1-year post-intervention with the pre-intervention comparison period (Goetzel et al., 2005)

A literature review by Mattke et al. (2007) evaluated the evidence for different types of disease management programs on quality, cost, and health outcomes for various chronic conditions. The authors identified 3 large-scale population-based studies, 10 meta-analyses, and 16 systematic reviews that contained 317 unique studies. They evaluated the effect of disease management on the following endpoints:

- Clinical processes of care such as adherence to guidelines and evidence-based practices.
- improvement in health and lifestyle behaviors such as exercise and medication adherence.
- Intermediate outcomes such as disease control, for example, glycosylated hemoglobin (A1C) control.
- Clinical outcomes such as mortality, self-reported symptoms and functional status, patient satisfaction, and quality of life.
- Healthcare utilization and financial outcomes.

The report concluded that there is consistent evidence that disease management improves the processes of care and appear to lead to better intermediate outcomes and improved disease control for CHF, CAD, CM, and depression. There was no consistent evidence for long-term improved health outcomes, although this may be a result of limited follow-up periods reported in most studies. The finding that received much attention in this study is that the evidence for disease management programs to reduce utilization and cost of care was inconclusive. Disease management was found to reduce hospitalization rates among patients with CHF and to result in higher utilization of outpatient care and prescription medications for patients with depression. There has been significant debate within the disease management industry on whether or not the claims of cost savings that are used by companies to promote their disease management programs are in fact supported by the evidence.

Norman (2008) suggested that the inconclusive results for cost savings should not deter the adoption of disease management due to the clear evidence of clinical improvements. He suggested focusing on fundamental questions regarding the quality of disease management programs, such as: What are the benefits? Are benefits predictable and long lasting? What contexts, populations, and other factors are related to benefits? Can benefits be achieved in a cost-effective manner and are cost savings possible? In the behavioral health arena research on depression disease management has followed the model suggested by Norman and is revealing new insights on clinical benefits and cost savings. The association between behavioral conditions and increased medical health service utilization and cost is exemplified by research on depression. Total healthcare costs are 50–100% greater for outpatients with depression than those without and these increased costs are predominantly due to higher utilization of medical services than behavioral (Henk et al., 1996; Simon et al., 1995; Unutzer et al., 1997). Improvement in depression is associated with decreased medical care utilization (Simon et al., 2000, 2002). Systematic reviews of the literature have shown that depression disease management improves the quality of care and can be cost-effective relative to usual care (Katon et al., 1995, 1999; Katzelnick et al., 2000; Simon et al., 2000).

The Stepped Care Toolbox and Resources for Each Step

An illustrative example of the stepped care toolbox in managed care depression disease management is a study by Wang et al. (2007) of a depression outreach treatment program on workplace outcomes. Patients were adult employees and enrollees of United Behavioral Health. Patient identification consisted of a two-step process. Phase one was completion of an HRA, a chronic condition checklist, screen for psychological distress and work performance questions. Patients with positive depression screen scores were contacted by letter and telephone to complete a phase two interview assessing depression using the Quick Inventory of Depression Symptoms Self-Report (QIDS-SR) (Rush et al., 1996) and the World Health Organization Health and Productivity Questionnaire (HPQ) (Kessler et al., 2003), a structured measure of four dimensions of work functioning: (1) work hours (absenteeism), (2) job performance, (3) job turnover, and (4) critical workplace incidents. Patients assigned to the treatment condition were contacted by phone by a licensed master's level mental healthcase manager and completed the PHQ-9, prior treatment history and motivation for treatment. Patients were followed with regular phone contacts for ongoing assessment. Patients who experienced significant depressive symptoms after 2 months were offered a structured eight-session cognitive-behavioral psychotherapy program with weekly telephone sessions of 30–40 min using the workbook.

Patients with significant depression severity were referred to in-person psychotherapy and medication evaluation. Patients who declined referrals were provided a brief motivational intervention and received continued follow-up contacts by the case manager. A psychoeducational cognitive-behavioral-based workbook designed to facilitate condition self-management was mailed to each patient. Patients who accepted in-person treatment were also followed by case managers who provided ongoing assessment of depressive symptoms, treatment adherence, and barriers to treatment. Feedback was provided to providers and a United Behavioral Health psychiatrist was available for consultation. For patients receiving only one mode of treatment a second was added if significant depression continued after 2 months.

The results of the study combining data across 6- and 12-month assessments demonstrated that the intervention group had significantly lower QIDS self-report scores, higher job retention, and more hours worked than the usual care groups. These results demonstrated both improved clinical and workplace outcomes. While a formal return on investment analysis was not conducted the financial value of the improved workplace outcomes expressed as recovered hiring, training, and salary costs suggest that employers would experience a positive return on investment from outreach and enhanced treatment of depressed workers. While this study did not include a web-based intervention, it is an illustration of a typical stepped care, evidence-based approach to depression disease management that managed care vendors have incorporated into their web-based disease management models.

E-Health, Stepped Care Managed Care Research

Kaiser Permanente, an integrated care delivery system, partnered with HealthMedia, a company that specializes in e-health, stepped care behavior change interventions to evaluate web-based weight management programs. In an initial study (Rothert et al., 2006) a web-based expert system weight management program was compared with a web-based information-only materials condition. All participants completed the same web-based assessment. The tailored expert system condition used HealthMedia Balance, a 6-week self-help weight management program. Balance uses a software algorithm to link baseline assessment content to an individually tailored weight management plan focused on healthy nutrition, physical activity, energy expenditure, cognitive attributions, body image, and social support. Tailored action plans were delivered at weeks 1, 3, and 6 of the program. E-mails were sent to alert participants to new materials, and follow-up e-mails were designed to reinforce health improvement activities, address barriers to progress, and provide self-monitoring tools and support. The information-only group had access to the standard educational resources on the Kaiser Permanente member web site. The web site was comprehensive and easily navigable, covering topics such as definitions of healthy weight, preparation for weight management, facts about diets, and weight management strategies. Baseline and 3- and 6-month data were collected using web-based questionnaires. Participants received multiple e-mail reminders to complete questionnaires. A total of 30% of the participants completed the 3-month survey and 20% responded to the 6-month survey. The study found that participants in the web-based expert system reporting significantly greater weight loss than the information-only condition were more likely to have read web-based information completely and to have found the information helpful, easy to understand, and relevant (Rothert et al., 2006). The high rate of non-response to the two follow-up questionnaires is a significant limitation of this study.

A more recent study by Kaiser Permanente and HealthMedia on web-based weight loss was designed to evaluate the problem of participation by studying the impact of (1) recruitment methods and patient characteristics related to (2) enrollment, (3) engagement, and (4) continued participation. Health plan overweight members with or without chronic illness (diabetes and CAD) were recruited from three HMOs for an Internet-based HealthMedia weight loss program using two different recruitment methods: (1) personal letters from the prevention directors in each HMO and (2)announcements in member newsletters. Participants were assigned to one of four interventions comprised of a combination of three HealthMedia programs: (1) the 6-week Balance weight loss program only; (2) balance plus an 8-week nutrition program called Nourish; (3) balance plus a concurrent goal-setting program called Achieve, and (4) balance plus Nourish plus Achieve. Follow-up contacts were made at 3, 12, and 18 months post-enrollment. The Achieve goal-setting program uses individual performance information based on progress with the Balance program, such as attributions for failure, motivation, and self-efficacy, to determine follow-up questions and subsequent goals. Nourish is a nutrition program similar in design to Balance. Assessment data are collected to tailor nutrition advice based on the individual profile. It is comprised of a nutrition guide, three tailored newsletters, and e-mail messages delivered over an 8-week period.

The two experimental recruitment conditions, personal letters and newsletters and flyers, were based on members recruited from three health plans. The subjects included members selected from HMO registries for diabetes, CAD, and overweight members from a hyperlipidemia registry with no known CAD. The letters were signed by physician leaders from the appropriate health plan and contained instructions for logging on to the HealthMedia programs for weight management. The newsletters and flyers included a brief description of the program and log on instructions. A total of 1,402 members out of a pool of 79,378, approximately 5%, enrolled in the general population and 909 out of 18,779 from the chronic illness group, 2.4%. As predicted, personalized letters produced higher enrollment rates than member newsletters. Members with diabetes or CAD were more likely to enroll than those without chronic conditions. Males, those over age 60, smokers, and individuals estimated to have higher medical expenses were all less likely to enroll. As with other e-health studies, the overall enrollment and participation rates were low, with substantial attrition. The authors reported that adding the Achieve and Nourish components to the Balance intervention created adherence problems. While almost all participants viewed the initial Balance program, few viewed the Achieve and Nourish programs.

An example of the Transtheoretical Model (TTM)-based expert system is a study by Johnson et al. (2006) on antihypertensive medication adherence. Participants were identified through the HMO pharmacy database based on failure to fill prescribed antihypertensive medication prescriptions as scheduled or discontinued. Recruitment letters were mailed to 11,333 members. Members could decline participation or be removed from the study by their physicians. Out of the 11,333 members 1,499 (13.2%) were excluded by providers, 2,710 (24%) were screened out due to eligibility criteria, and 2,718 (24%) refused participation, resulting in a total of 1,227 members enrolled, or 11% of those who received the introduction letters. Baseline assessments were mailed to the remaining members followed by telephone calls to members who did not return the assessment. Subjects were randomly assigned to intervention or control groups with follow-up assessments at 6-month intervals (baseline, 6, 12, and 18 months). At each assessment members who did not complete the form by mail were called and the assessment was completed by phone.

The intervention was the Pro-Change Program for high blood pressure medication, based on the TTM, a computer-generated, individualized, stage-matched expert system intervention and a stage-based manual for adherence to antihypertensive medication. The system provided normative printed intervention reports based on the patient assessment with individualized feedback on (1) the stage of change, (2) decisional balance, (3) process of change, (4) self-efficacy, and (5) suggested strategies for change. The self-help manual guided the individual to the process of change most appropriate for the current stage of change. The manual was organized by stage and included stage-matched exercises to help subjects understand and take action on the strategies recommended in their individual feedback reports. The reports, in turn, referred participants to sections in the manual that were most appropriate for them.

Retention was 71.6% at 6 months, 63.2 % at 12 months, and 63.3% at 18 months. One measure of intervention effectiveness, the percentage of individuals in the action or maintenance stage of change, showed that significantly more individuals in the intervention group were in the action or maintenance stage compared to the control group at 12- and 18-month assessments. In addition the intervention group scored significantly lower on a nonadherence measure at the 12- and 18-month assessments.

The results of these two studies by Kaiser Permanente and HealthMedia and the study by Johnson et al. (2006) demonstrate that web-based programs for behavioral conditions are effective for the participants who do enroll and complete the program. The limitation illustrated by these studies is that enrollment, participation, and completion in web-based behavior change programs are relatively low. The problem of patient engagement in web-based behavior change programs is receiving increased attention.

The Challenge of Engagement

A central challenge of DM programs is retaining patients in the program after enrollment. There is consensus that at least 6 months of participation in disease management is necessary for behavioral changes addressing lifestyle and disease management to take effect (Linden et al., 2003). The predominant reason for patient non-participation is patients who enroll but then discontinue before completing the program (MacStravic, 2007). Another problem is how participation is defined in disease management. It is common for opt out programs that once a member is enrolled, he or she must take actions, such as contact the disease manager, to actively discontinue enrollment from the program. A patient could be listed as participating by this definition but never actively take part in the intervention. The participation for disease management programs is low to begin with, such as 29% enrolled at 1 year in a study by Lynch et al. (2006). The combination of low participation and completion, combined with low enrollment, can result in annual retention rates as low as 11% (Lynch et al., 2006).

Prochaska and Prochaska (2005) propose that impact, defined as the participation rate time efficacy of the intervention, is critical to evaluate disease management effectiveness. For example, if a best practice for smoking cessation produces 30% abstinence and an intervention demonstrates 5% participation, the impact is 1.5%. If an alternative practice that produces 20% abstinence achieves 75% participation its impact is 15%. The practice that seems less effective had 10 times the impact on the target behavior in terms of maximum impact in disease management. The expert system algorithms designed to match intervention to patient assessment results increasingly include algorithms designed to improve impact. It is anticipated that continued refinement of expert systems by vendors such as Pro-Change and HealthMedia will lead to improvements in engagement and impact.

Other approaches are also emerging that demonstrate improved patient engagement. One is the use of incentives for patient participation in disease management programs. These incentives are funded by partnerships between health plans, vendors, and employer groups and include cash incentives, paid time off work, or a small reduction in employee participation for activities such as completing a health risk assessment or participating in a behavior change program targeting healthy behaviors and chronic illness (Schult et al., 2006).

Another approach is to combine web-based disease management programs with existing health and wellness programs and to include in-person support for participation in the program. A study conducted by Highmark Inc. (Highmark), a company that employs 12,000 workers and serves as a Blue Cross Blue Shield health insurance provider in Pennsylvania, began a comprehensive health promotion program for its employees. The Highmark Wellness program offered HRA's, online programs in nutrition, weight management, stress management and tobacco cessation, on-site nutrition and tobacco cessation coaching, biometric screenings, health campaigns, and employee use of fitness centers (Naydeck et al., 2008). Condition management services were offered to those with asthma, diabetes, CAD, CHF, and COPD. The overall participation in the program was very high based on the 81% of employees who participated in any component of the program in each of the 4 years of studies. The focus of this study was on ROI, so only a subset of the sample that met eligibility criteria for computation of ROI were analyzed and reported on. Return on investment was calculated based on growth curve analyses that compared medical claims for program participants compared to risk-matched nonparticipants for the years 2001–2005. The difference between groups was used to define savings with ROI computed by subtracting program costs from savings. The results of multivariate models estimated healthcare expense as $176 lower for participants, inpatient expenses were lower by $182. Four-year savings based on comparison of intervention expenses resulted in an ROI of $1.65 for every dollar spent on the program, demonstrating that a comprehensive health promotion program that relies on e-health web tools in combination of biotmetrics, coaching and on-site support, can lower the rate of healthcare cost increases and produce a positive ROI (Naydeck et al., 2008). While the results of this study did not measure participation in terms of enrollment, participation, and completion, it did appear to have high levels of participation and demonstrated a ROI.

A study by Wylie-Roset et al. (2001) of a computerized weight loss program in a managed care setting examined a cognitive-behavioral approach for lifestyle modification for three interventions: a workbook alone, the addition of computerized tailoring, and the addition of both computers and staff consultation. This study included overweight individuals in a freestanding HMO setting. The intervention was a stepped care model using the workbook to address motivation and behavioral goals for lifestyle change based on the Transtheoretical Model of behavior change. The result showed improved results with increasing levels of treatment intensity: the mean 12-month weight losses were 2.2, 4.7, and 7.4 pounds, 0.4, 0.9, and 1.2 BMI, and the respective costs per participant $12.33, 41.99, and $133.74. Components of the intervention correlated with weight loss included increased computer use, self-monitoring, walking and decreased energy and fat intake. Staff counseling achieved the most weight loss at a higher cost. Overall 81% of the participants completed the 12-month study. The dropout rates were similar for all three intervention groups. The results of this study demonstrated that increased intensity of intervention from only workbook to tailored computer program to staff consultation did lead to increasingly positive outcomes. Interestingly, there were no significant differences in participation, which was uniformly high.

Micco et al. (2007) compared the 12-month weight loss outcomes of an Internet-only behavioral weight loss treatment with the same program with the addition of a monthly in-person meeting. The Internet-only group participated in online lessons and met weekly in small groups in an online chat room. Participants were instructed to review the weekly and submit electronically homework assignments to their facilitator before each meeting. The dietary intervention combined calorie goals and self-monitoring with exercise. Behavior therapy was delivered in the online lessons and homework and reviewed in the next group chat discussion. The lesson topics included stimulus control, relapse prevention, problem solving, and social support. The chats were described as very interactive with the therapist guiding the discussion and participants joining in for discussion. Each week participants submitted e-journals to the therapist who reviewed them and provided feedback on maintaining nutritional and activity balance. E-mail communication tended to be brief and non-scripted. Participants received automated positive reinforcement for every lesson completed or self-monitoring entry that was made. The Internet plus in-person group received the same Internet intervention as above, plus they met once a month in-person. The results showed no significant differences between the Internet-only and Internet plus in-person group meeting interventions and the subjects in each group losing approximately 7 kg over 6 months. In addition there were no significant differences in participation/attrition between the treatment groups in the number of participants who completed all three assessments (63 vs. 62% for Internet-only and Internet plus in-person). This is the first study to demonstrate weight loss with an Internet-only intervention that showed weight loss similar to in-person weight loss programs. In term of engagement this study is of interest in that it demonstrated good participation rates in the Internet-only condition with the addition of a therapist facilitating regular group chat meetings.

A study by Frazee et al. (2008) combined telephonic disease management with a model that integrated worksite-based primary care and pharmacy services with telephonic intervention in a direct effort to improve rates of case identification and outreach, enrollment, participation, and completion. The integrated disease management worksite-based clinician program is designed to leverage the patient's trust in primary care and worksite in-person clinicians to facilitate participation in a traditional telephonic intervention. Frazee et al. (2008) compared participation rates for individuals assigned to telephonic and integrated disease management over 12 months.

The intervention targeted patients with diabetes, coronary artery disease, and hypertension using a stepped care model. Cases were identified by claims-based predictive modeling, geographic proximity to worksite-based primary care and pharmacy, and stratified based on costs to identify the patients with the highest avoidable costs. The recruitment process for both groups was the same except that the integrated group was reviewed to classify which patients received care from the worksite primary care office and these patients received direct contact by health center staff that explained the benefits of the program and invited the patient to enroll. Then both groups received traditional telephonic disease management follow-up contact for ongoing assessment of progress on condition self-management goals. The results of the study showed that the integrated program patients had significantly higher contact and enrollment rate and higher engagement and retention than telephonic disease management. Seventy-six percent of integrated program patients were retained at 12 months post-enrollment compared to only 19% for those enrolled in the telephonic program which had similar geographic proximity to their primary care physician. The integrated disease management program with face-to-face support from a clinician clearly improved enrolment, retention, and completion relative to a traditional telephonic program. It is assumed that a longer duration of patient active involvement in behavioral change interventions will result in improved clinical outcomes. In addition, improving enrollment, retention, and completion rates will in turn improve the likelihood of demonstrating both the clinical and cost of care improvements necessary to demonstrate a return on investment. While this study did not include an web-based intervention it is of interest in showing that the presence of a trusted clinician was related to significantly higher engagement in a traditional telephonic disease management program.

The Research and Development Agenda

The use of population-based, disease management interventions with e-health tools is a rapidly growing area in managed behavioral care. The clinical benefits of disease management programs based on collaborative care and traditional telephonic depression disease management are well established. The evidence for cost savings for disease management of depression and other conditions remains inconclusive. In line with Norton's (2008) recommendation to ask the right questions about disease management there is emerging evidence of cost savings for depression disease management when the cost savings for employer workplace productivity are included in the analysis. In spite of the controversy over cost savings or ROI for disease management programs the vendors promoting these products continue to develop new contracts with health plans and employer groups and further refine their products.

The design of disease management programs that have incorporated web-based e-health tools is an excellent example of evidence-based stepped care. Disease management programs are based on stepped care principles such as screening and assessment that progress from relatively brief measures, such as the PHQ-9, to structured assessment of detailed symptoms and functioning. The addition of workplace productivity has contributed to improved ability to demonstrate cost savings for employer groups. The interventions in disease management also follow stepped care principles of offering the least resource-intensive intervention that will best meet the patient's needs followed by increasing intensity if the patient does not make expected progress. The introduction of expert system design in web-based condition self-management tools is now offered with no formal involvement of a care manager in delivering the intervention.

The pace of technological innovation and product development underway in managed behavioral care approaches to Internet-based behavior change and disease management interventions is significant and outpaces the published research available at the time of this publication. A visit to the web sites for Pro-Change (www.prochange.com) or HealthMedia (www.healthmedia.com) illustrates new products and continued focus on patient engagement, expert systems, tailored messages, and interventions. A review of the web site for OptumHealth$_{SM}$ Behavioral Health (www.optumhealth.com), formerly United Behavioral Health, previews a new product called BrainHealth Strategies, a web-based expert system. The focus of managed behavioral care continues to be on efficiency and cost-effectiveness of population-based stepped care interventions. The focus on web-based interventions reflects the traditional focus of managed care to deliver the lowest cost interventions with the greatest impact on clinical improvement and cost savings.

The central question around web-based behavioral health interventions in managed behavioral healthcare is not if they will work, but rather can sufficient numbers of target patients enroll, participate, and complete the program to make these programs cost-effective for the health plans and employer groups that are the payers. The combination of continued refinement in expert systems design and the likely incorporation of facilitated chat rooms as in the design by Micco et al. (2007) show promise for continued improvement in patient engagement. On the other hand, it appears that the presence of a clinician in-person improves patient engagement, as in the study by Frazee (2008). It is likely that Internet-based interventions will increasingly be utilized by clinicians in primary care and worksite programs as a component of integrated behavioral care.

To date managed care has been reluctant to adopt disease management interventions that require care manager co-location in primary care or medical settings. In part this is due to the traditional managed care focus on remote, telephonic, and now web-based disease management as a more cost-effective intervention. In part it is due to long-standing reimbursement barriers for behavioral health clinicians in primary care. Research on both remote and co-located disease management programs using e-health interventions will continue with a focus on what works for whom, under what conditions, and in which settings. Managed care adoption of co-located disease management will likely be determined by the extent that research demonstrates a consistent advantage for co-located disease management, especially in the area of patient engagement, or that payment barriers are reduced through reform of primary care payment mechanisms. In the interim it is likely that both models will coexist and perhaps benefit mutually, as managed care programs involve co-located clinicians in disease management programs and co-located clinicians identify and refer patients with chronic conditions to available disease management programs.

References

Bandura A. Self-efficacy mechanism in human agency. Am Psychol. 1982;37:122–47.
Boles M, Pelletier B, Lynch W. The relationship between health risks and work productivity. J Occup Environ Med. 2004;46:737–45.
Burton WN, Conti D, Chen C. The role of health risk factors and disease on worker productivity. J Occup Environ Med. 1999;4:547–57.
Burton WN, Chen CY, Conti DJ, Schultz AB, Edington DW. The association of medical conditions and presenteeism. J Occup Environ Med. 2006;48:252–63.
Collins JJ, Baase CM, Sharda CE, et al. The assessment of chronic health conditions on work performance, absence, and total economic impact for employers. J Occup Environ Med. 2005;47:547–57.
Frazee SG, Sherman B, Fabius R, Ryan P, Kirkpatrick P, Davis J. Leveraging the trusted clinician: increasing retention in disease management through integrated program delivery. Popul Health Manag. 2008;11:247–54.

Goetzel RZ, Ozminkowski RJ, Billagra VG, Duffy J. Return on investment in disease management: a review. Health Care Financ Rev. 2005;26:1–19.

Henk HJ, Katzelnick DJ, Dobak KA, Greist HH, Jefferson JW. Medical costs attributed to depression among patients with a history of high medical expenses in a health maintenance organizations. Arch Gen Psychiatry. 1996;53:899–904.

Hodgman SB. Predictive modeling and outcomes. Prof Case Manag. 2008;13:19–23.

Hudson LR, Pope JE. The role of health-risk appraisals in disease management. Manag care interface. 2006;19:43–5.

Johnson SS, Driskell M, Johnson J, Prochaska JM, Zwick W, Prochaska JO. Efficacy of a transtheoretical model-expert system for antihypertensive adherence. Disease Manag. 2006;9(5):291–301.

Kathol R, Clarke D. Rethinking the place of the psyche in health: toward the integration of healthcare systems. Aust N ZJ Psychiatry. 2005;39:826–35.

Katon R, Unutzer J. Collaborative care models for depression: time to move from evidence to practice. Arch Inter Med. 2006;166:2304–6.

Katon W, VonKorff M, Lin E, Walker E, Simon G, Bush T, Robinson P, Russo J. Collaborative management to achieve treatment guidelines: impact on depression in primary care. JAMA. 1995;273:1026–31.

Katon W, VonKorff M, Lin, Simon G, Walker G, Unutzer J, Bush T, Russo J, Ludman E. Stepped collaborative care for primary care patients with persistent symptoms of depression. Arch Gen Psychiatry. 1999;56:1109–15.

Katzelnick DJ, Simon G, pearson S, Manning W, Helstead C, Henk H, Cole SM, Lin EHG, Taylor LH, Kobak KA. Arch Fam Med. 2000;9:345–51.

Kessler RC, Barber C, Beck A et al. The world health organization health and work performance questionnaire (HPQ). J Occup Environ Med. 2003;45:156–74.

Kroenke K, Spitzer RL, Williams JB. The PHQ-9: validity of a brief depression severity measure. J Gen Inter Med. 2001;16:606–13.

Linden A, Adams JL, Roberts N. An assessment of the total population approach for evaluating disease management program effectiveness. Disease Manag. 2003;10:247–51.

Loeppke R, Humel PA, Lofland JH. Health-related workplace productivity measurement: general and migraine-specific recommendations from the ACOEM expert panel. J Occup Environ Med. 2003;45:349–59.

Loeppke R, Hymel P. Good health is good business. J Occup Environ Med. 2006;48:533–7.

Loeppke R, Taitel M, Richling D, Parry T, Kessler RC, Hymel P, Konicki D. Health and productivity as a business strategy. J Occup Environ Med. 2007;49:712–21.

Lynch WD, Chen CY, Bender J, Edington DW. Documenting participation in an employer-sponsored disease management program: selection, exclusion, attrition, and active engagement as possible metrics; 2006.

Mattke S, Seid M, Ma S. Evidence for the effect of disease management: is $1 billion a year a good investment? Am J Manag Care. 2007;13:670–6.

MacStravic S. The challenge of participation in disease management. Disease Manag. 2007;10:247–51.

MacStravic S. Evaluating disease management results: individuals and cohorts vs. populations. Disease Manag. 2007;10:185–8.

Matheson D, Psacharopoulos D, Wilkins A. Realizing the promise of disease management: payer trends and opportunities in the United States. www.bcg.com/publications/files/Realizing_the_Promise_of_Disease_Management_Feb06.pdf.; 2006.

Micco N, Gold B, Buzzell P, Leonard H, Pintauro S, Harvey-Berino J. Minimal in-person support as an adjunct to internet obesity treatment. Ann Behav Med. 2007;33(1):49–56.

Myette TL. Integrated management of depression: improving system quality and creating effective interfaces. J Occup Environ Med. 2008;50:482–91.

Naydeck DL, Pearson JA, Ozminkowski FJ, Day BT, Goetzel RZ. The impact of the high-mark employee wellness programs on 4-year healthcare costs. J Occup Environ Med. 2008;50(2):146–56.

Norman GK. Disease management outcomes: are we asking the right questions yet? Popul Health Manag. 2008;11:183–7.

Partnership for Solutions. Chronic Conditions: making the case for ongoing care. Available at: www.partnershipforsolutions.org/DMS/files/chronicbook2004.pdf. Accessed February 28, 2009.

Prochaska JO, Prochaska JM. An update on maximum impact practices from a transtheoretical approach. In: Best Practices in the Behavioral Management of Chronic Disease. Los Altos, CA: Institute for Disease Management; 2005. p. 1–16.

Prochaska JO, Redding CA, Evers KE. The transtheoretical model of behavior change. In Glanz K,, Lewis FM, Rimer BK, editors. Health behavior and health education: theory, research and practice. 3rd ed. Jossey-Bass; 2008. p. 97–121.

Rothert K, Strecher VJ, Doyle SA, Caplan WM, Joyce JS, Jimison HB, Karm LM, Mims AD, Roth MA. Web-based weight management programs in an integrated health care setting: a randomized, controlled trial. Obesity. 2006;14(2):266– 72.

Rush AJ, Guillion CM, Basco MR, Jarrett RB, Trivedi MH. The inventory of depressive symptomatology (IDS): psychometric properties. Psychol Med. 1996;26:477–86.

Schult TM, McGovern PM, Dowd B, Pronk NP. The future of health promotion/disease prevention programs: the incentives and barriers faced by stakeholders. J Occup Environ Med. 2006;48:541–8.

Simon GE, VonKorff M, Barlow W. Health care costs of primary care patients with recognized depression. Arch Gen Psychiatry. 1995;52:850–6.

Simon GE, VonKorff M, Rutter C, Wagner E. A randomized trial of monitoring, feedback, and management of care by telephone to improve depression treatment in primary care. Br Med J. 2000;320:550–4.

Simon GE, Revicki D, Heiligenstein J, Grothaus L, VonKorff M, Katon W, Hylan TR. Recovery from depression, work productivity, and health care costs among primary care patients. Gen Hosp Psychiatry. 2000;22:153–62.

Simon GE, Chisholm D, Treglia M, Bushnell D. Course of depression, health services costs, and work productivity in an international primary care study. Gen Hosp Psychiatry. 2002;24: 328–35.

Stewart WF, Ricci KA, Chee E, Hahn SR, Morganstein D. Cost of lost productive work time among US workers with depressions. JAMA. 2003;289:3135–44.

Unutzer J, Patrick DL, Simon G, Brembowski D, Walker E, Rutter C, Waton, W. Depressive symptoms and the cost of health services in HMO patients age 65 and over: a four year retrospective study. JAMA. 1997;277:1618–23.

Velicer WG, DiClemente CC. Understanding and intervening with the total population of smokers. Tob Control. 1993;2:95–96.

Von Korff M, Tiemans B. Individualized stepped care of chronic illness. West J Med. 2000;172:133–7.

Wagner EH, Austin BT, Von Korf M. Organizing care for patients with chronic illness. Millbank Quart. 1996;74:511–44.

Wagner EH. What will it take to improve care for chronic illness? Effect Clin Pract. 1998;1:2–4.

Wagner EH, Austin BT, David C et al. Improving chronic illness care: translating evidence into action. Health Affairs. 2001;20:64–78.

Wagner EH, Davis C, Schaefer J, Von Korff M, Austin B. A survey of leading chronic disease management programs: are they consistent with the literature? J Nurs Care Quality. 2002;16(2):67–80.

Wang PS, Simon GE, Avorn J, Azocar F, Ludman E, McCulloch J, Petukhova MZ, Kessler RC. Telephone screening, outreach, and care management for depressed workers and impact on clinical and work productivity outcomes: a randomized controlled trial. JAMA. 2007;298: 1401–11.

Wu S, Green A. Projection of Chronic Illness Prevalence and Cost Inflation. RAND Health. Sanda Monica, California: RAND Corporation; 2000.

Wylie-Rosett J, Swencionis C, Ginsberg M, Cimino C, Wassertheil-Smoller S, Caban A, Segal-Isaacson CJ, Marting T, Lewis J. J Am Dietet Assoc. 2001;101:1155–62.

Chapter 15
Cultural Considerations in Stepped-Care and E-Health Interventions

Joaquin Borrego and Chelsea Klinkebiel

Introduction

The Unites States continues to experience a rapid demographic change with regard to culturally diverse (i.e., ethnic and racial minority) populations. As examples, people of Asian-origin heritage (e.g., Chinese, Japanese, Korean) have increased by over 200% (Leong et al., 2003) and people of Latino origin (e.g., Mexican, Puerto Rican, Dominican) have experienced a growth rate eight times faster than Caucasians (U.S. Bureau of the Census, 2000) in the last couple of decades. In fact, Latinos have surpassed African-Americans as the largest ethnic minority group in the United States. Given this trend with Asians, Latinos, and other ethnic and racial minority groups, it is expected that ethnic minorities will constitute the majority of the US population in the next few decades. Part of this rapid shift in demographics is driven by the continued high immigration patterns with some of these groups.

These trends pose a challenge for mental health providers as ethnic and racial minority groups have historically not fared well in our mental health system. For example, ethnic and racial minority groups continue to underutilize mental health services (U.S. DHHS, 2001), receive mental health services of lesser quality (U.S. DHHS, 2001), and these groups are generally not satisfied with the quality of mental health services received (Alegria et al., 2002). This inequity is of great concern considering racial and ethnic minorities are disproportionately affected by risk factors for mental health problems (e.g., living in poverty, exposure to violence) and are overrepresented in homeless and incarcerated populations (DHHS, 2001). Reasons for this lower rate of treatment seeking may include mistrust of health professionals due to experiences of racism and discrimination (DHHS, 2001). In addition, racial and ethnic minorities may experience stigma related to receiving therapy that may reduce the desire to seek treatment (Nadeem et al., 2007; Yang et al., 2008), as well as clinician bias, which may lead to misdiagnosis or providing a lower quality of treatment (Snowden, 2003). Adding to these barriers are language differences that

J. Borrego (✉)
Department of Psychology, Texas Tech University, Lubbock, TX 79409, USA
e-mail: joaquin.borrego@ttu.edu

W.T. O'Donohue, C. Draper (eds.), *Stepped Care and e-Health*,
DOI 10.1007/978-1-4419-6510-3_15, © Springer Science+Business Media, LLC 2011

limit the number of mental health professionals that may be available. This information points to a traditional mental health system that has not been prepared to meet the mental heath needs of ethnic and racial minority populations in the United States (McCabe et al., 1999; U.S. DHHS, 2001).

Although rates of psychological distress seem to be similar between ethnic and racial minority groups and Caucasians living in the United States, what is different is that the former group has less access to traditional mental health services and there is less availability of high quality mental health services for this population (U.S. DHHS, 2001). This clear need for quality mental health services paired with less availability and access creates a disparity in our system. Given the mental health disparities just noted, it is crucial for our mental health system to continue to find ways of adequately meeting the mental health needs of these populations (American Psychological Association, 2003). Efforts to increase access to care for ethnic minorities include the recruitment of ethnic minority practitioners, as well as the implementation of community programs to encourage ethnic minority individuals to seek treatment (Snowden et al., 2006). However, minority individuals also face financial and practical obstacles when receiving treatment, such as healthcare costs and lower insurance coverage, as well as geographic location barriers and lack of transportation that make receiving needed health services difficult and inconvenient (Brown et al., 2000; Frist, 2005; Woodward et al., 1992). Instead, viable options may be the use of stepped-care and e-health approaches when working with ethnic and racial minority populations and other underserved groups.

A stepped-care approach has the potential of addressing much of what has plagued traditional mental health services (e.g., one-on-one psychotherapy with a professional), namely adopting a stepped-care approach can address issues related to access and availability. More specifically, a stepped-care approach can expand the breadth of services offered to ethnic and racial minority groups by decreasing the need or demand for mental health providers and by offering these groups a menu of services in different settings.

Although stepped-care and e-health services seem promising, they are still in their infancy with regard to being used with ethnic and racial minority populations. This chapter is intended to be practical in nature by raising issues that may be useful to consider as well as possible ways of addressing these concerns when considering using a stepped-care approach with ethnic and racial minority populations. The chapter will first highlight why a stepped-care and e-health approach to addressing the mental health needs of ethnic and racial minority populous makes sense. This is followed by information regarding cultural factors that may be considered when using these approaches with these populations.

An Argument for a Stepped-Care Approach

As noted above, stepped-care and e-health approaches show promise in increasing access and availability of mental health services for ethnic and racial minority populations. As has been well documented, ethnic and racial minority groups continue to underutilize traditional mental health services. This underutilization of mental health services is compounded by less availability of services and less access to quality services. Part of this is driven by the fact that our mental health system is not adequately staffed with professionals that can implement services that are perceived as culturally appropriate. In addition, this is driven by the fact that our system does not have a sufficient number of mental health professionals who are able to provide services in a different language other than English. As was stated above, there continues to be a large influx of people from different countries where English is not the primary language (e.g., Mexico, Japan, Turkey).

Although these approaches are promising, there are still issues that need to be addressed when applying this approach and technology with these populations. The next sections highlight issues related to technology, health literacy, and e-health literacy.

Minorities and Technology

While the use of e-health may provide greater access of mental health information to minority populations, it is very important to examine the disparities that also exist in access to technology, specifically the Internet. The gap that exists between users and non-users of the Internet is referred to as the *Digital Divide*. Previous research has shown that along with age, socioeconomic status, and geographic location, race and ethnicity are associated with differences in access and use of Internet technology (Chen and Wellman, 2003). Recently, studies have shown that although the amount of Internet users in all US racial and ethnic groups is increasing, the gap in usage among these groups still remains (Lenhart et al., 2003; Rojas et al., 2004). In a 2005 study, the US Department of Commerce reported that 65% of Whites and 63.1% of Asians were Internet users, compared to only 45.6% of African-Americans and 37% of Hispanics. A similar trend was reported 2 years later by the U.S. Census Bureau (2007), with 69% of White Americans, 73% of Asians, 51% of African-Americans, and 48% of Hispanics living in households with Internet access. While it has been predicted that this gap will narrow due to a higher percentage of new Internet users being racial and ethnic minorities (National Telecommunication and Information Administration, 2002), many factors, such as income, education, and language, interplay to influence the access and use of computers and the Internet.

One of the major factors related to not going online is income (Chen and Wellman, 2003; Day et al., 2005). In a 2002 study, Reddick and Boucher reported that household Internet access had increased across all income levels; however, only 35% of lower income households and 46% of lower middle income households had Internet access, compared to 60% of upper middle income households and 81–83% of upper income households. Moreover, cost is more likely to be reported as a reason for not having Internet access by African-Americans, Hispanics, and those in low-income groups (Lenhart et al., 2003; Reddick and Boucher, 2002). It has been predicted that disparities due to income will decrease as Internet access and computers become a "necessity" instead of a "luxury" (Kim et al., 2007, p. 283).

Indeed, in a recent study, Horrigan (2009) found that low-income individuals were among a population subgroup that showed a significant increase in household broadband use. However, this study also reported that African-Americans showed the slowest growth in broadband adoption. In addition, it was found that although the overall adoption rate increased, so did the cost of broadband. Given that minority populations are overrepresented in lower income groups, concern is warranted about access to health information via the Internet due to cost barriers. Although a contributing factor, income does not account for all of the racial and ethnic differences in Internet use. Previous research has shown that at each income level, African-Americans and Latinos show significantly lower rates of computer ownership and Internet access, which suggests that other factors need to be considered (Fairlie, 2005).

Education is another important aspect to consider when examining access and use of computers and the Internet. Studies have shown that level of education is related to the household presence of a computer and Internet connection, and that individuals in lower education groups are less likely to utilize the Internet (Day et al., 2005; Lenhart et al., 2003; Wilson, 2003). It has been proposed that differences in education may explain a large part of the gap in Internet use between white and racial and ethnic minority Americans. In a 2007 study examining Internet use among Latino populations, Fox and Livingston reported that although the rate of Internet use was equally low for White, African-American, and Hispanic individuals with less than a high school diploma, over 40% of Latinos had not completed a high school degree, compared to 12% of Whites and 21% of African-Americans. Conversely, while the rates of Internet use are uniformly high for college graduates of these minority groups, much fewer Latinos had completed a college degree (10%) when compared to Whites (28%) and African-Americans (20%). Similar findings by Fairlie (2005) suggest that lower educational levels account for differences in household Internet use rates between African-Americans and white Americans. In addition to household Internet use, education may also influence the extent to which individuals have access to computers in job settings, with individuals at higher education levels having more access to a computer at work (Hoffman and Novak, 1998).

Discrepancies in education level may impact more than just physical access to the Internet. Low literacy levels may prevent individuals from understanding and obtaining meaningful information from the Internet. Furthermore, research has shown that individuals in higher education levels are more knowledgeable about the Internet than those with less education (Hargittai and Hinnant, 2008). Therefore, minority individuals in lower education groups may lack the skills necessary to utilize computers and navigate through Internet information and computer programs. These disparities in both access and skills related to utilization warrant concern that racial and ethnic minorities in lower education groups may fall behind and be unable to effectively utilize the Internet to obtain vital mental health information.

Language has also been strongly associated with Internet utilization. In a 2007 study examining Latino use of the Internet in the United States, Fox and Livingston found that 78% of English dominant and 76% of bilingual Latinos were online, compared to only 32% of Latinos who were Spanish dominant. This discrepancy may be explained by the large proportion of English-dominant content that exists on the Internet (Wilhelm, 2000). The fact that much of the content available online is only in English may create a disadvantage to any racial and ethnic minority individuals that prefer to obtain information in a language other than English.

In addition to physical and social access factors, the attitudes and perceptions that racial and ethnic minority individuals hold about computers and the Internet may also affect utilization rates and the way these technologies are used. It has been proposed that populations who do not utilize computer technology will be more likely to express disinterest in using it (Stanley, 2003). However, other research has shown that racial and ethnic minorities who are non-users are more likely to cite lack of access to technology as reasons for non-use, while whites are equally or more likely to cite that they are simply not interested (Fox and Livingston, 2007; Lenhart et al., 2003). Furthermore, Lenhart et al. (2003) found that non-users who believed they would eventually go online were more likely to be black or Hispanic, while those who believed they never would were more likely to be white. Minority individuals also perceive the Internet as being a useful source of information at a percentage similar to that of white individuals (Porter and Donthu, 2006). These statistics suggest that racial and ethnic minority individuals may be very likely to utilize the Internet to receive health information. Therefore, efforts to provide e-health information to minorities should focus on access related to income, education, and language barriers.

Health Literacy and E-Health Literacy

It has been estimated that 90 million Americans lack the literacy skills required to understand health information and utilize the healthcare system (Institute of Medicine, 2004). This type of literacy, known as *health literacy*, is defined as "the degree to which individuals have the capacity to obtain, process, and understand basic health information and services needed to make appropriate health decisions" (Institute of Medicine, 2004, p. 32). Research has shown that demographic factors associated with low health literacy include racial and ethnic minority status (Arnold et al., 2001; Gazmararian et al., 1999; Rudd, 2007), and although individuals with low health literacy are more likely to be White and native-born US citizens, racial and minority groups are overrepresented in low health literacy groups (Institute of Medicine, 2004). This relationship between race/ethnicity and health is a complex one, and contributing factors include education, language, and culture. Populations that are most vulnerable to not understanding health information are those with limited education and low English proficiency (Andrulis and Branch, 2007).

It is imperative to consider education and reading level when examining the health literacy of individuals utilizing the Internet to obtain health information. The 2003 National Assessment of Adult Literacy reported that US adults who had not completed high school and were not currently enrolled in school had lower average health literacy than adults with higher levels of education or adults who were currently enrolled in high school, with nearly half of those who did not complete high school scoring at a level below basic health literacy (Kutner et al., 2006). Given that gaps in education still remain between racial and ethnic groups, with African-Americans, Hispanics, and Native American/Alaskan Natives less likely to attain high school and college education than Whites and Asians/Pacific Islanders (KewalRamani et al., 2007), literacy levels may challenge minority individuals in obtaining and using health information. In a 2001 study analyzing health information available on the Internet, Berland et al. (2001) found that the reading level of health information on English-language web sites ranged from 10th grade to graduate school level, with an average reading level of 13.2. Reading levels of health information on Spanish-language web sites were also examined and ranged from grades 7 to 13, with an average reading level of 10th grade. This is of great concern, considering that a large percentage of the US population cannot read above the eighth grade level (Kirsch et al., 1993). In order to provide health information that can be understood by many different populations, it will be necessary to ensure that health information accessed through e-health is available to individuals in a wide range of literacy levels. Although years of education may be an indicator of the degree of literacy an individual may have, it does not guarantee an exact literacy level (Kirsch et al., 1993), nor is it the only demographic factor that should be considered when examining how individuals understand health information. For example, immigrants to the United States who have attained a high level of education in their native country but have limited English skills may experience great difficulty in comprehending English-language health information (Van Servellen et al., 2003).

Language and culture are also vital factors to consider when evaluating how racial and ethnic minority individuals understand health information. Due to the fact that the majority of health-related sites are available only in English (Kalichman et al., 2001), populations with limited English literacy due to language barriers may be unable to access much of the online health information that they need. The translation of health information into other languages may help improve access; however, simply translating material will likely be insufficient in improving understandability. For example, material written at a high reading level still may not be comprehensible to individuals in low literacy levels, even when written in their native language and therefore should also be simplified (Andrulis and Brach, 2007; Elder et al., 2009). Additionally, material directly translated from English may not be well understood if the cultural context of the language is not taken into consideration. For instance, abstract terms used in mental health information, such as "trauma" or "developmental delay," as well as words used to describe emotional states may be confusing to speakers of different languages if the meanings of these terms vary from the definitions that exist in English (Fontes, 2008). A direct translation of materials may not be sufficient as what is needed across translations is *construct equivalence* of terms. Additionally, the perception of mental illness may vary due to cultural factors. For example, members of Asian cultures have been found to report more somatic symptoms in depression than members of Western cultures (Kleinman, 1986, cited in Tsai et al., 2001). Therefore, individuals' views of what constitutes depression may vary, depending on cultural factors. Information presenting educational material on mental health disorders should be culturally sensitive and include symptoms unique to certain cultures in order to aid understanding. In addition to unique symptomology, members of racial and ethnic minority groups may also display disorders distinctive to their specific culture. These disorders are known as culture-bound syndromes and are defined as "locality-specific patterns of aberrant behavior and troubling experience that may or may not be linked to a particular DSM-IV diagnostic category" (DSM-IV-TR, 2000). A well-known culture-bound syndrome is *ataque de nervios,* a disorder prevalent among Latino cultures, primarily Caribbean Latino groups. Symptoms described by the DSM-IV include uncontrollable shouting, attacks of crying, trembling, heat in the chest rising into the head, and verbal or physical aggression. Other symptoms that may occur include dissociative experiences, seizure-like or fainting episodes, and suicidal gestures. Though the symptoms of *ataque de nervios* appear to match up most closely with panic attacks, most cases lack characteristic symptoms of panic disorder, such as acute fear and apprehension (DSM-IV-TR, 2000). This illustrates the fact that certain racial and ethnic minority groups may have unique mental health experiences and therefore need educational information that is specific to them.

While health literacy can greatly assist individuals in understanding mental health information, the use of e-health may require additional abilities that come with accessing health information using the Internet. In a 2006 article, Norman and Skinner proposed a model of e-health literacy made up of six distinct literacy skills. In addition to general literacy and health literacy, they posit that e-health users also need to possess information literacy, media literacy, computer literacy, and scientific literacy. With this new skill set, more demands may be placed on populations already experiencing difficulty in accessing and understanding health information.

Due to the fact that accessing e-health information requires the use of computers, individuals need to be literate in this technology. *Computer literacy* is essential in using computers to find health information and includes the ability to access e-health resources as well as adapt to new technology (Norman and Skinner, 2006). As described earlier, physical access barriers to computer and the Internet, such as cost could potentially provide fewer opportunities for some racial and ethnic minorities to attain high levels of computer literacy. In addition, social access barriers such as limited education and limited English proficiency may prevent underserved populations from developing needed skills related to technology.

Closely related to computer literacy, Norman and Skinner define *information literacy* as the ability to locate resources in order to find information on a topic, use ideal search terms, and select the results that are most relevant to the topic. This skill is especially relevant for finding information on the Internet with search engines or within health information web sites. In a 2004 study, Birru et al. (2004) evaluated Internet use by low literacy adults and found that participants experienced difficulty in information seeking, with participants experiencing difficulty in generating search terms that were specific enough, following links in the search engine, finding health information at a reading level that was low enough, as well as interpreting which information was useful and appropriate for their search question. Zarcadoolas et al. (2002) found similar results in a comparable study, in which individuals in low literacy levels used the Internet to maneuver through web sites to obtain information. Most participants in the study had previously accessed a computer and most reported being comfortable using a computer. However, a majority of the participants encountered difficulty when using the Internet. These difficulties included finding appropriate results with search words, due to incorrect spelling and inappropriate categorical links being chosen. Additionally, participants had difficulty understanding and using features such as pull-down menus and active graphics. Hispanic participants in the study also encountered an additional difficulty when they were not able to identify that the misspelling of search terms was the reason they were not able to access a web site. These results highlight the fact that persons with low literacy, whether due to low education attainment or limited English proficiency, may encounter a number of obstacles when using the Internet to search for health information and, therefore, may be at a disadvantage.

Another form of literacy that Norman and Skinner consider crucial to e-health literacy is *media literacy*, which they define as the ability to think critically about both media content and media context. This includes considering the "social and political context" of information, as well as considering the "marketplace, audience relations, and how media forms in themselves shape the message that gets conveyed" (Norman and Skinner, 2006, "Media Literacy," para. 1). The skill set involved with media literacy is essential for individuals to be able to determine which information is most applicable to them, as well as to recognize biases. In 2001, LaChausse examined the media literacy skills and attitudes of migrant Hispanic farm workers in relation to tobacco advertising in the form of billboards along the US/Mexican border. Results showed that media literacy skills among participants were low, with only 16% reporting that they always thought about the truthfulness of the messages and 67% reporting that they never did. In addition, those who indicated that they had seen the tobacco billboards were more likely to believe that most Americans smoke than those who reported not seeing the billboards. The ability to recognize how potentially harmful information is targeted at certain populations may help to prevent negative health consequences. Additionally, because many web sites with medical information may contain inaccuracies (Berland et al., 2001), the ability to critically evaluate Internet material is vital in ensuring that health information used by individuals is credible. In a 2004 study, Benotsch et al. (2004) examined the use of the Internet to obtain health information by patients with HIV. Participants were directed to two web pages containing HIV treatment information. One was a page from a well-known medical journal and published by the American Medical Association (AMA) that listed drug treatment options for HIV. The other was a web page describing a cure for AIDS made with chemicals extracted from goat serum. They found that trusting the less credible source was predicted by, being less knowledgeable about HIV, lower literacy levels, and poorer reading comprehension. The implications of this study suggest that low-income and low-literacy individuals, as well as those who use e-health with limited prior knowledge of health information may be vulnerable to misinformation about health topics.

Norman and Skinner propose that e-health users need to be able to distinguish between what is and what is not credible health information. This ability is contained within another type of literacy known as *scientific literacy*, which Norman and Skinner define as the ability to understand the process of science, including the "nature, aims, methods, applications, limitations, and politics of creating knowledge in a systematic manner ("Scientific Literacy," para. 1)." The knowledge of the underlying science that creates health information can help individuals to achieve greater comprehension and understanding, as well as help individuals to avoid misleading information (Royal Society, 1985; cited in Laugksch, 2000). An alarming statistic, however, shows that scientific literacy in the United States is fairly low and that nearly two-thirds of Americans do not have a complete understanding of the scientific process (National Science Board, 2004). Scientific literacy is a complex skill that is often fostered and focused on during formal education years. Therefore, populations with limited formal education may not attain scientific literacy and may be more likely to use and rely on information that is not credible.

As stated above, there are numerous issues to consider when working with underserved populations such as overall literacy and more specific computer and e-health literacy. The next sections briefly highlight relevant issues of where these populations can be accessed as well as assessment issues related to acculturation and language preference and proficiency.

Consumer Preferences

Although it has been documented that ethnic and racial minority groups have historically underutilized traditional mental heath services, this does not mean that they do *not* utilize mental health services at all. Research suggests that some groups, such as Latinos, are likely to seek mental heath services from physicians (Vega et al., 2001). Given this information, mental health providers can work with physicians and other health providers (e.g., nurses) who have initial contact with ethnic minority groups through clinics in initially disseminating information about psychological distress and means to address this and other problems.

Acculturation

An individual's level of acculturation is a factor that should be considered when deciding on how best to deliver an intervention via the Internet or other means. Acculturation is a psychological and sociocultural process by which an individual from one culture comes into contact with, engage, and acquire aspects of a new culture (Berry, 2003). It has been well established that acculturation can impact language acquisition, language preference, beliefs, attitudes, behaviors, and values. Given this, it may be important for mental health professionals to assess a person's level of acculturation before deciding which intervention format is best warranted. Individuals higher in acculturation may not have to have services adapted as much as someone who is low on acculturation. Please refer to Zane and Mak (2003) for a list and description of currently available acculturation scales for different ethnic and racial minority groups.

Language

There are many people living in the United States who do not have access to quality mental health services because the availability of services in their preferred language is nonexistent or offered on a limited basis. In addition, there may be problems with language match. As an example, there may be a client of Asian origin (e.g., Korean) who gets paired with an Asian-origin (e.g., Chinese) mental health professional but may not be able to communicate with each other due to language differences. This may be compounded by the fact that even though a therapist may be familiar with a certain language (e.g., Spanish), they may not be proficient enough to carry out therapy for a complete hour in that language. When assessing for language proficiency, it is not sufficient to simply assess on whether a client is bilingual. As an example, if working with a Latino client, the mental health professional may be interested in knowing which of these five descriptors fits the client best: monolingual Spanish, bilingual but more proficient in Spanish, equally bilingual in Spanish and English, bilingual but more proficient in English, and monolingual English. Clients can say that they are bilingual when prompted but one may be more proficient in Spanish while another client may be more proficient in English.

Translation

The accurate translation of document and information is crucial to the delivery of mental services to people who prefer to use or are more proficient in their native language. We advocate a *double translation* (also known as back translation) method as a way of assuring that the information disseminated is similar to the information that is available in English. The double translation method involves a bilingual individual translating the material from English to the target language (e.g., Spanish, Japanese). The second step is to have a different bilingual individual take the information that was translated into Spanish or Japanese and translating back into English. At the point, a third person would compare the original document in English with the translated document to see if there are any discrepancies regarding specific words or terminology. If there are discrepancies, the three-member group discusses the best terminology to use in that context. At times, an additional round of double translation may be necessary to get the translated information as close to the original information in English. In addition to this approach, mental health professionals need to assure that the information presented and the language used to present this information need to be simplified.

Conclusions

When used as a first stage of stepped care, the use of computerized treatment in place of standard face-to-face contact has potential advantages for ethnic minorities, including access to treatment that traditionally may come only from a specialist (and a long waiting list; Williams, 2008). Therefore, the use of e-health in a stepped-care model may help to eliminate gaps that exist between demand for and availability of mental health professionals (Green and Iverson, 2009; Bower and Gilbody,

2005). The use of computer technology in a stepped-care approach also may be an important development in reducing healthcare costs. By eliminating therapist–client contact in the first step and adding this contact in later steps, if needed, the use of e-health and computerized treatment in stepped care is more cost-effective than standard treatment (Barnett et al., 2008; Newman et al., 1999).

The access to treatment for individuals facing geographic limitations (i.e., rural populations) has been addressed with the implementation of technologically assisted therapy programs, such as telepsychiatry. This method of using videoconferencing to connect practitioners and clients has been shown to be effective and well accepted by clients, including members of ethnic minority groups (Monnier et al., 2003; Shore et al., 2008; Ruskin et al., 1998). With the implementation of e-health, a new opportunity exists to eliminate other barriers, such as stigma, as well as financial limitations, such as healthcare costs. The dissemination of mental health information through the Internet and through computer-based treatment programs has the potential to provide greater access for populations unable or not wanting to participate in traditional face-to-face treatment with a clinician. This diversification in the way that treatment is delivered helps patients to quickly access mental health information in the privacy of their own home. Additionally, computerized therapy allows for access of information about mental health without clinician bias (Hester and Miller, 2006). Table 15.1 provides a summary of Internet sites that have mental health-related information specific for ethnic, racial, and linguistic minority groups.

Although this approach holds significant promise, mental health professionals should also proceed with caution as there is limited information regarding the availability of mental health-related literature in different languages that is easy to access. Since stepped-care and e-health approaches are not as widespread as other traditional mental health approaches (e.g., individual therapy), it may be useful for mental health professionals to conduct a pre-treatment orientation with the client to educate and inform the client on why a stepped-care approach is being implemented. The client may have misconceptions or certain expectations about what mental health services should look like so it would be useful to spend sufficient time explaining the rationale of a stepped-care approach.

Other challenges mental health professionals may face are difficulties to access computers and computer literacy. It may be useful for mental health professionals to be aware of different community programs that may offer computer literacy and related programs. In addition, a person does not have to have a computer at home to necessarily access information on the web. Most public libraries offer free access to the Internet. In addition, community centers may also offer free access to computers and the Internet. This may be appealing to clients as community centers are strategically placed in certain neighborhoods that are usually easier to get to than psychology clinics, etc.

As a last point, it may be beneficial to collaborate with medical professionals in primary care settings. As discussed earlier, ethnic minority populations usually only access medical services through primary care settings. Collaborating with medical personnel (e.g., doctors, nurses) may be beneficial as it may help with credibility for the mental health professional and it would also add to the credibility of a stepped-care approach that includes e-health interventions.

Table 15.1 Mental health web sites targeting different ethnic, racial, and linguistic groups

Program name	Description	Target population	Language	Web site
CDC	*Alcoholism*: gives links for different topics. Mostly about drinking while pregnant. Also provides external links about alcoholism in general	Spanish-speaking Latinos	English and Spanish	http://www.cdc.gov/spanish/prevencion/alcohol.html
CDC	*Autism spectrum disorders*: includes information about symptoms, rates of ASD, and suspected causes. Also gives external links for more information	Spanish-speaking Latinos	English and Spanish	http://www.cdc.gov/ncbddd/spanish/spautism.htm
CDC	*ADHD*: information about the rate of ADHD and symptoms	Spanish-speaking Latinos	English and Spanish	http://www.cdc.gov/ncbddd/Spanish/spadhd.htm
CDC	*Mental retardation*: includes a definition and information about rates and causes	Spanish-speaking Latinos	English and Spanish	http://www.cdc.gov/ncbddd/Spanish/spmr.htm
CDC	*Addiction*: CDC links include information about alcohol, tobacco, and HIV related to injectable drugs. Also includes external links to information about many other drugs	Spanish-speaking Latinos	English and Spanish	http://www.cdc.gov/spanish/prevencion/drogas.html
CDC	*Suicide*: information includes rates, suicide in older adults, younger adults, and adolescents, and prevention	Spanish-speaking Latinos	English and Spanish	http://www.cdc.gov/ncipc/factsheets/suicidio.htm

Table 15.1 (continued)

Program name	Description	Target population	Language	Web site
CDC	*Violence*: information includes juvenile violence and workplace violence. External links include information about IPV and child maltreatment	Spanish-speaking Latinos	English and Spanish	http://www.cdc.gov/spanish/prevencion/violencia.html
CDC	*Adolescent health*: gives information about stress, family relationships, and acculturation	Spanish-speaking Latinos	English and Spanish	http://www.cdc.gov/spanish/especialesCDC/AdolescentesLatinos/
NIMH	*Anxiety disorders*: topics included in one booklet are panic disorder, obsessive-compulsive disorder, post-traumatic stress, phobias, and generalized anxiety	Spanish-speaking Latinos	English and Spanish	http://www.nimh.nih.gov/health/publications/espanol/trastornos-de-ansiedad/index.shtml
NIMH	*Generalized anxiety disorder*: A separate easy-to-read booklet that includes information about what it is, when it begins, and treatment. Also includes a self-test. Only available in PDF	Spanish-speaking Latinos	English and Spanish	http://www.nimh.nih.gov/health/publications/espanol/trastorno-de-ansiedad-generalizada-una-enfermedad-real/index.shtml
NIMH	*Panic disorder*: A separate easy-to-read booklet that includes information about what it is, when it begins, and treatment. Also includes a self-test	Spanish-speaking Latinos	English and Spanish	http://www.nimh.nih.gov/health/publications/espanol/trastorno-de-panico-una-enfermedad-real/index.shtml

Table 15.1 (continued)

Program name	Description	Target population	Language	Web site
NIMH	*PTSD*: A separate easy-to-read booklet that explains what it is, when it begins, and treatment	Spanish-speaking Latinos	English and Spanish	http://www.nimh.nih.gov/health/publications/espanol/trastorno-de-estres-postraumatico-facil-de-leer/index.shtml
NIMH	*OCD*: A separate easy-to-read booklet that explains what it is, when it begins, and treatment	Spanish-speaking Latinos	English and Spanish	http://www.nimh.nih.gov/health/publications/espanol/cuando-pensamientos-indeseados-toman-control-trastorno-obsesivo-compulsivo/index.shtml
NIMH	*Social phobia*: A separate easy-to-read booklet that explains what it is, when it begins, and treatment. Also includes a self-test	Spanish-speaking Latinos	English and Spanish	http://www.nimh.nih.gov/health/publications/espanol/fobia-social-una-enfermedad-real/index.shtml
NIMH	*Bipolar disorder*: easy-to-read information about what it is, what causes it, and treatment	Spanish-speaking Latinos	English and Spanish	http://www.nimh.nih.gov/health/publications/espanol/trastorno-bipolar-facil-de-leer/index.shtml
NIMH	*Depression*: includes information about depression in both women and men. Includes easy-to-read versions	Spanish-speaking Latinos	English and Spanish	http://www.nimh.nih.gov/health/publications/espanol/depression-listing.shtml
NIMH	*Schizophrenia*: includes information about what it is, how it is diagnosed, suicide related to schizophrenia, treatment, and medications	Spanish-speaking Latinos	English and Spanish	http://www.nimh.nih.gov/health/publications/espanol/esquizofrenia/index.shtml
DHHS	*Addiction and drug abuse*: link on DHHS web site takes viewer to NIDA. Available in Spanish	Spanish-speaking Latinos	English and Spanish	http://www.drugabuse.gov/infofacts/Explicacion-Sp.html

Table 15.1 (continued)

Program name	Description	Target population	Language	Web site
DHHS	*African-Americans*: link on DHHs web site takes viewer to NLM. Includes health information and some mental health information specifically about African-Americans, such as depression, bipolar disorder, drug abuse and addiction, and suicide	African-Americans	English and Spanish	http://www.nlm.nih.gov/medlineplus/africanamericanhealth.html
DHHS	*Alcoholism*: Link on DHHS web site takes viewer to NLM	Spanish-speaking Latinos	English and Spanish	http://www.nlm.nih.gov/medlineplus/spanish/alcoholism.html
DHHS	*Substance abuse and dependence*: A short PDF file that includes information about the signs of abuse and dependence, drugs most often abused, and resources for treatment	Spanish-speaking Latinos, Asian, Bosnian, Indian, Russian, Somalian, French-speaking, Portuguese- speaking, and hearing-impaired populations	American Sign Language, Bosnian, Chinese (simplified and traditional), French, Hindi, Japanese, Korean, Portuguese, Russian, Somali, Tagalog, and Vietnamese	http://www.nlm.nih.gov/medlineplus/languages/alcoholism.html#ASL
DHHS	*American Indians*: link on DHHs web site takes viewer to NLM—includes health information and some mental health information specifically about American Indians, such as drug abuse and addiction and suicide	Native Americans	English and Spanish Also includes a PDF document about inhalants in Navajo	http://www.nlm.nih.gov/medlineplus/nativeamericanhealth.html

Table 15.1 (continued)

Program name	Description	Target population	Language	Web site
DHHS	*Asian-Americans*: link on DHHs web site takes viewer to NLM—includes health information and some mental health information specifically about Asian-Americans, such as smoking and suicide	Asian-Americans	English and Spanish. Only documents in Chinese or Korean are about bone health and hepatitis B	http://www.nlm.nih.gov/medlineplus/asianamericanhealth.html
DHHS	*Child abuse*: link on DHHS web site takes viewer to Child Welfare Information Gateway. Includes information on reporting suspected abuse, the Child Welfare System, child abuse and neglect prevention, and resources for help with personal crises	Spanish-speaking Latinos	English and Spanish	http://www.childwelfare.gov/spanish
DHHS	*Domestic violence*: DHHS link takes viewer to NLM.	Spanish-speakingLatinos, Arabic, Bosnian, Russian, and Somali populations	English and Spanish. Also includes a video and a short PDF file about DV in Arabic, Bosnian, English Russian, Somali, and Spanish	http://www.nlm.nih.gov/medlineplus/domesticviolence.html

Table 15.1 (continued)

Program name	Description	Target population	Language	Web site
DHHS	*Drinking and alcohol*: DHHS link takes viewer to NLM	Spanish-speaking Latinos	English and Spanish. Also includes a document on aging, medicine, and alcohol in Chinese, Korean, Russian, and Vietnamese	http://www.nlm.nih.gov/medlineplus/spanish/alcohol.html
DHHS	*Drug abuse and addiction*: DHHS link takes viewer to NIDA. Includes information on hallucinogens, cocaine, club drugs, steroids, heroine, inhalants, marijuana, prescription drugs, MDMA, methamphetamines, nicotine, PCP, and Ritalin. Also includes info on prevention and treatment	Spanish-speaking Latinos	English and Spanish	http://www.nida.nih.gov/nidaespanol.html
DHHS	*Eating disorders*: DHHS link takes viewer to NLM. Includes information on diagnosis/symptoms, treatment, and prevention	Spanish-speaking Latinos	English and Spanish	http://www.nlm.nih.gov/medlineplus/spanish/eatingdisorders.html
DHHS	*Hispanics/Latinos*: DHHS link takes viewer to NLM page about Hispanic/Latino health. Includes some mental health information, such as depression and suicide	Hispanics/Latinos	English and Spanish	http://www.nlm.nih.gov/medlineplus/spanish/hispanicamericanhealth.html

Table 15.1 (continued)

Program name	Description	Target population	Language	Web site
NLM NIH	*Adolescent mental health*: includes information about stress, family, relationships, and mental disorders	Spanish-speaking Latinos	English and Spanish	http://www.nlm.nih.gov/medlineplus/spanish/teenmentalhealth.html
NLM NIH	*Children's mental health*: includes information about depression, anxiety, conduct disorders, and ADHD, which each have separate pages	Spanish-speaking Latinos	English and Spanish	http://www.nlm.nih.gov/medlineplus/spanish/childmentalhealth.html
NLM NIH	*Bipolar Disorder*: includes information about risk factors, symptoms, and treatment. Also includes easy-to-read information	Spanish-speaking Latinos	English and Spanish	http://www.nlm.nih.gov/medlineplus/spanish/bipolardisorder.html
NLM NIH	*Situational Depression*: Includes information about symptoms, prevalence, and treatment	Spanish-speaking Latinos	English and Spanish	http://www.nlm.nih.gov/medlineplus/spanish/seasonalaffectivedisorder.html
NLM NIH	*Anxiety*: includes information about panic disorder, OCD, PTSD, phobias, and generalized anxiety	Spanish-speaking Latinos	English and Spanish	http://www.nlm.nih.gov/medlineplus/spanish/anxiety.html
NLM NIH	*Antidepressants*: Includes information on how antidepressants work, different types of medications, side effects, and benefits and risks of taking antidepressants	Spanish-speaking Latinos	English and Spanish	http://www.nlm.nih.gov/medlineplus/spanish/antidepressants.html

Table 15.1 (continued)

Program name	Description	Target population	Language	Web site
NLM NIH	*Autism:* includes information on different levels of the autism spectrum, signs of autism, and information about education	Spanish-speaking Latinos	English and Spanish	http://www.nlm.nih.gov/medlineplus/spanish/autism.html
NLM NIH	*Depression:* includes information about symptoms and treatment, as well as information about other related mental disorders	Spanish-speaking Latinos	English and Spanish	http://www.nlm.nih.gov/medlineplus/spanish/depression.html
NLM NIH	*Postpartum depression:* includes information about risk factors, symptoms, and treatment	Spanish-speaking Latinos	English and Spanish	http://www.nlm.nih.gov/medlineplus/spanish/postpartumdepression.html
NLM NIH	*Stress:* includes information about different types of stress, symptoms, and treatment	Spanish-speaking Latinos	English and Spanish	http://www.nlm.nih.gov/medlineplus/spanish/stress.html
NLM NIH	*Mental health:* gives basic information on mental health and also includes specific information for Latinos	Spanish-speaking Latinos	English and Spanish	http://www.nlm.nih.gov/medlineplus/spanish/mentalhealth.html/

References

Alegria M, Canino G, Rios R, Vera M, Calderon J, Rusch D, Ortega A. Inequalities in use of specialty mental health services among Latinos, African Americans, and non-Latino whites. Psychiatr Serv. 2002;53:547–55.

American Psychiatric Association. Diagnostic and statistical manual of mental disorders, Revised 4th ed. Washington, D.C.: Author; 2000.

American Psychological Association. Guidelines on multicultural education, training, research, practice, and organizational change for psychologists. Am Psychol. 2003;58: 377–402.

Andrulis DP, Brack C. Integrating literacy, culture, and language to improve health care quality for diverse populations. Am J Health Behav. 2007;31(1):122–33.

Arnold CL, Davis TC, Berkel HJ, Jackson RH, Nandy I, London S. Smoking status, reading level, and knowledge of tobacco effects among low-income pregnant women. Prevent Med. 2001;32(4):313–20.

Barnett PG, Wong W, Hall S. The cost-effectiveness of a smoking cessation program for out-patients in treatment for depression. Addiction. 2008;103(5):834–40.

Benotsch EG, Kalichman S, Weinhardt LS. HIV–AIDS patients' evaluation of health information on the internet: the digital divide and vulnerability to fraudulent claims. J Consult Clin Psychol. 2004;72(6):1004–11.

Berland GK, Elliot MN, Morales LS, Algazy JI, Kravitz RL, Broder MS et al. Health information on the internet: accessability, quality, and readability in English and Spanish. JAMA. 2001;285(20):2612–21.

Berry JW. Conceptual approaches to acculturation. In: Chun KM, Organista PB, editors. Acculturation: advances in theory, measurement, and applied research. Washington, DC: American Psychological Association; 2003. p. 17–37.

Birru MS, Monaco VM, Lonelyss C, Drew H, Njie V, Bierria T et al. Internet usage by low-literacy adults seeking health information: an observational analysis. J Med Internet Res. 2004;6(3):e25. Retrieved September 25, 2009 from http://www.jmir.org.

Bower P, Gilbody S. Stepped care in psychological therapies: access, effectiveness and efficiency. Br J Psychiatry. 2005;186(1):11–7.

Brown ER, Ojeda VD, Wyn R. Levan R. Racial and ethnic disparities in access to health insurance and health care (Rep No. 104). Los Angeles, California: UCLA Center for Health Policy Research; 2000.

Chen W, Wellman B. Charting and bridging digital divides: comparing socio-economic, gender, life stage, and rural-urban internet access and use in eight countries. AMD Global Consumer Advisory Board, Retrieved September 17th 2009 from http//www.amd.com/us_en/assets/content_type/DownloadableAssests/FINAL_REPORT_CHARTING_DIGI_DIVIDES.pdf; 2003.

Day JC, Janus A, and Davis J. Computer and internet use in the United States: 2003. Retrieved September 17th 2009 from the U.S. Census Bureau Web site: www.census.gov/prod/2005pubs/p23-208.pdf-2005-10-27;2005.

Elder JP, Ayala GX, Parra-Medina D, Talavera GA. Health communication in the Latino community: issues and approaches. Ann Rev Public Health. 2009;30:227–51.

Fairlie RW. Are we really a nation online? Ethnic and racial disparities in access to technology and their consequences. Retrieved September 17th 2009 from http://www.ecs.org/html/Document.asp?chouseid=6676; 2005.

Fontes LA. Interviewing clients across cultures. New York: Guilford Press; 2008.

Fox S, Livinston G. Latinos online: hispanics with lower levels of education and english proficiency remain largely disconnected from the internet. Washington, DC: Pew Hispanic and Pew Internet Project. (ERIC Document Reproduction Service No. ED495954); 2007.

Frist WH. Overcoming disparities in U.S. health care. Health Affairs. 2005;24(2): 445–451.

Gazmararian JA, Baker DW, Williams MV, Parker RM, Scott TL, Green DC et al. Health literacy among Medicare enrollees in a managed care organization. JAMA. 1999;28(6):545–51.

Green KE, Iverson KM. Computerized cognitive-behavioral therapy in a stepped care model of treatment. Prof Psychol-Res Pr. 2009;40(1):96–103.

Hargittai E, Hinnant A. Digital inequality: differences in young adults' use of the internet. Communication Res. 2008;35(5):602–21.

Hester RK, Miller JH. Computer-based tools for diagnosis and treatment of alcohol problems. Alcohol Res Health. 2006;29(1):36–40.

Hoffman DL, Novak TP. Bridging the digital divide: the impact of race on computer access and internet use. Nashville, TN: Vanderbilt University (ERIC Document Reproduction No. ED421563); 1998.

Horrigan JB. Home broadband adoption 2009: broadband adoption increases, but monthly prices do too. Retrieved from Pew Internet and American Life Project Web Site: http://pewinternet.org/Reports/2009/10-Home-Broadband-Adoption-2009.aspx; 2009.

Institute of Medicine. Health literacy: a prescription to end confusion. Washington, D.C.: The National Academies Press; 2004.

Kalichman SC, Benotsch E, Weinhardt L, Detwiler SM, Fogel J, Alber SM et al. Quality of health information on the internet. JAMA. 2001;285(20):2612–21.

KewalRamani A, Gilbertson L, Fox M, Provasnik S. Status and trends in the education of racial and ethnic minorities (NCES 2007-039). Washington, DC: U.S. Department of Education; 2007.

Kim YC, Jung JY, Ball-Rokeach SJ. Ethnicity, place, and communication technology: effects of ethnicity on multi-dimensional internet connectedness. Inform Technol People. 2007;20(3):282–303.

Kirsch IS, Jungeblut A, Jenkins L, Kolstad A. Adult literacy in America: a first look at the national adult literacy survey (NCES 1993–275). Washington, DC: National Center for Education Statistics, U.S. Department of Education; 1993.

Kutner M, Greenberg E, Jin Y, Paulsen C. The health literacy of America's adults: results from the 2003 national assessment of adult literacy (NCES 2006–483). U.S. Department of Education. Washington, DC: National Center for Education Statistics; 2006.

LaChausse RG. Attitudes toward tobacco advertising among Hispanic migrant farm workers. J Immigrant Health. 2001;3(2):107–110.

Laugksch RC. Scientific literacy: a conceptual overview. Sci Educ. 2000;84(1):71–94.

Lenhart A, Horrigan J, Rainie L, Allen K, Boyce A, Madden M, et al. (2003). The ever-shifting internet populations: A new look at internet access and the digital divide. Retrieved September 17th from Pew Internet and American Life Project Web Site: http://www.pewinternet.org/reports/toc.asp?Report_88; 2003.

Leong FTL, Kohout J, Smith J, Wicherski M. A profile of ethnic minority psychology. In: Bernal G, Trimble JE, Burlew AK, Leong FTL, editors. Handbook of racial and ethnic minority psychology. Thousand Oaks, CA: Sage Publications; 2003. p. 76–99.

McCabe K, Yeh M, Hough R, Landsverk J, Hurlburt M, Culver S, Reynolds B. Racial/ethnic representation across five public sectors of care for youth. J Emotion Behav Disord. 1999;7: 72–82.

Monnier J, Knapp RG, Frueh BC. Recent advances in telepsychiatry: an updated review. Psychiatric Serv. 2003;54(12):1604–9.

Nadeem E, Lange JM, Edge D, Fongwa M, Belin T, Miranda J. Does stigma keep poor young immigrant and U.S.-born Black and Latina women from seeking mental health care? Psychiatric Serv. 2007;58(12):1547–54.

National Science Board. Science and technology: public attitudes and understanding. In: Science and Engineering (chap. 2). Retrieved September 24, 2009 from http://www.nsf.gov/statistics/seind04/c7/c7i.htm; 2004.

National Telecommunication and Information Administration. A nation online: how Americans are expanding their use of the internet. Retrieved September 17th 2009 from http://www.ntia.doc.gov/reports/anol/index.html; 2002.

Newman MG, Consoli AJ, Taylor CB. A palmtop computer program for the treatment of generalized anxiety disorder. Behav Modif. 1999;23(4):597–619.

Norman CD, Skinner HA. EHealth literacy: essential skills for consumer health in a networked world. J Med Internet Res. 2006;8(2):e9. Retrieved September 22, 2009 from http://www.jmir.org.

Porter CE, Donthu N. Using the technology acceptance model to explain how attitudes determine internet usage: the role of perceived access barriers and demographics. J Business Res. 2006;59(9):999–1007.

Reddick A, Boucher C. Tracking the dual digital divide. EKOS Research Associates, Inc. Retrieved September 17th 2009 from http://www.hrsdc.gc.ca/eng/hip/lld/olt/Skills_Development/OLTResearch/digital-divide_e.pdf; 2002.

Rojas V, Straubhaar J, Roychowdhury D, Ozlem O. Communities, cultural capital, and the digital divide. In: Bucy EP, Newhagen JE, editors. Media access: social and psychological dimensions of new technology use. Mahwah, NJ: Erlbaum; 2004. p. 107–30.

Rudd RE. Health literacy skills of U.S. adults. Am J Health Behav. 2007;31(1):8–18.

Ruskin PE, Reed S, Kumar R, Klink MA, Siegel E, Rosen M et al. Reliability and acceptability of psychiatric diagnosis via telecommunication and audiovisual technology. Psychiatr Serv. 1998;49(8):1086–8.

Shore JH, Brooks E, Savin D, Orton H, Grigsby J, Manson SM. Acceptability of telepsychiatry in American Indians. Telemed e-Health. 2008;14(5):461–6.

Snowden LR. Bias in mental health assessment and intervention: theory and evidence. Am J Public Health. 2003;93(2):239–43.

Snowden LR, Masland M, Ma Y, Ciemens E. Strategies to improve minority access to public health services in California: Description and preliminary evaluation. J Community Psychol. 2006;34(2):225–35.

Stanley LD. Beyond access: psychosocial barriers to computer literacy. Inform Soc. 2003;19(5):407–16.

Tsai JL, Butcher JN, Muñoz RF, Vitousek K. Culture, ethnicity, and psychopathology. In: Sutker PB, Adams HE, editors. Comprehensive handbook of psychopathology. 3rd ed. New York: Kluwer Academic/Plenum Publishers; 2001. p. 105–29.

U.S. Bureau of the Census. Overview of the race and Hispanic origin. Retrieved July 6, 2009, from http://www.census.gov/prod/2001pubs/cenbr01-1. pdf.; 2000.

U.S. Bureau of the Census. American community survey. Rockville, M.D.; 2004.

U.S. Department of Health and Human Services. Mental health: Culture, race, and ethnicity—a supplement to mental health: A report of the surgeon general. Rockville, MD: Author; 2001.

Van Servellen G, Brown JS, Lombardi E, Herrera G. Health literacy in low-income Latino men and women receiving antiretroviral therapy in community-based treatment centers. AIDS Patient Care and STDs. 2003;17(6):283–98.

Vega W, Kolody B, Aguilar-Gaxiola S. Help seeking for mental health problems among Mexican Americans. J Immigrant Health. 2001;3(3):133–40.

Wilhelm AG. Democracy in the digital age: challenges to political life in cyberspace. New York: Routledge; 2000.

Williams C, Martinez R. Increasing access to CBT: stepped care and CBT self-help models in practice. Behav Cogn Psychoth. 2008;36:675–83.

Wilson KR, Wallin JS, Reiser C. Social stratification and the digital divide. Soc Sci Comput Rev. 2003;21(2):133–43.

Woodward AM, Dwinell AD, Arons BS. Barriers to mental health care for Hispanic Americans: a literature review and discussion. J Ment Health Administration. 1992;19(3): 224–36.

Yang LH, Phelan JC, Link BG. Stigma and beliefs of efficacy towards traditional Chinese medicine and western psychiatric treatment among Chinese-Americans. Cult Div Ethnic Min Psychol. 2008;14(1):10–18.

Zane N, Mak W. Major approaches to the measurement of acculturation among ethnic minority populations: a content analysis and an alternative empirical strategy. In: Chun KM, Organista PB, Marín G, editors. Acculturation: advances in theory, measurement, and applied research. Washington D.C.: American Psychological Association; 2003. p. 44–53.

Zarcadoolas C, Blanco M, Boyer JF, Pleasant A. Unweaving the web: an exploratory study of low-literate adults' navigation skills on the World Wide Web. J Health Communication. 2002;7: 309–24.

Subject Index

Note: The letters 'f' and 't' following the locators refer to figures and tables respectively.

A

Acculturation, 291, 295t
Achieve (goal-setting program), 272
ADIS-IV, *see* Anxiety Disorders Interview Schedule for DSM-IV (ADIS-IV)
Agoraphobia, 49–50, 52–53, 55, 61–63, 65–66, 68–71
American Academy of Pediatrics (AAP), 137–138, 141, 143–145, 204–205
American Medical Association (AMA), 290
Antiandrogens, 257
Antidepressant medication, 32, 35–36, 48, 57, 167–168, 237
Antisocial Behavior in School: Evidence-Based Practices (2nd ed.), 184
Anxiety, 45–58
    assessment/triage, 45–47
    bibliotherapy, 53–54
    computer-based intervention/e-health, 54
    consumer preferences and cultural sensitivity, 56
    dissemination agenda, 57–58
    group therapy, 54–55
    individual therapy, 55
    inpatient treatment, 56
    medication, 55
    psychoeducation, 53
    research and development agenda, 57
    stepped care options
        consumer preferences, 47–49
        outcome data, 49–52
        quality improvement outcomes, 52
    triage agenda, 56–57
    watchful waiting, 52–53
Anxiety Disorders Association of America (ADAA), 53
Anxiety Disorders Interview Schedule for DSM-IV (ADIS-IV), 45

Anxiety Disorders Interview Schedule Revised, 63, 100
Anxiety Sensitivity Index, 63
Applied behavior analysis, 206–207, 211
Asperger's disorder, 203–204
Assessment and triage, 7
    autism, 217
    chronic disease, 171–172
    grief, 236–237
    panic disorder, 72
Assessment and triage, anxiety, 56–57
    benzodiazepine medications, 57
    clinical severity, 56
    computer-assisted treatment, 56
    individual or group therapy sessions, 57
    patient treatment preference, 56
    self-administered bibliotherapy, 56
    side effect symptoms, 57
    treatment delivery options, 56
Assessment and triage, ODD, 196–197
    early intensive treatment, 196
    minimal interventions, 196
    online screening protocols, 197
    treatment recommendations, 196
Assessment and triage, PTSD, 80–82, 91
    CAPS, 80
    cost and physical barriers, 91
    IES (15-item self-report scale), 81
    PTSD self-report assessments, 13 measures, 80t
    self-monitoring and e-health, 91
    SPRINT scores (8-item clinical interview), 81–82
    TSQ (10-item self-report measure), 81
    Web-based administration of assessments, 81

W.T. O'Donohue, C. Draper (eds.), *Stepped Care and e-Health*,
DOI 10.1007/978-1-4419-6510-3, © Springer Science+Business Media, LLC 2011